Physical Activity and the Abdominal Viscera

T0136371

Physical Activity and the Abdominal Viscera is the first book to examine the response of the visceral organs to acute and chronic physical activity, in cases of both health and disease. Bringing together a previously disparate body of research, Professor Roy Shephard sets out the physiology, function during exercise, pathology of disease, and role of physical activity in preventing and managing disease in the visceral organs.

Working systematically through the viscera, the book first identifies the response to exercise and pathologies of the liver, gall bladder and biliary tract, then goes on to examine the function of the kidneys and bladder, and finally covers issues including the spleen, sickle cell disease and prostate cancer.

Providing a clear and well-structured guide to the relationship between the visceral organs and physical activity, *Physical Activity and the Abdominal Viscera* is a vital reference text for academics and upper-level students in sports medicine and clinical exercise physiology, and for health professionals in preventive medicine.

Roy J. Shephard is Professor Emeritus of Applied Physiology in the Faculty of Kinesiology & Physical Education at the University of Toronto, Canada. He was Director of the School of Physical and Health Education (now the Faculty of Kinesiology & Physical Education) at the University of Toronto for 12 years (1979–1991), and he served as Director of the University of Toronto Graduate Programme in Exercise Sciences from 1964–1985.

Routledge Research in Physical Activity and Health

The *Routledge Research in Physical Activity and Health* series offers a multi-disciplinary forum for cutting-edge research in the broad area of physical activity, exercise and health. Showcasing the work of emerging and established scholars working in areas ranging from physiology and chronic disease, psychology and mental health to physical activity and health promotion and socio-economic and cultural aspects of physical activity participation, the series is an important channel for groundbreaking research in physical activity and health.

Physical Activity and the Gastro-Intestinal Tract
Responses in health and disease
Roy J. Shephard

Technology in Physical Activity and Health Promotion
Edited by Zan Gao

Physical Activity and the Abdominal Viscera
Responses in Health and Disease
Roy J. Shephard

Physical Activity and the Abdominal Viscera
Responses in Health and Disease

Roy J. Shephard

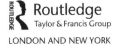

Routledge
Taylor & Francis Group

LONDON AND NEW YORK

First published 2018
by Routledge
2 Park Square, Milton Park, Abingdon, Oxon OX14 4RN

and by Routledge
711 Third Avenue, New York, NY 10017

Routledge is an imprint of the Taylor & Francis Group, an Informa business

British Library Cataloguing in Publication Data
A catalogue record for this book is available from the British Library

Library of Congress Cataloging in Publication Data
Names: Shephard, Roy J., author.
Title: Physical activity and the abdominal viscera : responses in health and disease / Roy J. Shephard.
Description: Milton Park, Abingdon, Oxon ; New York, NY : Routledge, 2017. | Series: Routledge research in physical activity and health | Includes bibliographical references and index.
Identifiers: LCCN 2017009052 | ISBN 978-1-138-74138-6 (hardback) | ISBN 978-1-315-17593-5 (ebook)
Subjects: LCSH: Abdomen—Diseases. | Viscera—Diseases. | Physical fitness. | Exercise.
Classification: LCC RC944 .S52 2017 | DDC 617.5/5—dc23
LC record available at https://lccn.loc.gov/2017009052

ISBN: 978-1-138-74138-6 (hbk)
ISBN: 978-1-315-17593-5 (ebk)

Typeset in Times New Roman
by FiSH Books Ltd, Enfield

Contents

Tables

Preface

In the early 20th century, sports scientists began their investigations with a cycle ergometer or a motor driven treadmill, and an interest in establishing the energy expenditures of athletes by the technique of indirect calorimetry. Many reports appeared on the maximal oxygen consumption developed by various classes of competitor, along with information on their peak levels of ventilation, heart rate and cardiac output. During the 1960s, it was recognized that vigorous aerobic activity made a valuable contribution to population health, helping to counter the growing epidemics of cardiovascular disease and obesity. A vast literature thus developed on the responses of the muscles and the cardio-respiratory system to acute and chronic physical activity.

The muscles certainly provide the immediate motive force for an active individual, and the cardio-respiratory system plays an essential role in delivering oxygen and nutrients to the working muscles. However, sustained physical activity would be impossible without the contribution of the viscera to maintaining the constancy of the milieu intérieur. The fluid needed to dissipate heat, the energy provided by ingested fats and carbohydrates, and the essential amino acids needed for muscle hypertrophy are all delivered to the body via the gastro-intestinal tract. Critical steps in the provision of the prime energy source of glucose to the active muscles (glycolysis and gluconeogenesis) depend upon metabolic processes within the liver, and the regulation of fluid balance and the excretion of the unwanted by-products of metabolism depend upon the healthy functioning of the kidneys and urinary tract. A clear understanding of the impact of exercise upon the viscera is thus important in optimizing athletic performance, in developing tactics to prevent chronic disease and in enhancing the individual's overall health.

Two recent textbooks of exercise physiology included short chapters on the gastro-intestinal tract,[1, 2] Lambert[3] and Poortmans and Zembraski[4] contributed articles on the gastro-intestinal and renal systems, respectively, to a recent history of exercise physiology, and a Swedish text of preventive physical activity[5] included brief contributions on gastro-intestinal disease, renal disease and cancer. However, the 1990 consensus conference on physical activity, fitness and health[6] made scant reference to the viscera, and the *Olympic Textbook of Science in Sport*[7] offers only brief comments on liver glycogen and colon cancer, with no substantive mention of gastro-intestinal function, the liver or the kidneys. I had planned to provide a brief overview of the topic for the *Year Book of Sports Medicine*, beginning in 2013,[8] but this initiative was thwarted when this particular *Year Book* ceased publication. Nevertheless, the time was ripe to summarize existing knowledge on the physiology of the gut and the abdominal viscera and its application to preventive medicine. A first volume, looking at physical activity and the function of the gastro-intestinal tract was thus published.[9] The present text complements this volume with information on physical activity and the abdominal viscera.

Each chapter considers first the normal physiological responses to exercise, and then examines how these responses are modified by repeated exercise sessions, whether the moderate bouts of activity typical of the community fitness centre or the intensive programmes of the international competitor. Implications for health promotion and preventive medicine are also reviewed. It is recognized that although moderate physical activity typically enhances health, excessive exercise can impair both competitive performance and health. Adverse effects are particularly likely if a competitive athlete pushes exercise to the point where most of the cardiac output is directed to the claims of the muscles (for nutrients and oxygen) and the skin (for heat dissipation), leaving the viscera dangerously deprived of their normal blood supply. It is important to define the tipping point where exercise begins to have adverse effects, relating this threshold to the individual's age, fitness and health. Further, the potential benefits of moderate activity will not be realized unless people persist with their prescribed activity, so there is also a need to document factors affecting compliance with exercise programmes in various types of visceral disorder.

Our narrative begins with the liver. Here, the chemical processing of carbohydrate, fats and protein takes place. These vital biochemical reactions are substantially modified by acute and chronic physical activity, and excessive physical activity can adversely affect function. Further, habitual physical activity can reduce the risk of various pathologies, including the metabolic syndrome, non-alcoholic fatty liver disease, hepatic inflammation, cirrhosis and hepato-cellular carcinoma. This chapter is followed by a discussion of the gall bladder and biliary tract, noting that function can be modified by both acute physical activity and aerobic training, and that an active lifestyle can modify the risks of developing gallstones, cholecystitis and gall bladder cancer.

The next section of the text addresses the excretion of waste products via the kidneys and urinary tract. It considers the significance of temporary manifestations of renal dysfunction (exercise-induced microproteinuria and microhaematuria), as well as the potential for developing acute renal failure during exhausting exercise. It points also to the danger of chronic renal damage from an excessive intake of creatine and non-steroidal anti-inflammatory drugs. Further, it explores the place of rehabilitation programmes for patients undergoing dialysis or receiving renal transplants, and it discusses the role of regular physical activity in reducing the risk of renal cancer and kidney stones. A specific chapter examines the risks of contact sport for an athlete with a single kidney. A chapter on the bladder looks at the influence of impact sports upon stress incontinence; it also directs attention to exercise haematuria and considers the possible value of habitual physical activity in relation to cancer of the urinary bladder.

The final section of the book looks at the spleen and the prostate gland. Changes in splenic volume with exercise are reviewed and their practical significance for circulatory and immune function are considered. Subsequent chapters explore the clinical issues of restriction of exercise participation in those affected by infectious mononucleosis and sickle cell disease. The final two chapters consider the practical significance of physical activity in the prevention and management of chronic prostatitis, benign prostate hyperplasia and prostate cancer.

Two areas that are not discussed in detail are the fat stores and immune function. Both body fat and the immune system might well be considered as "internal organs". Interactions between habitual physical activity and fat accumulation are certainly very important in the context of the prevention of obesity, diabetes, hypertension and other forms of chronic disease, and there is growing evidence that exercise can cause a favourable modulation of immune function. The topic of physical activity and the metabolic syndrome receives brief discussion in the context of hepatic function (Chapter 1) and the impact of physical activity upon the immune system is noted in the context of changes in splenic volume (Chapter 7). However, the effects of physical activity upon obesity and immune function are both large topics, and have already been covered in some detail by other books,[10, 11] so that in the interests of providing a compact account I have not allocated space to a detailed discussion of these issues.

As the writing of this book has progressed, I myself have learned much about a badly neglected area of exercise science and health promotion, with relevance not only to the maximizing of human performance, but also the prevention and clinical management of some major clinical problems. I hope that this will also be your experience.

Roy J. Shephard,
Brackendale, BC, Canada, 2017

References

1. Gisolfi CV. The gastrointestinal system. In: *Exercise physiology: People and ideas.* Tipton, CM, (ed.). New York: Oxford University Press, 2003, pp. 475–495.
2. Murray R, Shi X. The gastrointestinal tract. In: *ACSMs advanced exercise physiology.* Tipton CM, (ed.). Philadelphia, PA: Lippincott, Williams and Wilkins, 2006, pp. 357–369.
3. Lambert GP. The gastrointestinal system. In: *History of exercise physiology.* Tipton CM, (ed.). Champaign, IL: Human Kinetics, 2014, pp. 405–422.
4. Poortmans, JR, Zambraski E. The renal system. In: *History of exercise physiology,* Tipton CM, (ed.). Champaign, IL: Human Kinetics, 2014, pp. 507–524.
5. Professional Associations for Physical Activity (Sweden). *Physical activity in the prevention and treatment of disease* (English translation). 2nd ed. Stockholm: Sweden, 2010, pp. 1–621.

6. Bouchard C, Shephard RJ, Stephens T. *Physical activity, fitness and health.* Champaign, IL: Human Kinetics, 1992, pp. 1–1085.

7. Maughan RJ. *The Olympic textbook of science in sport.* Oxford, UK: Wiley-Blackwell, 2009, pp. 1–426.

8. Shephard RJ. Physical activity and the visceral organs. In: Shephard RJ, Cantu RC, DesMeules F et al. (eds). *Year book of sports medicine, 2013.* Philadelphia, PA: Elsevier, 2013, pp. xvi–xxviii.

9. Shephard RJ. *Physical activity and responses of the gastro-intestinal tract in health and disease.* Abingdon, UK: Taylor & Francis, 2017.

10. Bray GA. *A guide to obesity and the metabolic syndrome. Origins and treatment.* Boca Raton, FL: CRC Press, 2011, pp. 1–360.

11. Shephard RJ. *Physical activity, training and the immune response.* Carmel, IN: Cooper Publishing, 1997, pp. 1–463.

1   Responses of liver to acute and chronic physical activity

Introduction

With a mass of between 1.4 and 1.7 kg, the human liver is the largest of the viscera. Galen considered it the most important organ in the body, responsible for the formation of three of the body's four "humours", the blood, yellow bile and black bile.[1] It has a wide range of biological functions, including not only the secretion of bile, but also the synthesis of various proteins, amino acids, glycogen, cholesterol, triglycerides, hormones and vitamins, the metabolism of proteins, fats and carbohydrates, the storage of iron and copper, the regulation of glycogen storage and blood volume, and the elimination of various toxins from the body by a combination of metabolism and excretion. It also ensures an adequate blood level of the metabolites needed to maintain vigorous physical activity and to allow the synthesis of new muscle and brain tissue.[2-5] However, major consensus texts on physical activity, fitness and health[6, 7] have provided little information as to how its function is modified by either an acute bout of physical activity or by regular endurance training. The main focus of available literature has been upon physical activity in the context of pathologies such as acute hepatitis and fatty liver (steatosis).[8]

The present chapter considers the physiological and pathological responses of the liver to acute and chronic physical activity. The text spans the population spectrum from very sedentary individuals to elite endurance athletes, assessing the level of physical activity that promotes optimal hepatic function, and examining possible dangers of excessive physical activity. In the interests of simplicity, the reader is referred to a recent review for details of the complex biochemical and molecular processes underlying these responses.[9] Specific clinical issues relating to the metabolic syndrome, non-alcoholic fatty liver disease, hepatic inflammation, hepatic cirrhosis and hepato-cellular carcinoma are deferred to Chapter 2.

Acute hepatic responses to moderate endurance activity

In the healthy individual, the liver makes an important contribution to maintaining the constancy of the body's internal environment (what the classical

French physiologist Claude Bernard[10] termed the "milieu intérieur").We will here look at the favourable changes in carbohydrate, lipid and protein metabolism that are induced by an optimal volume of moderate endurance activity, and will consider briefly biochemical triggers and molecular processes underlying the hepatic responses.

Carbohydrate metabolism

Under resting conditions, the human liver normally contains 100–150 g of glycogen. This store is important to performance, providing a reserve of carbohydrate that can stabilize blood glucose levels during a prolonged bout of physical activity. Studies using stable isotopes have demonstrated an increased output of glucose from the liver during exercise.[11] The resulting rise of blood glucose contributes to an increase in the rate of glucose oxidation during physical activity. It also causes a temporary suppression of appetite, an important tactic for the clinician who includes regular exercise as a component of any weight-loss programme.

The rate of glucose usage is closely matched to the individual's work-rate,[12, 13] but during moderate and vigorous physical activity (50–85% of an individual's maximal oxygen intake, $\dot{V}O_{2max}$), liver-derived glucose contributes less to the body's total energy requirement than oxidation of the larger glycogen reserves found in skeletal muscle.[12] The breakdown of hepatic glycogen (glycolysis) may initially lead to an outflow of lactate from the liver, but subsequently an increased glucose output is the main manifestation. As activity continues, the liver takes up lactate produced by the skeletal muscles,[14] glycerol and amino acids (released from skeletal muscle through the action of cortisol), using these substances as substrates to synthesize glucose (the process of gluconeogenesis).[15–17] The hepatic metabolism of lactate is important not only in providing a fuel for gluconeogenesis, but also in controlling the decrease of blood pH that inhibits performance as the muscle production of lactate increases.

Depending upon a person's recent diet and training status, liver and muscle glycogen reserves together suffice for 90–180 minutes of vigorous aerobic exercise.[18] The athlete can increase these resting glycogen stores both by endurance training and by the ingestion of a high carbohydrate diet for several days (the process of "carbohydrate loading"). For the first hour or more of physical activity, blood glucose levels are maintained predominantly by the breakdown of hepatic glycogen.[3] However, as activity continues, there is a progressive increase in the relative contribution of hepatic gluconeogenesis. During very prolonged activity, there is still a substantial rate of hepatic gluconeogenesis,[19] but this is no longer sufficient to maintain homeostasis. Once hepatic and muscle glycogen reserves have been exhausted, the blood glucose concentration falls, unless the work-rate is reduced.[11]

The glycogen reserves of the liver must be replenished following exercise. Storage is regulated by the hormone insulin. This acts on the hepatocytes, up-regulating the enzyme glycogen synthase to increase the rate of glycogen synthesis. The process is dependent upon GTPase ADP-ribosylation factor-related protein 1 (ARFRP1). This protein regulates the secretion of insulin-like growth factor-1 and sorting of the glucose-transporter GLUT-2, contributing to both normal tissue growth and the glycogen synthesis needed to rebuild liver glycogen stores.[20]

Lipid metabolism

The influence of exercise upon hepatic lipid metabolism is important to the understanding and prevention of fatty infiltration of the liver. Hormonal responses to endurance exercise, particularly the secretion of catecholamines, cause a mobilization of free fatty acids (FFAs) from fat depots in various parts of the body, and there is also a reduction of hepatic re-esterification of fatty acids, thus increasing the net availability of FFA in the circulation.[21, 22] Given that much of the total blood flow is redistributed from the viscera to the working muscles during vigorous physical activity, the majority of circulating FFAs are redirected to the contracting muscles, and the liver rapidly loses its dominant role in clearing circulating fatty acids from the blood stream. Muscular oxidation of the circulating FFAs accounts for most of the whole-body fat that is metabolized during physical activity, although during intense exercise triglycerides already stored within the muscle fibres also make a small contribution to the total energy expenditure.[12]

Under resting conditions, the liver accounts for about 40% of circulating fatty acid uptake, substantially exceeding the uptake by skeletal muscle (~15%).[23, 24] A portion of the fatty acid uptake is oxidized by the liver,[25, 26] and a part is re-esterified to triglycerides.[27, 28] The latter are either stored in the liver, or are secreted as very low density lipoprotein triglycerides (VLDLs). During physical activity, the hepatic uptake of FFAs drops sharply, now accounting for less than a quarter of the total FFA that is cleared from the circulation.[22] If the oxygen supply to the working muscles is good, the VLDL particles could in principle be oxidized by skeletal muscle.[29] However, one report found that the hepatic release of VLDL triglycerides was unchanged during 90 minutes of exercise at 58% of $\dot{V}O_{2max}$,[30] and in another study 60 minutes of cycle ergometry at 60% of $\dot{V}O_{2max}$ had no influence upon the release of VLDLs in sedentary women.[31] Thus, the current consensus is that hepatic VLDL triglycerides make only a trivial contribution to whole-body fat metabolism during exercise.[32]

Animal data suggest that the ability of the liver to synthesize triglycerides is decreased during exercise. One study was performed on obese Zucker rats, an in-bred species that has a high rate of fat synthesis; this investigation found a decrease in hepatic fatty acid synthase mRNA and thus of the enzyme needed for fatty acid synthesis in response to a bout of exhausting exercise.[33] A second report used Sprague-Dawley rats which had been starved and then refed;[34] treadmill running to exhaustion again decreased hepatic fatty acid synthase activity in these animals. However, a review of animal experiments concluded that laboratory exercise had no significant effect upon the liver content of total lipids, phospholipids or cholesterol in normally fed rats;[35] presumably, an excessive intake of food is also a factor in fatty infiltration of the liver.

Following a bout of vigorous physical activity, a combination of persistently high concentrations of circulating fatty acids and an up-regulation of the hepatic enzymes involved in triglyceride synthesis tends to replenish the fat content of the liver. Thus, Johnson et al.[36] noted that endurance-trained men showed small but significant increases in proton magnetic resonance spectroscopy estimates of hepatic triglyceride content both 30 minutes and 4 hours after 90 minutes of cycle ergometry at 65% of $\dot{V}O_{2peak}$. Likewise, Hu et al.[21] observed that in mice, high levels of circulating fatty acids were induced by a prolonged (60–90 min.) period of exercise, and this led to an increase of hepatic triglycerides three–four hours following exercise. Again, a single four-hour bout of swimming up-regulated hepatic stearyl CoA desaturase, with a resultant increase in hepatic triglyceride content.[37]

Protein metabolism

Sustained physical activity can augment the hepatic synthesis of a number of proteins, including albumin and insulin-like growth factor binding protein (IGFBP). This response is important to the anabolic response to regular exercise. The IGFBP binds IGF-1, allowing growth hormone to act continuously upon nearby cells in the liver, and thus to produce more IGF-1, in what is termed a paracrine action.

Isotope infusion studies in humans have demonstrated increases in both the fractional (6%) and the absolute synthesis (16%) of albumin six hours after completing a session of vigorous interval exercise.[38] In rats, an increase in hepatic IGFBP-1 mRNA expression was also observed for up to 12 hours following vigorous treadmill running. This response likely reduces blood levels of IGF-1, and thus curtails muscle glucose uptake immediately post-exercise, preventing hypoglycemia,[39] although it also has the paracrine effect of augmenting hepatic synthesis of IGF-1, as noted above.

If muscle and liver glycogen reserves have been depleted by very prolonged physical activity, the liver plays an important role in sustaining the glucose supply by forming glucose from amino acids. The necessary amino acids are released from skeletal muscle in response to the action of catabolic hormones such as cortisol. One study found that arterial concentrations of the amino acid alanine rose 20–25% with mild exertion, and by 60–95% at heavier work rates; 8–35% increases were also seen in the arterial concentrations of other amino acids, including isoleucine, leucine, methionine, tyrosine and phenylalanine.[40] From differences in blood concentrations between the hepatic artery and the hepatic vein, it can be deduced that even during mild and moderate physical activity, humans increase the splanchnic blood stream uptake of alanine by 15–20%.[40] The use of these amino acids in gluconeogenesis is evidenced by increased concentrations of urea nitrogen in the sweat.[41]

Triggers of hepatic responses to physical activity

The relative importance of blood-borne factors (changes in the temperature and volume of blood flow, circulating hormones, cytokines and metabolite concentrations) and direct influences (for example, local hypoxia and a depletion of high energy phosphates) in triggering acute hepatic responses to physical activity remains unclear. If the dominant trigger could be determined, it might become possible to tailor the exercise stimulus to cause a selective modification of this factor, and thus maximize hepatic adaptations either to improve physical changes in liver metabolism performance or to enhance liver health. For instance, if a decrease in hepatic blood flow was found to be a primary determinant, a short bout of high-intensity exercise might be recommended rather than a prolonged period of low-to-moderate-intensity activity.

There seems no fundamental reason why triggers of altered hepatic metabolism should differ between humans and laboratory animals, but one issue in interpreting current evidence is that much of the available research has been conducted on rodents, where resting hepatic glycogen reserves are relatively much larger than in humans.[42, 43] The classical view has been that the exercise-induced stimulation of hepatic glucose metabolism is largely a consequence of an altered hormonal milieu, with an attenuated secretion of insulin[44] and rising glucagon concentrations.[45] The latter hormone stimulates hepatic glucagon receptors, and if physical activity continues for longer than 60–90 minutes, responses can be accentuated by a combination of declining plasma glucose concentrations[46] and depletion of hepatic glycogen reserves.[47, 48] A rising glucagon concentration boosts the liver's extraction of glucose precursors from the blood, speeds the conversion of these precursors into glucose[45] and also stimulates glycolysis.[49] The underlying biochemical sequence is a stimulation of hepatic glucagon receptors that increases concentrations of cyclic adenosine monophosphate (cAMP), with an activation of protein kinase A and an extracellular signal-regulated kinase (ERK)[50] that acts as an "on/off" switch. Glucagon also amplifies adenosine monophosphate kinase (AMPK) signalling,[51] thus inhibiting processes that use the energy stored in the ATP molecule, while at the same time stimulating processes that increase stores of ATP.

Somewhat surprisingly, moderate physical activity does not cause much change in peripheral venous glucagon levels. However, this may be because the concentrations measured in blood collected from the arm veins do not necessarily reflect hepatic glucagon levels.[52] During vigorous exercise, catecholamine secretion may also contribute to the increase in gluconeogenesis, either by providing the liver with additional substrate from adipose tissue lipolysis and increased peripheral lactate formation,[5] or by activating hepatic catecholamine receptors and thus the ERK on/off switch.[53] Against this last hypothesis, hepatic glucose output does not seem to be greatly affected by adrenoreceptor blockade.[54]

Some correlate of glycogen depletion, albeit changes in concentration of a metabolic substrate, a derivative of substrate oxidation, an energy-storing compound such as ATP, or an associated alteration in cell volume might also trigger a metabolic response more directly by acting on the hepatic afferent nerves.[55] In support of this hypothesis, studies in rats show that if glucagon secretion is suppressed by infusion of the hormone somastatin, an increased activity of the hepatic sympathetic nerves can be detected in terms of an augmented output of epinephrine and norepinephrine.[56] However, hepatic glucose release is unaffected by hepatic denervation alone,[44, 56] and section of the hepatic nerves does not curtail the increase of blood sugar seen in rats during a brief bout of exercise.[57]

Some of the changes of liver function that are seen during physical activity may occur independently of either hormones or the autonomic nerve supply. One possible trigger is the cytokine interleukin-6; this is released from muscle during exercise and appears to play an important role in regulating carbohydrate metabolism.[58] A number of pointers suggest an action of IL-6 upon the liver. IL-6 stimulation of hepatoma cells increases their glucose production and the injection of IL-6 into mice induces a small increase of hepatic phosphoenolpyruvate carboxykinase (PECPK), an enzyme involved in gluconeogenesis.[59] Exercised mice also show an increase of CXCL-I., a hepatic chemokine that attracts neutrophils and is involved in inflammation and wound healing. Muscle-derived IL-6 seems the trigger for secretion of this chemical messenger;[60] the full range of functions of CXCL-1 are unclear, but given its anti-inflammatory actions, it could well be responsible for some of the beneficial health effects associated with an adequate programme of habitual physical activity. Finally, IL-6 may mediate a very large increase of hepcidin, a hormone that inhibits iron uptake and causes a trapping of iron in hepatic cells and macrophages; an increase of hepcidin and a resulting anaemia is a problem encountered in some athletes following a prolonged and strenuous bout of training.[61, 62]

Physical activity might also modify liver function through an increased generation of reactive oxygen species, as in skeletal muscle.[63–65] Vigorous and prolonged physical activity (particularly if performed under hot and humid conditions) significantly restricts visceral blood flow,[17, 66] temporarily depriving the liver of an adequate oxygen supply,[67] and this could favour an increased formation of reactive oxygen species (ROS). The secretion of heat shock proteins is linked to the production of ROS, and the exercise-induced up-regulation and accumulation of heat shock proteins, as seen in several rat studies following an hour of exhausting treadmill running[64, 65, 68–70] might seem to support this hypothesis. However, other researchers have found little evidence of oxidative stress in the liver lipids and proteins of the rat following either acute[71] or chronic exhausting exercise,[72] with no clear changes in the activity of various antioxidant enzymes such as metallotheonine-1, heme oxygenase-1 and superoxide dismutase following a non-exhausting 60 minute run.[74, 81]

Thus, there remain several competing hypotheses as to what triggers the observed hepatic adaptations to physical activity: an alteration in the hormonal milieu (changes in the concentrations of insulin, glucagon and/or epinephrine), an effect upon afferent nerves through some correlate of glycogen depletion, a response to secretion of a cytokine such as IL-6 or an effect of oxidant stress.

Molecular changes in the liver with acute physical activity

Information on the molecular changes induced by acute exercise is based almost exclusively on studies of normally inactive rodents (Table 1.1). The changes are complex and details can be found elsewhere.[9, 81] Manifestations, all of which seem favourable to performance, include an up-regulation of enzymes involved in carbohydrate metabolism, a decreased expression of fat synthesizing enzymes and an up-regulation of systems protecting the liver cells against genetic mutation and heat shock. An analysis of the transcriptome (the total of RNA messengers) in mice hepatocytes following 60 minutes of moderate intensity exercise showed that while 352 transcripts were up-regulated, 184 were down-regulated. Many of the changes in messenger RNA affected the activity of genes of recognized importance for glycolysis, gluconeogenesis and fatty acid metabolism.[87] Physical activity also activated some of these same genes in skeletal muscle, but the response was generally more marked in the liver. The effect was transient, disappearing within a few hours of ceasing a given bout of physical activity.[74, 81]

An acute bout of exercise consistently leads to an up-regulation of gluco-neogenic and metabolic enzymes such as glucose-6-phosphatase, pyruvate dehydrogenase and phosphoenolpyruvate carboxykinase (PEPCK),[58, 74] a down-regulation of fat-synthesizing enzymes[33, 34] and the induction of metabolic regulators such as insulin receptor substrate.[74] Cortisol is normally implicated in the activation of hepatic PEPCK transcription. Thus, responses to physical activity are greatly attenuated in adrenalectomized animals and are absent in transgenic mice bred with deletion of the normal glucocorticoid regulatory unit.[77]

Hepatic responses to high-intensity and prolonged physical activity

High intensities of physical activity can reduce hepatic blood flow, and if exercise is prolonged, there is evidence of temporary derangements of hepatic function. However, recovery is rapid, and the changes usually have little clinical significance. We will look at the extent of reductions in local blood flow, and will review markers of impaired liver function that include histological changes, impaired pharmokinetics, markers of oxidative stress and altered blood levels of hepatic enzymes (Table 1.2). Long-lasting or permanent changes might deter athletes from participation in ultra-endurance events, but information to date suggests that liver function is typically normalized within a few days even after an event such as an ultra-marathon run.

Hepatic blood flow

Human hepatic blood flow is commonly estimated from the circulatory clearance of intravenously injected indocyanine dye. This technique suggests decreases of ~ 20% during brief vigorous effort and a much larger reduction of blood flow if

Table 1.1 A summary of the molecular changes seen in the liver with acute exercise

Author	Change	Biological effect
Anthony et al.[39]	Increased IGFBP-1 mRNA expression	May help to limit hypoglycaemia post-exercise
Banzet et al.;[58] Dohm et al.;[73] Hoene et al.;[74] Nizielski et al.[75]	Up-regulation of glucose-6-phosphatase, pyruvatedehydrogenase, phosphoenol pyruvate carboxylase	Increase of gluconeogenesis
Banzet et al.;[58] Helmrich et al.;[76] Hoene et al.[74]	Increase of perioxosome proliferator-activated receptor coactivator PGC-1	Increased levels of protein that regulates mitochondrial biogenesis
Fiebig et al.;[34] Griffiths et al.[33]	Reduced expression of lipogenic enzymes	Less fat synthesis
Friedman;[77] Ropelle et al.[78]	Increase of PEPCK gene and PECPK mRNA in mice, decrease of PECPK and glucose phosphatase in obese rats	Regulation of gluconeogenesis
Gonzalez and Manso[69]	Increased synthesis of heat shock protein molecular chaperones	Protection of proteins against stressors
Haase et al.[79]	Increased mRNA and cytochrome c protein	Improves oxidative potential
Hansen et al.[80]	Increased production of follistatin	Inhibits myostatin, facilitates muscle hypertrophy
Hoene et al.[74]	Induction of insulin-receptor substrate	Increases insulin binding, facilitates gluconeogenesis
Hoene and Weigert[81]	Changes in 352 gene transcripts	Many of the genes active in glycolysis, gluconeogenesis and fatty acid metabolism
Huang et al.[82]	Increase of adiponectin receptor 1, decrease of adiponectin receptor 2, increase of the transcription factor forkhead box O1	Regulation of gluconeogenesis
Kelly et al.[83]	Increased hepatic AMP-activated protein kinase activity	Regulation of carbohydrate and lipid metabolism; effect less in IL-6 knock-out mice
Khanna et al.[84]	Increased hepatic content of bound form of alpha-lipoic acid	Co-factor for many mitochondrial proteins active in metabolism
Lavoie et al.;[85] Leu and George[86]	Increased blood levels of insulin binding growth factor binding protein	Helps glucose regulation by neutralizing insulin-like effects of insulin-like growth factor-1; also counters apoptotic effect of p53

Table 1.1 continued

Author	Change	Biological effect
Ochiai and Manso[37]	Up-regulation of hepatic stearyl CoA desaturase	May protect against insulin resistance
Peeling;[61] Roecker et al.[62]	Increase of hepcidin	Inhibition of iron uptake; could contribute to athlete's anaemia

Notes: AMP = adenosine monophosphate. Co A = conezyme A. IGFBP-1 = insulin-like growth
factor binding protein 1. mRNA = messenger ribonucleic acid. PGC = perioxosome gamma
co-activator. PECPK = phosphoenolpyruvate carboxykinase

activity is prolonged or is undertaken in a hot environment.[88, 89] For any given duration of effort, there appears to be an inverse dose-response relationship between visceral blood flow and the intensity of physical activity, with indo-cyanine clearance decreasing by ~ 80% as the intensity of activity approaches the individual's $\dot{V}O_{2max}$.

The elimination of indocyanine depends upon both hepatic blood flow and the continued ability of the liver cells to excrete the dye in a normal fashion.[90] Thus, it has been argued that during heavy physical activity, in docyanine-based inferences regarding hepatic blood flow may be confounded because of impairments in the excretory capacity of the liver cells. Nevertheless, major exercise-related decreases in hepatic blood flow have been corroborated by other techniques. Thus, clearance of intravenous injections of sorbitol have indicated hepatic blood flow reductions of ~ 40% when exercising at 40% of $\dot{V}O_{2max}$,[91] of 60–70% at 60–70% of $\dot{V}O_{2max}$[92] and of 83% during near-maximal exercise.[93] Further, Fojt et al. demonstrated dramatic drops of oxygen saturation in the hepatic vein during prolonged physical activity,[94] much as would be expected if the oxygen extraction due to hepatic metabolism was unchanged, but local blood flow was greatly reduced. Nevertheless, the magnitude of changes remains somewhat contentious, particularly during short periods of vigorous exercise. Thus, using a radionuclide technique, Flamm et al.[95] found only a 25% decrease in hepatic blood content during brief but intense cycle ergometry (5 minutes at 75% and 5 minutes at 100% of maximal aerobic effort). Likewise, Froelich et al.[96] noted only a statistically non-significant 14% reduction of hepatic blood content during a short progressive cycle ergometer test to voluntary exhaustion.

The indocyanine and sorbitol-based human estimates of hepatic blood flow seem confirmed by animal studies where para-aminohippuric acid and sulphobromthalein were injected into a mesenteric vein, and blood samples were drawn from both portal and hepatic veins,[97] with the hepatic arterial blood flow calculated as the difference between these two readings. Further, application of an electromagnetic flow-probe to the portal vein of rats showed that there was a large

Table 1.2 Reports of adverse changes of liver function following participation in prolonged endurance exercise

Authors	Subjects	Exercise	Findings	Comments
Ultra-endurance exercise				
Bürger-Mendonça et al.[121]	6 male athletes	Half-triathlon	Comparison of blood samples before and after race; significant change in AST and ALP but not ALT	Moderate temperatures. All enzyme values remained within normal limits
De Paz et al.[122]	13 male runners, mean age 36 years	100 km race	Post-race increases in ALT +42%, AST+193%, GGT +56%, CK +2,000%	Cool conditions; serum bilirubin +106%. Also decrease of serum haptoglobins
Fallon et al.[123]	7 male, 2 female	1,600 km ultramarathon	Increases of ALT, AST, GGT, LDH, CK; ALT remains high when AST and CK falling	Temperatures 11–32 °C
Holly et al.[124]	6 male, 3 female triathlon competitors	Hawaiian Ironman competition	ASAT +700%, SGPT +262%, LDH +222% immediately after competition	Initial resting values high normal; enzymes marginally increased 5–6 days later
Kratz et al.[125]	32 male, 5 female runners, average age 49 years	Boston marathon	AST +265%, ALT +37%, CK +2,343% increased after race, 24 h > 4 h	Cool environment; bilirubin increased 60%, serum urea nitrogen increased 29%
Lippi et al.[126]	15 healthy males	21 km half-marathon	AST, LDH, CK increased 0–24 h following run	ALT not measured
Long et al.[127]	10 athletes	Short triathlon (10 km run, 20–40 km cycle, 1.0–1.5 km swim)	Modest increases of AST (30%) and LDH(53%)	Moderate temperatures; ALT not measured
Mena et al.[128]	Professional cyclists	800 km/ 6 days and 2,700 km/20 days with overnight rests	Increases of ALT, AST, ALP and (in longer race) LDH; partial return to normal with overnight rest	Cumulative increase of serum enzyme concentrations over race

Table 1.2 continued

Authors	Subjects	Exercise	Findings	Comments
Nagel et al.[129]	55 runners	1,000 km in 20 days	AST increased 500%, ALT 300%, GGT 600%, CK 2,000%; ALT remains high when AST and CK falling	Decreases in serum albumin and choline esterase (could reflect decreased synthesis or increase of IL-1)
Noakes and Carter[130]	13 athletes	160-km run	Increases of LDH 241%; AST 821%; CPK 1,732% in those completing event	Temperatures not stated; total bilirubin also increased twofold; ALT and GGT not determined
Noakes and Carter[131]	18 experienced, 5 novice competitors	56 km ultra-marathon	Greater rise of AST and CPK in novices, despite slower running speed	
Rama et al.[132]	7 well-trained male distance runners, mean age 37 years	100 km road race	GGT +19%, CK +3,121%	Cool conditions; ALT not measured
Richards et al.[133]	43 successful runners (28 M,16 F) vs. 10 who collapsed (9M, 1F)	14 km Sydney city to surf run	Casualties showed higher values for blood urea nitrogen, serum creatinine, uric acid and bilirubin	
Shapiro et al.[134]	26 untrained men	110 km march in 2 days	Increases in CK, AST and aldolase	Midday temperatures 30°C; ALT not measured. Increased enzyme levels only seen in those marching at 6 km/h
Smith et al.[135]	27 male, 7 female runners, aged 18–65 years	Marathon run	Significant increases in CK, AST, LDH immediately following event	ALT not determined; climate not specified
Suzuki et al.[136]	9 well-trained male triathletes	Ironman triathlon	Significant increases immediately and especially 24 h after race: ALT 185%; AST 759%; CK 2,680%; GGT −20%	Moderately warm conditions

Table 1.2 continued

Authors	Subjects	Exercise	Findings	Comments
Van Rensburg et al.[137]	23 male athletes, average age 33 years	Triathlon competition	Significant increases of AST, CK and LDH immediately post-race	ALT not measured; 4.5% decrease of body mass over event
Waskiewicz et al.[138]	14 male runners mean age 43 years	24 h ultra-marathon	Increased enzymes 24 h after run; ALT 350%, AST 1,354%, CK 1,204%, no change of GGT	Cool conditions
Wu et al.[139]	10 males, 1 female	24-h marathon	Blood enzymes tested immediately, 2 and 9 days after event. AST 1,344,630, −8%; ALT 237,259, 44%; LDH 286,205, 59%; no significant change of GGT	Moderately warm conditions; bilirubin increased immediately post-race

Other forms of exercise

Authors	Subjects	Exercise	Findings	Comments
Apple and McGue[140]	2 male runners	6 weeks of training for a marathon	ALT increased in 6 subjects; large increases of LDH and CK	
Beard et al.[141]	2 joggers with heat stroke		Reduced level of clotting factors produced by liver	
Bunch[142]	6 runners		Clinically "abnormal" levels of hepatic enzymes	
Fojt et al.[94]	6 male volunteers	Cycle ergometer exercise at 70–85% of maximal oxygen intake to exhaustion (26–60 min)	Hepatic vein shows increased content of ALT and other liver enzymes	
Hammouda et al.[143]	18 male football players	30 sec Wingate test	Small increases of CK 11%; AST 10%; ALT 16%; LDH 13%	

Table 1.2 continued

Authors	Subjects	Exercise	Findings	Comments
Kayashima et al.[101]	14 soldiers aged 24–36 years	80-km trek on limited diet over 4 days	Enzymes sampled immediately and after 8 days. Increases: AST 177, 152%; ALT 39, 234%; LDH 66, 8%; CK 208, −68%	Associated leucocytosis and bilirubinaemia immediately after exercise
Malinoski[144]	3 soldiers	Several days of strenuous training	Increases of ALT, AST and CK	
Nathwani et al.[145]	4 prison inmates	3 undertook vigorous squatting; 1 a long-distance run	Increases of AST, ALT, CPK and LDH	Liver damage unlikely since normal serum bilirubin and prothrombin times
Ohno et al.[146]	7 sedentary male students	Running 5 km,6 times/week for 10 weeks	50% decrease of resting GGT	
Pettersson et al.[147]	15 healthy men not used to weight-lifting	1 h of weight-lifting	AST, ALT, LDH, CK all remained elevated for 7 days post-exercise	Laboratory conditions
Takahashi et al.[148]	7 male rugby players, average age 21 years	2 successive Rugby sevens matches of 10 min duration, with 4-h inter-game interval	Increases of CK 42%; LDH 25%; AST 13%; but not ALT	Cool conditions

Animal data

Authors	Subjects	Exercise	Findings	Comments
Litvinova and Viru[149]	Male Wistar rats aged 10–12 weeks	10-h swimming with loading 10% of body mass	103% increase in hepatic ^{14}C urea content	Effect decreased by adrenalectomy

Notes: ALP = alkaline phosphatase; ALT = alanine transaminase; AST = aspartate transaminase; CK = creatine kinase; CPK = creatine phosphokinase; GGT = gamma-glutamyl transferase; LDH = lactate dehydrogenase; SGFT =serum glutamic pyruvic transaminase, also known as alanine amino transferase and progressive decrease of flow when animals exercised for 40 minutes at an oxygen consumption of 70 ml/(kg.min).[98]

Recovery of the normal hepatic blood flow is quite rapid even following heavy physical activity, and ultrasound studies suggest that for a few hours the local flow may even rise above normal levels. This response may reflect inflammation of the liver. Arguably, it also serves to replenish glycogen reserves and to speed normalization of circulating FFAs following exercise.[99]

Histological changes with physical activity

Histological changes associated with vigorous and/or exhausting physical activity could point to adverse effects of excessive physical activity, but studies have been conducted mainly in animals, and the findings are controversial. Sixty minutes of moderate intensity treadmill running has little effect upon the morphological characteristics of hepatic tissue.[100] However, this activity is enough to cause an acute inflammatory response, with an increase in the peripheral white cell count.[101] Moreover, the hepatocytes show a greater decrease in cell volume than can be attributed simply to glycogen depletion;[100] possibly, cell size is reduced due to a glucagon-induced decrease in cytoplasmic potassium ion content.

Rowell[17] suggested that activity of sufficient intensity to cause hepatic hypoxia predisposed to central lobular necrosis. Based on an extracellular fluid shift and a decrease of serum amino acids observed during a 23-hour ultra-marathon, Lehmann et al.[102] hypothesized that a decrease of intracellular volumes served as a signal leading to a catabolic degradation of various body cells, including the adverse changes in hepatocytes that others had reported.

A study of rats running for 60 minutes at 75% or 90% of $\dot{V}O_{2max}$ purported to show not only increased blood levels of hepatic enzymes, but also oedema and necro-inflammation of the liver tissue.[103] However, this conclusion was based upon only 24 animals divided between six controls and four other treatment groups. Moreover, only two of the four treatment groups showed necrotic changes, and interpretation of the liver histology was not conducted in a "blinded" fashion. The same criticism of a lack of "blinded" evaluation applies to other reports. Mitochondrial swelling in hepatocytes surrounding the hepatic venules was reported when rats ran for 100 or more minutes to exhaustion,[104] and 60–90 minutes of running to exhaustion was said to induce cancerous changes, necrosis and apoptosis of the hepatocytes.[105]

Impaired hepatic drug clearance

One practical measure of the extent of any activity-related changes in hepatic function is to monitor the clearance of drugs normally eliminated by the liver. Test agents fall into two basic categories: "low clearance" drugs such as acetamino-phen, antipyrine, diazepam, amylobarbitone and verapamil, where elimination depends largely upon hepatic enzyme activity and biliary excretion,[106] and "high clearance" drugs such as indocyanine, bromsulphthalein, sorbitol and lidocaine, where elimination reflects mainly hepatic blood flow.[89, 107]

The elimination of low-clearance drugs clearance in humans is largely unaffected by either moderate exercise[108–112] or by prolonged low to moderate intensity activity such as six–nine hours of marching,[113, 114] although there remains a need for further observations on very prolonged events such as ultra-marathon runs. In contrast, given the dramatic changes of blood flow noted above, it is not surprising that vigorous and/or prolonged physical activity reduces the elimination of high clearance substances.[111, 115]

Oxidant stress

Oxidant stress impairs the ability of the hepatocyte endoplasmic reticulum to fold and assemble proteins correctly. It can be caused by severe exercise and by aging. Significant oxidant stress may develop after rather than during physical activity,[64] and in order to determine the extent of such changes it is important to continue the search for markers of oxidant stress into the recovery period. As in skeletal muscle, oxidant stress is not always an "adverse" phenomenon; on occasion, it provides valuable signals, inducing adaptations of the liver to regular physical activity.[81]

Some[116–118] but not all human studies[119] have demonstrated transient oxidant stress following prolonged and/or vigorous exercise. However, human studies have not examined changes within the liver itself. Thus, Pinho et al.[116] found a variety of circulatory markers of such stress (increases of thiobarbituric reactive substances [TBARS], lipid hydroperoxide and protein carbonylation), along with up-regulation of superoxide dismutase and catalase, the enzymes breaking down reactive products, following participation in an Ironman triathlon. Neubauer et al.[117] made observations not only immediately after a triathlon, but also 1, 5 and 19 days later. They found that markers of oxidative stress had normalized within five days. Turner and associates[118] examined athletes after participating in a 223 km race. Their investigation noted DNA damage in peripheral blood mononuclear cells immediately after the run, with increased protein carbonylation persisting for seven days. Further, levels of the anti-oxidant reduced glutathione were still depressed at 28 days. In contrast, Margaritis et al.[119] found evidence of inflammation, including increased leucocyte counts, but no signs of oxidative stress following participation in a triathlon event.

Animal studies have provided more direct evidence that exhausting exercise can indeed cause oxidative stress within the liver tissue. As in the human study of Turner et al.,[118] the hepatic glutathione levels of rats fell following a bout of exhausting exercise, reflecting a large increase in oxidative metabolism and reduced stores of the normal buffer to reactive oxygen species.[120] Increased blood levels of malondialdehyde (MDA, a marker of lipid peroxidation), NOx and xanthine oxidase were seen in mice following 15 maximal sprints of 30 seconds. Temporary muscle damage was suggested by large increases in serum aminotransferases and lactate dehydrogenase (LDH), but there were no changes in levels of TBARS, superoxide dismutase or glutathione peroxidase in liver samples.[150] Relative to control animals, liver samples of aging rats that ran to exhaustion at 70–75% of their maximal oxygen intake showed increased neutrophil infiltration, along with higher levels of myeloperoxidase (an enzyme that is a marker of neutrophil infiltration) and MDA, with (paradoxically) reductions in levels of the anti-oxidant enzymes catalase and glutathione peroxidase.[151] Other studies of rats have found significant increases in measures of hepatic lipid peroxidation, with a substantial increase of MDA following 30 minutes[152] or 80 minutes of swimming to exhaustion.[153]

There is also a substantial rise in the temperature of hepatic tissue during exhausting exercise, and rodent studies have demonstrated an associated increase in concentrations of 70 kDa and 72 kDa heat shock proteins.[69, 70]

Serum enzyme levels

Clinicians frequently evaluate human hepatic function in terms of serum enzyme levels. Short periods of physical activity usually have little or no effect upon such indices,[143, 148] but in the hours following a marathon or triathlon competition, many investigators have found increased serum concentrations of amino-transferases, often accompanied by increased bilirubin levels and markers of inflammation such as IL-6 and C-reactive protein. Such findings have also been observed in laboratory animals after prolonged and vigorous physical activity.[103] However, the cause of these changes (hepatic injury, haemolysis or muscle injury) and their clinical significance has remained unclear. Confirmation of hepatic malfunction has been sought in a decreased synthesis of proteins such as albumin and choline esterase,[129, 139] although any reduction in the circulating concen-trations of these substances could also reflect the influence of increased serum concentrations of the cytokine interleukin-1.[129]

By catheterizing the hepatic vein, it is possible to show that the liver rather than muscle is the source of increased enzyme levels during exhausting exercise. Thus, Fojt et al.[94] noted that after 25–60 minutes of cycle ergometry at 70–85% of maximal oxygen intake, concentrations of enzymes as such lactate dehydro-genase, succinate dehydrogenase and creatine phosphokinase were greater in hepatic venous blood than in arterial blood. Moreover, local ischaemia was demonstrated by a hepatic venous oxygen saturation that dropped from a typical resting level of 75% to as low as 5% during the exercise bout.

Other measures of impaired liver function

Several pieces of biochemical evidence suggest that any exercise-induced distur-bances of liver function are usually short term and of relatively minor clinical significance. Nagel et al.[129] saw decreases in serum albumin and choline esterase over a 1000 km event, likely reflecting some transient decrease in hepatic synthesis of these proteins, and Beard[141] observed a decreased hepatic production of clotting factors in two runners who suffered from heat stroke. However, many investigations have noted an increase of bilirubin synthesis during and following competition. Thus, De Paz et al. reported a substantial increase in bilirubin levels following a 100 km race,[122] Noakes et al.[130] noted a large increase of bilirubin over a 160 km run, Wu et al.[139] observed an increase of bilirubin following a 24-hour marathon and Kratz et al.[125] found an increased excretion of both bilirubin and urea following participation in the Boston marathon. Nathwani et al[145] also commented on the normality of prothrombin times in their subjects following a bout of vigorous exercise.

Conclusions

Vigorous and/or prolonged physical activity can cause an inflammatory response in animal livers, but possible histological evidence of more permanent damage to the hepatocytes requires confirmation by blinded observations. Vigorous physical activity causes a slowing in the elimination of markers dependent on hepatic blood flow, but little change in the clearance of markers dependent on normal liver function. There is some evidence of oxidative stress in both humans and animals, and a transient appearance of hepatic enzymes in the serum with exhausting exercise. However, these changes are reversed within a few days. There is little evidence of either depressed protein synthesis or permanent hepatic damage; indeed, some of the changes that have been observed may be a necessary component of normal and positive hepatic adaptations to vigorous physical activity.

Chronic effects of moderate endurance activity

Carbohydrate metabolism

Strenuous endurance training increases an athlete's ability to sustain a higher work-rate during prolonged activity and to exercise for a longer time before the onset of fatigue. One factor contributing to this change is an improved ability to maintain blood glucose levels during prolonged effort. This is in part a consequence of an increased capacity for skeletal muscle to store glycogen and to oxidize fat at the expense of glucose. However, further adaptations likely include an increased storage of glycogen in the resting liver, and slower rates of both glycolysis and gluconeogenesis at any given absolute intensity of effort. Thus, Murakami et al.[154] found that after 12 weeks of treadmill training, the glycogen content of rats livers was increased by about 30%. Coggan et al.[155] required human volunteers to cycle for 45–90 minutes per day at 75–100% of peak oxygen intake, and at the end of 12 weeks they observed a substantially reduced rate of glycolysis and some reduction of gluconeogenesis at any given intensity of exercise. This probably reflected mainly a lesser secretion of epinephrine and norepinephrine during what had become a less challenging test exercise, but there were also higher insulin and lower glucagon concentrations, as also noted by Galbo et al.[156] Further, the availability of gluconeogenic precursors (lactate and glycerol) was reduced at any given intensity of exercise.[155]

Rodent investigations have shown some differences from human studies, probably because whereas gluconeogenesis accounts for some 20% of glucose production when humans undertake moderate exercise, in rats the figures range from 40–70%. Most but not all[157] rodent studies have observed increased activity of the enzymes and signalling molecules involved in carbohydrate and lipid metabolism following aerobic training.[158, 159] For example, Khanna et al.[84] trained rats by running them to exhaustion up a 10% grade at 2.1 km/h; this induced an increase in the hepatic content of the bound form of alpha-lipoic acid (lipoyl-lysine), an important co-factor in lipid metabolism. Both glycolytic and gluconeogenic responses to a given concentration of glucagon were also enhanced following training.[172, 173] Mechanisms underlying the increased response to glucagon apparently include an adjustment in the ratio of inhibitory to stimulatory guanine-nucleotide binding protein (G protein) and a resultant increase in activity of the "second messenger" adenyl cyclase.[172] The increased capacity for gluconeogenesis allows the trained animal to sustain higher work-rates and to maintain blood glucose levels for longer during a sustained bout of activity.[174] Moreover, the liver has an increased absolute capacity to metabolize lactate[175] and alanine,[176] with an associated increase of gluconeogenesis.[176, 177]

Lipid metabolism

The enhanced ability of the exerciser to metabolize fat following training is largely a function of enzymatic adaptations in skeletal muscle, and there is little evidence that the liver contributes to this response. Nevertheless, regular exercise is associated with alterations in lipid/lipoprotein metabolism and appears to reduce the storage of triglyceride in the liver.

The limited effect of training upon the hepatic metabolism of fat is perhaps understandable, given the apparently trivial contribution of the liver to fat oxidation during physical activity.[32] The hormones that contribute to the lipolysis of depot fat include epinephrine, norepinephrine, ghrelin, growth hormone, testosterone and cortisol, and plainly training blunts the response of several of these hormones to exercise. After training, the action of the growth hormones is countered by increasing circulating concentrations of insulin and insulin-like growth factor binding protein-1.[178] Blood glycerol and FFA concentrations are also lower at a given absolute exercise intensity,[246] thus reducing the available substrate for hepatic synthesis of triglycerides.

A substantial number of studies have examined associations between regular physical activity, liver fat content and liver mass. In general, liver fat content has been lower in more active individuals, but it is difficult to be certain exercise was responsible, since many studies have had no control group, and interventions have often included alterations of diet as well as increases of physical activity. Liver fat content has generally been determined by proton magnetic resonance spectrosopy, ultrasound, CT scan or biopsy, but habitual physical activity has usually been assessed by questionnaires of dubious validity, rather than by objective techniques, and when comparisons have been made, large discrepancies have been seen between subjective and objective estimates of habitual physical activity.[161]

Cross-sectional associations between habitual physical activity and amount of liver fat

Of 12 cross-sectional studies, 6 samples, often quite large, involved healthy individuals, and 6 smaller subject-groups had fatty livers (Table 1.3). Nine investigations relied on questionnaire assessments of habitual activity, but there were also studies using a Sense-wear arm-band,[161] an accelerometer[162] and a pedometer.[168] All reports except that of Kang et al.[165] found less fat accumulation and fewer pathological changes in the livers of individuals who engaged in greater amounts of physical activity, with benefit being seen with both aerobic and resistance exercise.[171] The negative report of Kang et al.[165] measured habitual physical activity using the Paffenbarger questionnaire, and they observed comparable levels of physical activity in those with and without evidence of the metabolic syndrome.

Cross-sectional cassociations between aerobic fitness and amount of liver fat

Eleven studies (mostly with relatively small samples, and some deliberately including obese subjects or individuals with fatty livers) have related aerobic fitness (generally measured as the peak effort attained on a treadmill or cycle ergometer test) to liver fat content (Table 1.4). All except two investigations with small sample sizes[183, 188] found less hepatic fat in individuals with higher levels of aerobic fitness.

Physical activity interventions and amount of liver fat

At least 36 studies have examined the impact of physical activity interventions upon liver fat content (Table 1.5). Unfortunately, many of the studies have lacked controls, and sometimes the interpretation of data has been compromised by the inclusion of dieting and other lifestyle measures as a part of the intervention. All 12 controlled investigations showed a reduction of liver fat in response to a physical activity programme, although in some cases the benefit was no greater than that which was obtained by a dietary intervention.

Animal studies of exercise training and amount of liver fat

Investigations of exercise and hepatic fat accumulation have often used animals that were fed high-fat diets or were genetic variants prone to obesity (Table 1.6). A further limitation of many animal studies is that controls have lived unnatural lives of physical inactivity and over-eating relative to their natural state. In consequence, differences in hepatic tissue mass between sedentary and exercised

Table 1.3 Influence of regular physical activity on fat content of human liver, as seen in cross-sectional comparisons

Author	Sample	Methodology	Results	Comments
Bae et al.[160]	72,359 Korean adults	Ultrasound, self-reported physical activity	Risk of fatty liver 0.53–0.72 if exercise for 30 min, 3 times/wk for 3 months	Active individuals also had reduced AST and ALT levels
Fintini et al.[161]	Children with fatty livers (n = 40) vs. obese (n = 30) vs. lean peers (n = 41)	Physical activity questionnaire & Sense-ware arm bands	Those with fatty livers devoted more time to sedentary pursuits, engaged in less physical activity	Questionnaire data did not agree well with Sense-ware data
Gerber et al.[162]	3,056 participants in the US NHANES survey of 2003–2006 aged >20 years	Fatty liver index based on BMI, waist circumference, triglycerides and GGT, accelerometer	Individuals with fatty liver index >60 units had lower accelerometer readings (29 counts/ min per day), and spent less time at all levels of activity	
Hattar et al.[163]	Hispanic children, aged 12.1 years; 20 fatty liver, 20 obese, 17 controls	Liver biopsy, retrospective physical activity questionnaire	Sedentary score >2 associated with stage 2–3 hepatic fibrosis	15% of children with fatty livers performed light exercise, vs. 35% of obese and 59% of non-obese children
Hsieh et al.[164]	3,331 adult Japanese men	Ultrasound, physical activity questionnaire	Fatty liver less prevalent in those exercising regularly >2 days/week than in sedentary men	Dose–response relationship (sedentary vs. those active 1, 2 and 3 days/week)
Kang et al.[165]	39 M, 52 F with fatty liver, age 48 years	Liver biopsy, physical activity questionnaire	No difference of histology with reported physical activity	
Kistler et al.[166]	302 men, 511 women with fatty liver	Liver biopsy, self-reported physical activity	Neither moderate nor total exercise associated with stage of hepatic fibrosis; however, those meeting recommended vigorous activity had reduced odds of fatty liver	

Table 1.3 continued

Author	Sample	Methodology	Results	Comments
Leskinen et al.[167]	16 same-sex middle-aged twin pairs discordant for activity	Proton magnetic resonance spectroscopy, physical activity questionnaire	Inactive twins had 3 times as much liver fat as active peers	Inactive twins also had greater body mass, fat mass, visceral fat and lower fitness
Newton et al.[168]	36 M, 36 F (36 with fatty liver, 36 controls)	Liver biopsy, pedometer	Those with fatty liver took 20% fewer steps/day	
Perseghin et al.[169]	114 M, 77 F aged 19–62 years	Proton magnetic resonance spectroscopy, physical activity questionnaire	Hepatic fat >5%) 25% in least active quartile, 2% in most active quartile	Association attenuated by adjustments for age, sex, BMI, insulin sensitivity and adiponectin
Tiikkainen et al.[170]	27 women with previous gestational diabetes	Proton magnetic resonance spectroscopy, physical activity questionnaire	Women with low fat exercised for 30 min 5 times/ week, those with >5% liver fat only 3 times/week	Fatty liver associated with insulin resistance
Zelber-Sagi et al.[171]	375 Israeli men and women, mean age 51 years	Abdominal ultrasound, physical activity questionnaire	Hepatic fat related to sports participation (odds ratio 0.66) and resistance exercise (0.61).	Hepatic fat only related to resistance exercise if adjusted for BMI; relationship non-significant if also adjusted for leptin or waist circumference

Note: ALT = alanine transaminase; AST = aspartate transaminase; BMI = body mass index; GGT = gamma-glutamyl transferase

Table 1.4 Influence of regular physical activity on fat content of human liver, as inferred from cross-sectional comparisons between individuals differing in aerobic fitness

Author	Sample	Methodology	Results	Comments
Church et al.[179]	218 men aged 33–73 years	CT scan, peak treadmill endurance time	Treadmill endurance time and BMI independently associated with fatty liver	Associations attenuated if abdominal fatness included in model
Hannukainen et al.[180]	Nine male monozygotic twin-pairs differing in habitual physical activity	Proton magnetic resonance spectroscopy, maximal oxygen intake on cycle ergometer	20% less visceral fat in more active twins	Hepatic uptake of free fatty acids lower in active twins
Haufe et al.[181]	Overweight and obese subjects (31 M, 108 F aged 40–50 years)	Proton magnetic resonance spectroscopy, peak oxygen intake on cycle ergometer	Negative correlation between aerobic fitness and hepatic fat, M > F	In men, correlation independent of visceral adipose tissue
Kantartzis et al.[182]	70 M, 100 F (50 with fatty liver)	Proton magnetic resonance spectroscopy, peak oxygen intake on cycle ergometer	Initial peak oxygen intake strongest predictor of reduction in hepatic fat with diet and physical activity	Authors conclude cardio-respiratory fitness determines liver fat content
Krasnoff et al.[183]	19 M, 18 F, average age 45.9 years	Liver biopsy, symptom-limited peak oxygen intake on treadmill	No relationship between peak oxygen intake and fatty liver	
Kuk et al.[184]	86 lean pre-menopausal women	CT scan, peak treadmill endurance time	Treadmill endurance lower in those with fatty liver	Liver fat not related to other metabolic risk factors
Leskinen et al.[167]	16 same-sex middle-aged twin pairs discordant for activity	Proton magnetic resonance spectroscopy, peak oxygen intake on cycle ergometer	Inactive twins had 3 times as much liver fat	Inactive twins also had greater bodymass, fat mass, visceral fat and lower aerobic fitness

Table 1.4 continued

Author	Sample	Methodology	Results	Comments
McMillan et al.[185]	293 men aged 29–78 years	CT scan and peak treadmill endurance time	Peak treadmill time weakly correlated with liver fat (r = −0.24)	
Nguyen-Duy et al.[186]	161 men aged 33–72 years	CT scan and peak treadmill endurance time	Peak treadmill time weakly correlated with liver fat (r = −0.26)	Probable overlap of sample with McMillan et al.[185]
O'Donovan et al.[187]	50 men aged 34–56, both obese and lean	Proton magnetic resonance spectroscopy, peak oxygen intake on cycle ergometer	Liver fat was greater in unfit	Relationship eliminated by introduction of waist circumference
Seppala-Lindroos et al.[188]	30 middle-aged men (15 with fatty liver)	Proton magnetic resonance spectroscopy, maximal oxygen intake	No significant difference of maximal oxygen intake between high and low fat groups [35.6 vs. 33.5 ml/(kg min)]	High liver fat defined as >3%, so that some relatively normal individuals included in high fat group

animals have varied widely between investigations. In the study of Yiamou-yiannis et al.,[247] rats that were fed *ad libitum* and given free access to a running wheel also ate more than controls, thus presenting with larger livers and increased values for total liver protein, mitochondrial and cytosolic protein tissue. Because of liver hypertrophy, the total activity of several enzymes involved in the break-down of foreign chemical substances was also increased, although the activity per gram of liver or per gram of hepatic protein remained unchanged.[247]

The physical activity intervention adopted in animal experiments has usually been enforced treadmill running or swimming, although two studies have examined the effects of resistance exercise.[230, 238, 239] Of 19 studies, 18 showed lower hepatic fat in the exercised group, the one exception being Yasari et al.[245] In terms of fat reduction, resistance exercise seemed as effective as aerobic activity, and perhaps because peak intensities of effort were higher, intermittent activity had a greater effect than continuous effort.[242]

Impact upon circulating lipids

The cardio-protective benefit of regular physical activity in modifying circulating lipids and lipoproteins is well documented, although delayed effects of recent

Table 1.5 Effects of regular physical activity on fat content of human liver, as seen in longitudinal studies of exercise training

Author	Sample	Methodology	Results	Comments
Albu et al.[189]	58 obese subjects, average age 59 years	CT scan, 175 min moderate aerobic exercise/ week + moderate energy restriction	18% decrease in hepatic fat	No control group
Bacchi and Moghetti;[190] Bacchi et al.[191]	31 overweight or obese individuals	Magnetic resonance imaging, 4 month programme; 60 min aerobic exercise at 60–65% heart rate reserve 3 times/week vs. 60 min resistance exercise at 70–80% 1RM 3 times/week	Hepatic fat reduced 33% (aerobic) vs. 26% (resistance programme)	No control group
Bonekamp et al.[192]	45 adults with type 2 diabetes mellitus, age 53 years	Proton magnetic resonance spectroscopy, 45 min of moderate aerobic exercise plus weight lifting, 3 times/week for 6 months, vs. controls	2.5% reduction in hepatic fat, effect persisted if adjusted for BMI or visceral fat	Dietary policy unclear
Chen et al.[193]	54 M and F Taiwanese with fatty livers, age 38–40 years	Ultrasound, 10 week diet + exercise (high-intensity cycle ergometry, 1 h twice/ week) vs. exercise alone vs. control	Liver fat decreased by either exercise or diet	
de Piano et al.[194]	58 obese adolescents, with or without fatty liver average age 16.5 years	Ultrasound, 1-year lifestyle intervention with aerobic (60 min at ventilatory threshold, 3 times/ week) or aerobic + resistance (3 sets of 6–20 reps for main muscle groups) training	Combined aerobic + resistance exercise more effective than aerobic exercise alone	No non-exercise control group
Devries et al.[195]	41 men and women, aged 38–40 years; half of sample lean, half obese	CT scan, 3 months of cycle ergometer training, 60 min/day, 3 times/week, progressing to 65% of maximal oxygen intake in women and 70% in men	Training did not alter liver attenuation on CT scan	No control group

Table 1.5 continued

Author	Sample	Methodology	Results	Comments
Eckard et al.[196]	56 adults aged 18–70 with fatty liver	Liver biopsy, 6 month programme; moderate exercise (30–60 min, 4–7 times/week, tracked by exercise log and pedometer) vs. exercise + low fat or moderate fat + low processed carbohydrates vs. standard care	All intervention groups improved, with no significant inter-group differences	
Fealy et al.[197]	13 obese subjects aged 58 years, sex not specified	Proton magnetic resonance spectroscopy, 1 week of walking, 60 min/day at 85% of maximal heart rate	Reduced markers of apoptosis, mediated through increase doxidative capacity and greater insulin sensitivity	No control group
Finucane et al.[198]	100 healthy older people (50 served as controls)	Proton magnetic resonance spectroscopy, 12 week cycle ergometer exercise, 60 min, 3 times/week vs. control group	Significant reduction of liver fat in intervention group	Increased predicted maximal oxygen intake, no change of body mass
Franzese et al.[199]	41 M, 34 F obese children aged 9.5 years	Ultrasound, 6 months of diet + exercise	Liver fat decreased with loss of weight	No control group
Goodpaster et al.[200]	130 severely obese adults (101 completed trial)	CT scan, 6 months, diet + exercise vs. diet	Both groups lost weight, exercised group lost more liver fat	
Grønbæk et al.[201]	117 obese children, average age 12.1 years	Ultrasound, 10 week period at a weight loss camp with daily hour of varied aerobic exercise	Reduction of fatty liver	No control group
Hallsworth et al.[202]	19 sedentary adults with fatty livers, aged 52 years experimental, 62 year controls	Proton magnetic resonance spectroscopy, 8 week resistance exercise (n = 11) vs. standard treatment (n = 8); physical activity monitored by Sense-wear arm band	13% reduction of liver fat with no change in body mass, total fat mass or visceral fat volume	Lipid oxidation, glucose control and insulin resistance all improved. Controls older

Table 1.5 continued

Author	Sample	Methodology	Results	Comments
Hickman et al.[203]	35 men and women (21 with hepatitis C virus), aged 44 years	Liver biopsy, 15 month programme of diet plus encouraging 150 minaerobic exercise per week	14 patients biopsied after 3–6 months of exercise showed lessening of liver fat	No control group
Jin et al.[204]	120 potential liver donors with fatty livers	Hepatic biopsy, dietary restriction + 10 weeks of exercise (3 × 20 min sessions of joggingor walking per week)	Histological improvement in 103 of 120 subjects	Improvement of steatosis with weight reduction >5% and cholesterol reduction >10%. No control group
Johnson et al.[205]	19 sedentary obese men and women	Proton magnetic resonance spectroscopy, 4 weeks of aerobic cycle ergometer exercise (30–45 min, 3 times/week) at intensity rising to 70% of peak oxygen intake	21% reduction of hepatic triglycerides	No control group
Kawaguchi et al.[206]	35 adults with fatty liver resistant to lifestyle counselling (12 trained, 23 controls)	Ultrasound, hybrid training (voluntary and electrical contraction of quadriceps and hamstrings, 19 min 2 times/week for 12 weeks	Liver fat decreased	Associated reduction of insulin resistance and small decrease of body mass. No control group
Koot et al.[207]	144 obese children, mean age 14.1 years	Ultrasound, 6 month programme, with 3 × 1 hour sessions of unspecified exercise/week plus changes in eating behaviour	Prevalence of fatty liver decreased from 31 to 12%	Changes related to decreased insulin resistance and 12% decrease of body mass. No control group

Table 1.5 continued

Author	Sample	Methodology	Results	Comments
Larson-Meyer et al.[208]	46 overweight men and women	Proton magnetic resonance spectroscopy, CT scan, 6-month study: dietary restriction + exercise (structured to increase energy expenditure 12.5%) vs. dietary restriction vs. low-calorie diet vs. control	Liver fat reduced in all 3 experimental groups	
Lazo et al.[209]	96 men and women with diabetes mellitus, aged 45–76 years, divided between lifestyle and education/support group	Proton magnetic resonance spectroscopy, weekly meetings to encourage dieting and progression to 175 min of moderate exercise per week for 1 year	Decrease in fatty liver 50.8% (intervention) vs. 22.8% (controls)	
Lee et al.[210]	48 obese adolescent boys divided into 3 groups	Proton magnetic resonance spectroscopy, 3 month trial, 3 sessions/week 60 min aerobic exercise (50% rising to 60–75% of maximal oxygen intake) or resistance exercise (60% of initial 1RM) or controls	Both types of exercise reduced hepatic lipids	Subjects instructed to follow weight maintenance diet; only resistance exercise increased insulin sensitivity
Nobili et al.[211]	37 boys, 16 girls, aged 5.7–18.8 years (plus 33 drop-outs)	Liver biopsy, diet plus physical activity for 24 months	Improvements of liver histology	No non-exercise control group
Oza et al.[212]	67 cases of fatty liver, only 22 completed treatment	CT scan, 6 month home-based diet + exercise (target of 23 MET-h/week physical activity + 4 MET-h/week of exercise	19/22 showed decreases of visceral fat	Poor compliance, no control group

Table 1.5 continued

Author	Sample	Methodology	Results	Comments
Promrat et al.[213]	Overweight or obese subjects randomized to lifestyle (20) or education (10) groups	Liver biopsy, 48-week intervention; weekly, then biweekly counselling aiming for 7–10% weight loss, exercise and altered behaviour	Histology improvement >3 points in 14/20 of intervention vs. 3/10 of control subjects	Improvements in hepatic condition associated with weight loss
Santomauro et al.[214]	36 obese children with fatty livers	Ultrasound, 1 year lifestyle approach, focusing on dieting and increased physical activity	Reduction or disappearance of fatty liver linked to increased physical activity and associated weight loss in 12 of 36 children	Weight loss main variable accounting for reduction of liver fat. No control group
Schäfer et al.[215]	48 with impaired glucose tolerance, 133 normal subjects	Proton magnetic resonance spectroscopy, 24-month diet + exercise at anaerobic threshold (Polar heart rate monitor)	Liver fat decreased 28%, visceral fat 8% in those with impaired glucose tolerance	Body mass decreased 3% in both groups. No non-exercise control group
Shah et al.[216]	18 obese subjects >65 years	Proton magnetic resonance spectroscopy, diet vs. diet + exercise (thrice weekly 90-min sessions of aerobic, resistance, flexibility and resistance training, with diet adjusted to achieve a similar energy deficit)	Both treatments reduced liver fat and insulin resistance to similar extent, but added exercise improved physical function	Body mass decreased 9–10% in both groups. No non-exercise control
Shojaee-Moradie et al.[217]	17 initially sedentary men (7 of 17 served as controls)	Proton magnetic resonance spectroscopy, exercised for 6 weeks. 60–85% of maximal aerobic power for 20 min, 3 times/week	No change of liver fat content, but decrease in hepatic insulin resistance	No control group

Table 1.5 continued

Author	Sample	Methodology	Results	Comments
Slentz et al.[218]	155 overweight adults aged 18–70 years	Computed tomography, 8 month training 3 days/week: aerobic (running 19 km/week at 75% aerobic power) vs. resistance vs. combined aerobic + resistance training	Aerobic training decreased hepatic fat 5.6%. No benefit from resistance training alone, combined therapy similar to aerobic training alone	No non-exercise controls
Sullivan et al.[219]	18 obese adults with fatty livers, average age 48 years	Proton magnetic resonance spectroscopy, 16-week exercise (45–55% peak oxygen intake, 30–60 min/day, 5 times/m week, n = 12) vs. control (n = 6)	Exercise reduced liver fat 10%, but no change in body mass or % body fat	No change in hepatic VLD secretion or VDL apoB-100 secretion
Tamura et al.[220]	14 patients with	Proton magnetic resonance spectroscopy, 2 week comparison, diet or diet + exercise (walking 60–90 min/day for an increase in energy expenditure of about 0.7 MJ/day)	Hepatic lipids decreased in both groups, but no added effect of exercise	Diet + exercise group younger than diet alone group
Thamer et al.[221, 222]	48 M, 64 F, average age 46 years	Proton magnetic resonance spectroscopy, diet + 3 h/week aerobic exercise monitored by Polar pulse-counter, average follow-up of 264 days	33% decrease of liver fat, despite little change in overall body fat	Decrease of liver fat associated with improved insulin sensitivity. No control group
Thomas et al.[223]	10 obese adults, age not stated	Proton magnetic resonance spectroscopy, diet + pedometer monitored recommendation of 10,000 steps/day	40% decrease of liver fat	Changes associated with body fat. No control group
Ueno et al.[224]	25 obese (10 served as controls)	Liver biopsy, restricted diet and walking or jogging for 3 months	Reduction of liver fat	No control group

Table 1.5 continued

Author	Sample	Methodology	Results	Comments
van der Heijden et al.[225]	15 obese and 14 lean adolescents	Proton magnetic resonance spectroscopy, 12 week aerobic programme (30 min sessions, 2 or 4 times/week at 70% of maximal oxygen intake)	Hepatic fat reduced in obese but not in lean subjects	No control group. Exercise increased hepatic and peripheral insulin sensitivity
van der Heijden et al.[225]	Obese adolescents (6 M, 6 F)	Proton magnetic resonance spectroscopy, 12 week resistance exercise (twice/week, all major muscle groups)	Hepatic fat content unchanged, but insulin sensitivity increased 24%	No control group. Body mass increased 2.6 kg

Notes: BMI = body mass index; CT = computed tomography

exercise sessions may contribute to some of the observed improvements in lipid and lipoprotein concentrations that have been attributed to training.[248, 249] Cross-sectional research shows that high density lipoprotein cholesterol (HDL-C) levels are higher in regular exercisers than in their inactive counterparts,[250] and circulating concentrations of HDL-C increase with exercise training.[251, 252] Similarly, exercise training can reduce circulating triglycerides and the secretion of hepatic VLDL triglycerides.[253] These benefits are associated with a decreased activity of hepatic lipase[254] and alterations in the levels of other hepatic enzymes that are involved in HDL-C remodelling (including cholesteryl ester transfer protein and lecithin cholesteryl acyl transferase).[255, 256] Inter-individual human differences in the response of hepatic lipase to training programmes have been traced to a polymorphism in the hepatic lipase gene LIPC −514C-T.[257]

Rodent investigations have provided insights into the molecular changes underlying training-induced changes in lipid and lipoprotein metabolism. Training reduces the hepatic levels of two enzymes central to the synthesis of fatty acids: acetyl-coenzyme A carboxylase and fatty acid synthase.[34, 258–260] Regular exercise also down-regulates the hepatic gene and protein content of stearoyl-CoA desaturase-1 (SCD-1), the rate-limiting enzyme in the biosynthesis of saturated-derived monounsaturated fats that are a major constituent of VLDL triglycerides. Further, there is a down-regulation of the microsomal triglyceride transfer protein that plays a key role in the assembly and secretion of VLDL lipoprotein,[261] and training increases levels of hepatic mRNA for the ATP-binding cassette transporter A-1 that plays a vital role in the membrane transport of HDL cholesterol and its remodeling in the plasma.[262]

Table 1.6 Effects of regular physical activity or fitness level on fat content of liver, as seen in animal experiments

Author	Animal model	Intervention	Results	Comments
Botezelli et al.[226]	Male Wistar rats initially aged 28 weeks fed on 60% fructose diet	Swimming 1 h/day at anaerobic threshold, starting at 28 or 90 days	Liver lipids reduced by either early or late onset training	Swimming improved insulin sensitivity. No control group
Cameron et al.[227]	Male Wistar rats fed high-fat/high carbohydrate diet or corn starch	8 weeks of treadmill running, 20 min/day increasing to 30 min/day, 5 days/week; 1 km/h, 0% incline	Liver mass and hepatic fat decreased in experimental group	Exercise decreased body fat, abdominal fat and blood glucose, improved blood lipid profile
Charbonneau et al.[228]	Female Sprague–Dawley rats initially 10 weeks old, fed high-fat diet	Treadmill exercise progressing to 60 min/day at 26 m/min, 10% slope	28% gain of hepatic fat with high-fat diet was completely reversed by exercise	Glucagon resistance of obese rats also prevented by exercise
Cintra et al.[229]	Obese mice fed high-fat diet	8 weeks of running (50 min/day 5 days/week at 1 km/h)	1.7-fold reduction of liver fat	Associated reduction of regulatory element-binding protein-1c
Colombo et al.[159]	Male diabetic fatty Zucker rats	5 weeks of treadmill running (1 h/day, 6 days/week, 20 m/min)	Liver fat decreased	Modification of many hepatic genes associated with lipogenesis and detoxification
Corriveau et al.[230]	Three groups of ovariectomized vs. one group of sham-operated rats	25% dietary restriction vs. dietary restriction + resistance exercise (weighted stair climbing 5 times/week)	Liver lipid accumulation not stopped by dietary restriction, but reversed by resistance exercise	Abdominal fat also reduced by resistance exercise
Gauthier et al.[231]	Female Sprague–Dawley rats initially 6 weeks old, fed high-fat diet	Treadmill exercise progressing to 60 min/day at 26 m/min, 10% slope	Liver triglyceride content substantially reduced by concomitant exercise relative to sedentary controls	

Table 1.6 continued

Author	Animal model	Intervention	Results	Comments
Gauthier et al.;[232] Yasari et al.[233]	Female Sprague–Dawley rats initially 6 weeks old fed high-fat diet	Treadmill exercise progressing to 60 min/day at 26 m/min, 10% slope introduced from 8th to 16th week of high-fat diet	Exercise decreased visceral fat 30%	Leptin concentrations also reduced by exercise
Hao et al.[234]	12 week ovariectomized female rats	Treadmill running (10–18 min/day at 0% grade for 15–60 days)	Exercise reduced hepatic fat relative to controls	Associated increase in HDL/total cholesterol ratio
Leite et al.[235]	Adult female Wistar rats, half of sample ovariectomized	Sedentary vs. resistance training (weighted ladder climbing), 4–9 climbs every 3 days	Exercise reduced liver fat content, less in ovariectomized than in intact animals	Other fat depots also reduced
Marques et al.[236]	C57/BL6 mice fed standard chow or very high-fat diet	Sedentary vs. 8 weeks treadmill running (60 min/day, 5 days/week at 1 km/h)	Hepatic fat content reduced by exercise	Exercise also reduced insulin resistance, cholesterol and triglycerides
Moura et al.[237]	60 day alloxan-treated diabetic Wistar rats	Swimming 1 h/day, 5 days/week for 44 days with load 3.5% body mass (below anaerobic threshold)	Hepatic fat content lower in swimmers than in sedentary peers	
Pighon et al.[238, 239]	Ovariectomized rats following 8 weeks of food restriction +	Normal feeding vs. food restriction vs. resistance training (weighted ladder climbing)	Resistance exercise and dieting both avoid regain of liver fat	

Table 1.6 continued

Author	Animal model	Intervention	Results	Comments
Rector et al.[240]	Hyperphagic, Otsuka Long–Evans Tokushima Fatty rats initially aged 4 wks	36-week voluntary wheel running vs. sedentary controls	Exercise prevented hepatic fat accumulation (also prevented by dietary restriction)	Exercise group showed greater benefits, including increased hepatic mitochondrial fatty acid oxidation, enhanced oxidative enzyme function and protein content, and suppression of hepatic lipogenic proteins
Schultz et al.[241]	Male C57BL/6 mice fed high-fat diet	Unweighted swimming progressing to 60 min/day	15% reduction of fatty liver relative to high-fat controls	
Sene-Fiorese et al.[242]	Male Wistar rats aged 90–120 days fed high-fat diet	min/day 90 swimming vs. 330 min/day swimming sessions	Intermittent exercise more effective than continuous in preventing hepatic fat accumulation	
Takeshita et al.[243]	Mice initially aged 6 weeks	Access to running wheel (covering 4.9 km/day) vs. sedentary control	Exercisers had lower liver weights and liver triglyceride content	Exercisers had lower plasma leptin and insulin-like growth factor-1 levels
Thyfault et al.[244]	Rats selected for high (1,514 m) and low (200 m) running capacity		Less fit rats had reduced mitochondrial content, reduced oxidative capacity, increased peroxisomal activity, and fatty liver	
Yasari et al.[245]	Female rats given high-fat diet from 6th to 8th week	Treadmill running progressing to 60 min/day at 26 m/min, 10% slope	Liver triglyceride content not affected by exercise	

Rats have shown changes in the composition of hepatic phospholipids following eight weeks of wheel training. These changes likely have implications for the membrane properties of the hepatocytes, cell signalling and gene expression, although details of such changes remain to be explored.[263]

Protein metabolism

An expansion of plasma volume is a well-recognized adaptation to regular physical training, and is important to the increase in aerobic performance. Increased expression of the hepatic albumin gene mRNA augments hepatic albumin synthesis, and rodent studies indicate that this can occur within as little as 12 days of the initiation of training.[264] Endurance training also increases the production of heat shock proteins in both the liver and other tissues,[265, 266] and decreases the secretion of appetite stimulating orixigenic proteins.[267]. An increased synthesis of IGF-1, stimulated by action of the pituitary growth hormone, is important to the muscle hypertrophy associated with training.[268]

Triggers of hepatic responses to training

Changes in the concentrations of several hormones (insulin, glucagon and oestrogen) and cytokines (IL-1-b, IL-6, IL-10 and IGF-1) and altered tissue sensitivity to these agents may all contribute to the changes of hepatic metabolism that are observed following a period of aerobic training.

In terms of carbohydrate homeostasis, an increased hepatic sensitivity to insulin has been observed in some animal studies. Regular exercise training reduces the hepatic mRNA level and protein content of hepatic PEPCK, thus contributing to enhanced insulin sensitivity.[269] Human studies have usually shown an enhanced hepatic insulin sensitivity following training, although this has not always been the response.[203] Gains of overall insulin sensitivity have been observed following the aerobic and resistance training of obese diabetic patients,[270] with 16 weeks of resistance training in adolescents,[271] with progressive resistance training of older men with type-2 diabetes mellitus,[272] with resistance training of obese adolescents[273] and with high-intensity interval training of obese mice.[274]

An increased availability of glucagon seems important to the reduction of liver fat content. The hepatic glucagon receptor density and glucocorticoid receptor count are increased in exercise-trained rats,[275] and exercise does not reduce liver fat in animals that lack glucagon receptors.[276] Hepatic oestrogen receptors also influence fat accumulation;[277] ovariectomy predisposes female rats to the development of fatty livers, with an increase of inflammatory biomarkers such as inhibitor-κB kinase β and interleukin-6, an increased activity of hepatic lipogenic enzymes such as sterol regulatory element-binding protein-1c, acetyl-CoA carboxylase (ACC) and stearoyl CoA desaturase), and a decreased expression of enzymes related to fat oxidation such as carnitine palmitoyltransferase and hydroxyacyl-CoA-dehydrogenase. With the exception of increases in ACC, regular physical activity can reverse the adverse changes associated with ovariectomy, at least in rats and mice.[238, 278, 279] Carnitine, an important co-factor for the oxidation of both long-chained fatty acids and carbohydrate, may also be important to the hepatic response, with regular exercise attenuating the reduction of carnitine palmitoyltransferase I activity that is induced by a high-fat diet,[280] and up-regulating the genes involved in hepatic carnitine synthesis and uptake.[281] Training also increases the gene expression of microsomal triglyceride transfer protein and diacylglycerol acyltransferase-2 in ovariectomized rats, further changes that lead to a reduction in hepatic triglyceride content.[282]

In terms of hepatic protein synthesis, some investigators have observed greater serum levels of IGF following aerobic training. This could reflect either an increased hepatic production of IGF[178] or an increased hydrolysis of the corresponding binding factor.[283] Resistance training also causes an early and sustained release of IGF-1.[284] However, such responses are not seen with a low fat diet; exercise training then increases serum concentrations of IGF-1 binding protein, thus decreasing circulating levels of free IGF-1, both in rats and in humans.[285, 286] Rodent studies have also suggested that regular aerobic exercise training may decrease levels of the inflammatory cytokines IL-6[287] and IL-1b[288] and increase levels of the anti-inflammatory cytokine IL-10, with an associated decrease in hepatic apoptosis during an experimental episode of bacterial sepsis.[288]

Role of oxidant stress

Most studies of mice, rats and dogs have shown moderate aerobic training as minimizing markers of oxidant stress,[289] and concentrations of hepatic glutathione transferase S activity and reduced glutathione are increased,[120, 290] with enhanced gene expression of unfolded protein response markers.[291] Further, the activities of hepatic antioxidant enzymes such as superoxide dismutase[292–294] and the corresponding signalling molecules[295] are increased. Nevertheless, a few investigators have found no change or even a decrease of anti-oxidant enzyme activity following heavy endurance training.[296] One problem in such investigations is that (unlike early observations on isolated hepatocytes[297]) there is sometimes little relationship between anti-oxidant enzyme levels as measured in the general circulation and local oxidant stress in the liver.[298, 299] In one study of rats, prolonged bouts of vigorous exercise (two hours of swimming/day for three months) led to a down-regulation of cytosolic aconitase, a key factor in cellular iron homeostasis,[300] possibly due to an increased production of NO and oxidative stress. Another report described a decrease in the mRNA for one anti-oxidant enzyme (hepatic superoxide dismutase), although there was an increase of mRNA for another anti-oxidant enzyme, catalase.[301]

Physical activity and functional activity of the liver

Ferreira[302] found a decrease of apoptotic cells in mice livers following seven weeks of treadmill training. It is unclear from studies of serum enzyme levels and pharmacokinetics how far human liver function is enhanced by regular low to moderate intensities of aerobic training. Nevertheless, the traditional clinical markers of impaired hepatic function (serum ALT and GGT levels) do show a negative correlation with habitual physical activity,[303–305] probably at least in part because a sedentary lifestyle predisposes to the development of a fatty liver.[306]

In terms of pharmacokinetics, some reports have shown little benefit from physical activity. Exercise training did not alter creatinine clearance in boxers;[307] nor did it change the elimination of propranolol in initially sedentary subjects.[308, 309] Likewise, cross-sectional comparisons showed no significant differences of aminopyrine metabolism, galactose elimination or indocyanine green clearance between endurance runners and relatively sedentary medical students.[310] Nevertheless, the majority of reports have suggested that hepatic function is enhanced by vigorous (but not exhausting) training.[107] Thus, the clearance of antipyrine (which depends almost exclusively on hepatic metabolism) was faster in athletes than in controls, with no difference between sprinters and endurance competitors.[311] Likewise, endurance runners had a faster clearance of antipyrine than sedentary but otherwise healthy men.[312]

Longitudinal evidence supports these cross-sectional inferences. Three months of exercise training increased the clearance of antipyrine and aminopyrine in previously sedentary students. Moreover, individual improvements in these indices correlated highly with gains in $\dot{V}O_{2max}$.[313] Three months of moderate intensity exercise (a thrice weekly mixture of aerobic and strength training) also increased antipyrine clearance in elderly women.[314]

Animal experiments generally confirm that regular moderate physical activity has beneficial effects upon hepatic function. Five weeks of training increased antipyrine clearance in mares,[315] and the livers of regularly exercised rats had a greater ability to metabolize and excrete certain chemicals not normally found in the body, such as naphthol and styrene products[247] and halothane.[316] In the study of halothane toxicity, hepatic glutathione levels were unchanged by ten weeks of treadmill exercise, and it remained unclear whether the more rapid clearance of halothane was due to enhanced anti-oxidant defence mechanisms or the associated decrease in hepatic fat.[316]

One factor that increases the liver's ability to eliminate some substances after training is an increased secretion of biliary transporters. Chronic exercise such as swimming or running augments the hepatic production of bile acids[317] and increases the availability of bile acid transporters.[318] These changes accelerate the biliary clearance (but not necessarily the blood stream clearance) of substances such as indocyanine green,[318] acetaminophen and antipyrine.[317]

Areas for further research

There remain several competing hypotheses as to what triggers the hepatic responses to an acute bout of exercise, and further research elucidating the underlying mechanisms might enable investigators to design exercise programmes that would enhance adaptations favourable to performance and hepatic health.

The magnitude of the decrease in hepatic blood flow during a bout of prolonged and vigorous exercise remains contentious, with the indocyanine technique suggesting large and potentially harmful reductions, and other techniques apparently showing much smaller changes (although as yet only evaluated over shorter periods of exercise). There is a need to repeat radionucleide studies following periods of vigorous exercise that are as long as those used in the indocyanine research. Confirmation is also required of the single study suggesting that hepatic enzyme release is increased by prolonged exercise. If this is indeed the case, the duration of the enzyme leakage needs to be determined. Information to date suggests that liver function is normalized within a few days of ceasing a demanding bout of endurance exercise, but if such changes prove to be long lasting or permanent, sports physicians may need to reconsider the wisdom of participation in ultra-endurance athletic events.

Evidence that regular physical activity reduces hepatic fat seems convincing, underlining the role of physical activity in countering fatty liver. However, there remains scope for further studies where the reduction in hepatic fat content is related to objective rather than subjective measures of habitual physical activity, providing clearer evidence on optimal patterns of physical activity. Further, it remains important to resolve the question as to how far regular physical activity enhances overall hepatic function.

Practical implications and conclusions

The liver plays a vital role in maintaining the constancy of the internal environment, with particular reference to blood glucose and pH. During an acute bout of physical activity, there is a release of glucose from the liver, initially by the breakdown of local glycogen reserves and (as these reserves are depleted) by the synthesis of glucose from lactate, glycerol and amino acids. These responses help to maintain a stable blood glucose in prolonged athletic endeavours. Triggers to hepatic adjustments include changes in the levels of hormones (particularly insulin, glucagon and adrenaline), altered afferent nerve input associated with some correlate of glycogen depletion, a response to the muscular release of IL-6, or an accumulation of reactive oxygen species. Under resting conditions, the liver is a major site for fatty acid uptake. Much of the fat is repackaged and secreted as VLDLs. However, during a prolonged bout of physical activity, possibly as a consequence of reduced hepatic blood flow and/or increased fatty acid uptake by muscle, the liver adopts a more 'passive' role, with no measurable change in its fat content. Albumin and IGF-1 levels are increased after an acute bout of exercise; they likely have growth-promoting effects on the active muscles and contribute to maintenance of a stable blood glucose. Prolonged or exhausting physical activity causes a dramatic decrease in blood flow to the liver. There may then be a short-term inflammation, with a reduced clearance of drugs, oxidant stress, increased concentrations of heat shock proteins and a release of hepatic enzymes. However, such disturbances usually resolve spontaneously within a few days.

After training, glycogenolysis and gluconeogensis are reduced at a given absolute work-rate, but liver glycogen storage and the hepatic capacity for glucose output are increased, thus enhancing performance potential. Training also appears to reduce the overall liver mass, with a reduction in its fat content and an increase of HDL-C levels. Hepatic concentrations of albumin and heat shock proteins increase, and levels of appetite-stimulating proteins decrease. Triggers for these changes likely include altered secretion of hormones (insulin, glucagon and estrogen) and a number of cytokines. Most cross-sectional and longitudinal research studies also suggest an improvement of hepatic function with training, as shown by a decreased fat content, reduced markers of oxidant stress and increased concentrations of anti-oxidant enzymes.

References

1. Shephard RJ. *An illustrated history of health and fitness, from pre-history to our post-modern world*. Cham, Switzerland: Springer, 2015.
2. Fritsche L, Weigert C, Haring HU, et al. How insulin receptor substrate proteins regulate the metabolic capacity of the liver – implications for health and disease. *Curr Med Chem* 2008; 15: 1316–1329.
3. Kjaer M. Hepatic glucose production during exercise. *Adv Exp Med Biol* 1998; 441: 117–127.
4. Wahren DG, Ekberg K. Splanchnic regulation of glucose production. *Annu Rev Nutr* 2007; 27: 329–345.
5. Wasserman DH, Cherrington AD. Hepatic fuel metabolism during muscular work: role and regulation. *Am J Physiol* 1991; 260: E811–E24.
6. Bouchard C, Shephard RJ, Stephens T, et al. *Exercise, fitness and health*. Champaign, IL: Human Kinetics Publishers, 1990.
7. Bouchard C, Shephard RJ, Stephens T. *Physical activity, fitness and health*. Champaign, IL: Human Kinetics Publishers, 1994.
8. Ritland S. Exercise and liver disease. *Sports Med* 1988; 6: 121–126.
9. Shephard RJ, Johnson N. Effects of physical activity upon the liver. *Eur J Appl Physiol* 2015; 115(1): 1–46.
10. Bernard C. *Leçons sur les phenomènes de la vie* [Lessons on the phenomena of life]. Paris, France: Ballière, 1878.
11. Ahlborg G, Felig P, Hagenfel L, et al. Substrate turnover during prolonged exercise in man – splanchnic and leg metabolism of glucose, free fatty-acids, and amino-acids. *J Clin Invest* 1974; 53: 1080–1090.
12. Romijn JA, Coyle EF, Sidossis LS, et al. Regulation of endogenous fat and carbohydrate metabolism in relation to exercise intensity and duration. *Am J Physiol* 1993; 265: E380–E91.
13. Bergstrom J, Hermansen L, Hultman E, et al. Diet, muscle glycogen and physical performance. *Acta Physiol Scand* 1967; 71: 140–150.
14. Wasserman DH, Connolly CC, Pagliassotti MJ. Regulation of hepatic lactate balance during exercise. *Med Sci Sports Exerc* 1991; 23: 912–919.
15. Shephard RJ. *Physiology & biochemistry of exercise*. New York, NY: Praeger Publications, 1982.
16. Nielsen HB, Febbraio MA, Ott P, et al. Hepatic lactate uptake versus leg lactate output during exercise in humans. *J Appl Physiol* 2007; 103: 1227–1233.

17. Rowell LB. Visceral blood flow and metabolism during exercise. In: Shephard RJ, (ed.). *Frontiers of fitness*. Springfield, IL: C.C. Thomas, 1971, pp. 210–232.

18. Terjung RL, Baldwin KM, Winder WW, et al. Glycogen repletion in different types of muscle and in liver after exhausting exercise. *Am J Physiol* 1971; 226: 1387–1391.

19. Suh SH, Paik IY, Jacobs K. Regulation of blood glucose homeostasis during prolonged exercise. *Mol Cells* 2007; 23: 272–279.

20. Hesse D, Jaschke A, Kanzleiter T, et al. GTPase ARFRP1 is essential for normal hepatic glycogen storage and insulin-like growth factor 1 secretion. *Mol Cell Biol* 2012; 32: 4363–4374.

21. Hu C, Hoene M, Zhao X, et al. Lipidomics analysis reveals efficient storage of hepatic triacylglycerides enriched in unsaturated fatty acids after one bout of exercise in mice. *PLoS ONE* 2010; 5(10): e13318.

22. Wolfe RR, Klein S, Carraro F, et al. Role of triglyceride fatty-acid cycle in controlling fat-metabolism in humans during and after exercise. *Am J Physiol* 1990; 258: E382–E389.

23. Jensen MD. Gender differences in regional fatty-acid metabolism before and after meal ingestion. *J Clin Invest* 1995; 96: 2297–2303.

24. Meek SE, Nair KS, Jensen MD. Insulin regulation of regional free fatty acid metabolism. *Diabetes* 1999; 48: 10–14.

25. Havel RJ, Kane JP, Balasse EO, et al. Splanchnic metabolism of free fatty acids and production of triglycerides of very low density lipoproteins in normotriglyceridemic and hypertriglyceridemic humans. *J Clin Invest* 1970; 49: 2017–2035.

26. Wolfe BM, Havel JR, Marliss EB, et al. Effects of a 3-day fast and of ethanol on splanchnic metabolism of FFA, amino-acids, and carbohydrates in healthy young men. *J Clin Invest* 1976; 57: 329–340.

27. Frayn KN, Amer P, Yki-Jarvinen H. Fatty acid metabolism in adipose tissue, muscle and liver in health and disease. *Essays Biochem* 2006; 42: 89–103.

28. Klein S, Peters EJ, Holland OB, et al. Effect of short-term and long-term beta-adrenergic-blockade on lipolysis during fasting in humans. *Am J Physiol* 1989; 257: E65–E73.

29. Kiens B, Richter EA. Utilization of skeletal muscle triacylglycerol during post-exercise recovery in humans. *Am J Physiol* 1998; 275: E332–337.

30. Børsheim E, Knardahl S, Høistmark AT. Short-term effects of exercise on plasma very low density lipoproteins (VLDL) and fatty acids. *Med Sci Sports Exerc* 1999; 31(4): 522–530.

31. Magkos F, Patterson BW, Mohammed BS, et al. Basal adipose tissue and hepatic lipid kinetics are not affected by a single exercise bout of moderate duration and intensity in sedentary women. *Clin Sci* 2009; 116: 327–334.

32. Helge JW, Watt PW, Richter EA, et al. Fat utilization during exercise: adaptation to a fat-rich diet increases utilization of plasma fatty acids and very low density lipoprotein-triacylglycerol in humans. *J Physiol* 2001; 537: 1009–1020.

33. Griffiths MA, Fiebig RG, Gore MT, et al. Exercise down-regulates hepatic lipogenic enzymes in food-deprived and refed rats. *J Nutr* 1996; 126: 1959–1971.

34. Fiebig RG, Hollander JM, Ji LL. Exercise down-regulates hepatic fatty acid synthase in streptozotocin-treated rats. *J Nutr* 2001; 131: 2252–2259.

35. Gorski J, Oscai LB, Palmer WK. Hepatic lipid metabolism in exercise and training. *Med Sci Sports Exerc* 1990; 22: 213–221.

36. Johnson NA, van Overbeek D, Chapman PG, et al. Effect of prolonged exercise and

pre-exercise dietary manipulation on hepatic triglycerides in trained men. *Eur J Appl Physiol* 2012; 112: 1817–1825.

37. Ochiai M, Matsuo T. Increased stearoyl-CoA desaturase index and triglyceride content in the liver of rats after a single bout of swimming exercise. *Biosci Biotech Biochem* 2012; 76: 1350–1355.

38. Yang RC, Mack GW, Wolfe RR, et al. Albumin synthesis after intense intermittent exercise in human subjects. *J Appl Physiol* 1998; 84: 584–592.

39. Anthony TG, Anthony JC, Lewitt MS, et al. Time course changes in IGFBP-1 after treadmill exercise and postexercise food intake in rats. *Am J Physiol* 2001; 280: E650–E6.

40. Felig P, Wahren J. Amino acid metabolism in exercising man. *J Clin Invest* 1971; 50(12): 2703–2712.

41. Lemon PW, Nagle FJ. Effect of exercise on protein and amino acid metabolism. *Med Sci Sports Exerc* 1981; 133(3): 141–149.

42. Baldwin KM, Reitman JS, Terjung RL, et al. Substrate depletion in different types of muscle and liver during prolonged running. *Am J Physiol* 1973; 225: 1045–1050.

43. Terjung RL, Baldwin KM, Winder WW, et al. Glycogen repletion in different types of muscle and in liver after exhausting exercise. *Am J Physiol* 1974; 226: 1387–1391.

44. Kjaer M, Engfred K, Fernandes A, et al. Regulation of hepatic glucose production during exercise in humans: role of sympathoadrenergic activity. *Am J Physiol* 1993; 265: E275–E83.

45. Wasserman DH, Spalding JA, Lacy DB, et al. Glucagon is a primary controller of hepatic glycogenolysis and gluconeogenesis during muscular work. *Am J Physiol* 1989; 257: E108–E117.

46. Trimmer JK, Schwarz JM, Casazza GA, et al. Measurements of gluconeogenesis in exercising men by mass isotopomer distribution analysis. *J Appl Physiol* 2002; 93: 233–241.

47. Peterson KF, Price TB, Bergeron R. Regulation of net hepatic glycogenolysis and gluconeogenesis during exercise: impact of type I diabetes. *J Clin Endocrinol Metab* 2004; 89: 4656–4664.

48. Wahren JP, Ahlborg G, Jorfeldty L. Glucose metabolism during leg exercise in man. *J Clin Invest* 1971; 50: 2715–2725.

49. Wasserman DH, O'Doherty RM, Zinker BA. Role of the endocrine pancreas in control of fuel metabolism by the liver during exercise. *Int J Obesity Relat Metab Disord* 1995; 19 (Suppl. 4): S22–S30.

50. Jiang Y, Cyress AM, Muse ED, et al. Glucagon receptor activates extracellular signal-regulated protein kinase 1/2 via cAMP-dependent protein kinase. *Proc Natl Acad Sci USA* 2001; 98: 10102–10107.

51. Berglund ED, Lee-Young RS, Lustig DG, et al. Hepatic energy state is regulated by glucagon receptor signaling in mice. *J Clin Invest* 2009; 119: 2412–2422.

52. Wasserman DH, Lacy DB, Bracy DP. Relationship between arterial and portal vein immunoreactive glucagon during exercise. *J Appl Physiol* 1993; 75: 724–729.

53. Christensen NJ, Galbo H. Sympathetic nervous activity during exercise. *Annu Rev Physiol* 1983; 45: 139–153.

54. Coker RH, Krishna MG, Lacy DB, et al. Role of hepatic alpha- and beta-adrenergic receptor stimulation on hepatic glucose production during heavy exercise. *Am J Physiol* 1997; 273: E831–E8.

55. Lavoie J-M. The contribution of afferent signals from the liver to metabolic regulation during exercise. *Can J Physiol Pharm* 2002; 80: 1035–1044.

56. van Dijk G, Balkan B, Lindfeldt J, et al. Contribution of liver nerves, glucagon and adrenaline to the glycemic response to exercise in rats. *Acta Physiol Scand* 1994; 150: 305–313.
57. Lindfeldt J, Balkan B, van Dijk G, et al. Influence of peri-arterial hepatic denervation on the glycemic response to exercise in rats. *J Autonom Nerv Syst* 1993; 44: 45–52.
58. Banzet S, Koulmann N, Simler N, et al. Control of gluconeogenic genes during intense/prolonged exercise: hormone independent effect of muscle-derived IL-6 on hepatic tissue and PEPCk mRNA. *J Appl Physiol* 2009; 107: 1830–1839.
59. Fritsche L, Hoene M, Lehmann R, et al. IL-6 deficiency in mice neither impairs induction of metabolic genes in the liver nor affects blood glucose levels during fasting and moderately intense exercise. *Diabetologia* 2010; 53: 1732–1744.
60. Pedersen L, Pilegaard H, Hansen J, et al. Exercise-induced liver chemokine CXCL-1 expression is linked to muscle-derived interleukin-6 expression. *J Physiol* 2011; 589: 1409–1420.
61. Peeling P. Exercise as a mediator of hepcidin activity in athletes. *Eur J Appl Physiol* 2010; 110: 877–883.
62. Roecker L, Meier-Buttermilch R, Brechtel L, et al. Iron-regulatory protein hepcidin is increased in female athletes after a marathon. *Eur J Appl Physiol* 2005; 95: 569–571.
63. Davies KJ, Quintanilha AT, Brooks GA, et al. Free radicals and tissue damage produced by exercise. *Biochem Bipophys Res Commun* 1982; 107: 1198–1205.
64. Koyama K, Kaya M, Ishigaki T, et al. Role of xanthine oxidase in delayed lipid peroxidation in rat liver induced by acute exhausting exercise. *Eur J Appl Physiol* 1999; 80: 28–33.
65. Liu J, Yeo HC, Overvik-Douki E, et al. Chronically and acutely exercised rats: biomarkers of oxidative stress and endogenous antioxidants. *J Appl Physiol* 2000; 89: 21–28.
66. Wade OL, Bishop JM. *Cardiac output and regional blood flow.* Oxford, UK: Blackwell Scientific, 1962.
67. Shephard RJ. Are the abdominal viscera important to the sport physician? 1. Esophagus, stomach, intestines, spleen and pancreas. In: Shephard RJ, et al. (ed.). *Year book of sports medicine, 2013.* Philadelphia, PA: Elsevier, 2013, pp. xv–xxviii.
68. Davies KJA, Quintanilhat AT, Brooks GA, et al. Free radicals and tissue damage produced by exercise. *Bicohem Biophys Comm* 1982; 107(4): 1198–1205.
69. Gonzalez B, Manso R. Induction, modification and accumulation of HSP70s in the rat liver after acute exercise: early and late responses. *J Physiol* 2004; 556: 369–385.
70. Salo DC, Donovan CM, Davies KJ. HSP70 and other possible heat shock or oxidative stress proteins are induced in muscle, heart and liver during exercise. *Free Radic Biol Med* 1991; 11: 239–246.
71. Bejma J, Ramires P, Ji LL. Free radical generation and oxidative stress with ageing and exercise: differential effects in the myocardium and liver. *Acta Physiol Scand* 2000; 169: 343–351.
72. Ogonovszky H, Sasvári M, Dosek A, et al. The effects of moderate, strenuous and overtraining on oxidative stress markers and DNA repair in the rat liver. *Can J Appl Physiol* 2005; 30: 186–195.
73. Dohm GL, Kasperek GJ, Barakat HA. Time course of changes in gluconeogenic enzyme activities during exercise and recovery. *Am J Physiol* 1985; 249: E6–E11.
74. Hoene M, Lehmann R, Hennige AM, et al. Acute regulation of metabolic genes and insulin receptor substrates in the liver of mice by one single bout of treadmill exercise. *J Physiol* 2009; 587: 241–252.

75. Nizielski SE, Arizmendi C, Shteyngarts AR, et al. Involvement of transcription factor C/EBP-beta in stimulation of PEPCK gene expression during exercise. *Am J Physiol* 1996; 270: R1005–R12.

76. Helmrich SP, Ragland DR, Leung RW, et al. Physical activity and reduced occurrence of non-insulin dependent diabetes mellitus. *N Engl J Med* 1991; 325: 147–152.

77. Friedman JE. Role of glucocorticoids in activation of hepatic PEPCK gene transcription during exercise. *Am J Physiol* 1994; 266: E560–E566.

78. Ropelle ER, Pauli JR, Cintra DE, et al. Acute exercise modulates the Foxo1/PGC-1alpha pathway in the liver of diet-induced obesity rats. *J Physiol* 2009; 587: 2069–2076.

79. Haase TN, Ringholm S, Leick L, et al. Role of PGC-1 in exercise and fasting-induced adaptations in mouse liver. *Am J Physiol* 2011; 301: R1501–R1509.

80. Hansen J, Brandt C, Nielsen AR, et al. Exercise induces a marked increase in plasma follistatin: evidence that follistatin is a contraction-induced hepatokine. *Endocrinology* 2011; 152: 164–171.

81. Hoene M, Weigert C. The stress response of the liver to physical exercise. *Ex Immunol Rev* 2010; 16: 163–183.

82. Huang H, Iida KT, Sone H, et al. The regulation of adiponectin receptor expression by acute exercise in mice. *Exp Clin Endocrinol Diabetes* 2007; 115: 417–422.

83. Kelly M, Keller C, Avilucea PR, et al. AMPK activity is diminished in tissues of IL-6 knockout mice: the effect of exercise. *Biochem Biophys Res Comm* 2004; 320: 449–454.

84. Khanna S, Atalay M, Lodge JK, et al. Skeletal muscle and liver lipoyl-lysine content in response to exercise, training and dietary alpha-lipoic acid supplementation. *Biochem Mol Biol Internat* 1998; 46: 297–306.

85. Lavoie JM, Fillon Y, Couturier K, et al. Evidence that the decrease in liver glycogen is associated with the exercise-induced decrease increase in IGFBP-1. *J Appl Physiol* 2002; 93: 798–804.

86. Leu JI, George DL. Hepatic IGFBP-1 is a prosurvival factor that binds BAK, protects the liver from apoptosis, and antagonizes the proaptotic actions of p53 at mitochondria. *Genes Dev* 2007; 21: 3095–3109.

87. Hoene M, Franken H, Fritsche L, et al. Activation of the mitogen-activated protein kinase (MAPK) signalling pathway in the liver of mice is related to plasma glucose levels after acute exercise. *Diabetologia* 2010; 53: 1131–1141.

88. Rowell LB. *Human circulation: regulation during physical stress.* New York, NY: Oxford University Press, 1986.

89. Rowell LB, Blackmon JR, Bruce RA. Indocyanine green clearance and estimated hepatic blood flow during mild to maximal exercise in upright man. *J Clin Invest* 1964; 43: 1677–1690.

90. Daemen MJAP, Thijssen HHW, van Essen H, et al. Liver blood flow measurement in the rat: the electromagnetic versus the microsphere and clearance methods. *J Pharmacol Methods* 1989; 21: 287–297.

91. Busse M, Nordhusen D, Tegtbur U, et al. Sorbitol clearance during exercise as a measure of hepatic and renal blood flow. *Clin Sportsmed Internat* 2003; 1: 1–8.

92. Kemme MJ, Burggraaf J, Schoemaker RC, et al. The influence of reduced liver blood flow on the pharmacokinetics and pharmacodynamics of recombinant tissue factor pathway inhibitor. *Clin Pharmacol Ther* 2000; 67: 504–511.

93. Schoemaker RC, Burggraaf J, Cohen AF. Assessment of hepatic blood flow using continuous infusion of high clearance drugs. *Br J Clin Pharmacol* 1998; 45: 463–469.

94. Fojt E, Ekelund L-G, Hultman E. Enzyme activities in hepatic venous blood under strenuous physical exercise. *Pflüg Arch* 1976; 361: 287–296.

95. Flamm SD, Taki J, Moore R, et al. Redistribution of regional and organ blood volume and effect on cardiac function in relation to upright exercise intensity in healthy human subjects. *Circulation* 1990; 81: 1550–1559.

96. Froelich JE, Strauss HW, Moore RH, et al. Redistribution of visceral blood volume in upright exercise in healthy volunteers. *J Nucl Med* 1988; 29: 1714–1718.

97. Katz M, Bergman EN. Simultaneous measurements of hepatic and portal venous blood flow in the sheep and dog. *Am J Physiol* 1969; 216: 946–952.

98. Yano L, Yano H, Taketa K. Electromagnetic determination of portal venous flow in rats during exercise. *Internat Hepatol Comm* 1996; 5: 184–190.

99. Hurren NM, Balanos GM, Blannin AK. Is the beneficial effect of prior exercise on postprandial lipaemia partly due to redistribution of blood flow? *Clin Sci* 2011; 120: 537–548.

100. Latour MG, Brault A, Huet PM, et al. Effects of acute physical exercise on hepatocyte volume and fuction in rat. *Am J Physiol* 1999; 276: R1258–R1264.

101. Kayashima S, Ohno H, Fujioka T, et al. Leucocytosis as a marker of organ damage induced by chronic strenuous physical exercise. *Eur J Appl Physiol* 1995; 70: 413–420.

102. Lehmann M, Huonker M, Dimeo F, et al. Serum amino acid concentrations in nine athletes before and after the 1993 Colmar ultramrathon. *Int J Sports Med* 1995; 16(3): 155–159.

103. Praphatsorn P, Thong-Ngam D, Kulaputana O, et al. Effects of intense exercise on biochemical and histological changes in rat liver and pancreas. *Asian Biomed* 2010; 4: 619–625.

104. Yano H, Kinoshita S, Yano L. Acute exercise induces mitochondrial swelling of hepatocytes surrounding the terminal hepatic venule in rat liver acinus. *Jpn J Phys Fitness Sports Med* 1997; 46: 49–54.

105. Huang CC, Yang S-C, Chan C-C, et al. Ganoderma tsugae hepatoprotection against exhaustive exercise-induced liver injury in rats. *Molecules* 2013; 18: 1741–1754.

106. Khazaeinia T, Ramsey AA, Tam YK. The effects of exercise on the pharmacokinetics of drugs. *J Pharm Pharmaceut Sci* 2000; 3: 292–302.

107. Døssing M. Effect of acute and chronic exercise on hepatic drug metabolism. *Clin Pharmacokinet* 1985; 10: 426–431.

108. Balasubramian K, Mawer GE, Simons PJ. The influence of dose on the distribution and elimination of amylobarbitone in healthy subjects. *Br J Pharmacol* 1970; 40: 578–579.

109. Klotz U, Lücke C. Physical exercise and disposition of diazepam. *Br J Clin Pharmacol* 1978; 5: 349–350.

110. Swartz RD, Sidell FR, Cucinell SA. Effects of physical stress on the disposition of drugs eliminated by the liver in man. *J Pharmacol Exp Therap* 1974; 188: 1–7.

111. Mooy J, Arends B, Kaminade JV, et al. Influence of prolonged submaximal exercise on the pharmacokinetics of verapamil in humans. *J Cardiovasc Pharmacol* 1986; 8: 940–942.

112. Loniewski I, Sawrymowicz M, Pawlik A, et al. Lack of effect of physical exercise on pharmacokinetics of acetaminophen tablets in healthy subjects. *Acta Pol Pharmaceut* 2001; 58: 141–144.

113. Theilade P, Hansen JM, Skovsted L, et al. Effect of exercise on thyroid parameters and on metabolic clearance rate of antipyrine in man. *Acta Endocrinol* 1979; 92: 271–276.

114. Fabbri A, Bianchi G, Zoli M, et al. Effect of physical exercise on one-sample antipyrine clearance. *Ital J Gastroenterol* 1991; 23: 74–76.
115. van Griensven JM, Burggraaf KJ, Gerloff J, et al. Effects of changing liver blood flow by exercise and food on kinetics and dynamics of saruplase. *Clin Pharmacol Therap* 1995; 57: 381–389.
116. Pinho RA, Silva LA, Pinho CA, et al. Oxidative stress and inflammatory parameters after an Ironman race. *Clin J Sports Med* 2010; 20: 306–311.
117. Neubauer O, König D, Kern N, et al. No indications of persistent oxidative stress in response to an ironman triathlon. *Med Sci Sports Exerc* 2008; 40: 2119–2228.
118. Turner JE, Hodges NJ, Bosch JA, et al. Prolonged depletion of antioxidant capacity after ultraendurance exercise. *Med Sci Sports Exerc* 2011; 43: 1770–1776.
119. Margaritis I, Tessier F, Richard MJ, et al. No evidence of oxidative stress after a triathlon race in highly trained competitors. *Int J Sports Med* 1997; 18: 186–190.
120. Sen CK, Marin E, Kretzschmar M, et al. Skeletal muscle and liver glutathione homeostasis in response to training, exercise, and immobilization. *J Appl Physiol* 1992; 73: 1265–1272.
121. Bürger-Mendonça M, Bielavsky M, Barbosa FCR. Liver overload in Brazilian triathletes after half-ironman competition is related to muscle fatigue. *Ann Hepatol* 2008; 7: 245–248.
122. De Paz JA, Villa JG, Lopez P, et al. Effects of long-distance running on serum bilirubin. *Med Sci Sports Exerc* 1995; 27: 1590–1594.
123. Fallon KE, Sivyer G, Sivyer K, et al. The biochemistry of runners in a 1600 km ultramarathon. *Br J Sports Med* 1999; 33: 264–269.
124. Holly RG, Barnard RJ, Rosenthal M, et al. Triathlete characterization and response to prolonged strenuous competition. *Med Sci Sports Exerc* 1986; 18: 123–127.
125. Kratz A, Lewandrowski KB, Siegel AJ, et al. Effect of marathon running on hematologic and biochemical laboratory parameters, including cardiac markers. *Am J Clin Pathol* 2002; 118: 856–863.
126. Lippi G, Schena F, Montagnana M, et al. Significant variation of traditional markers 3of liver injury after a half-marathon run. *Eur J Int Med* 2011; 22(5): e36–38.
127. Long D, Blake M, McNaughton L, et al. Hematological and biochemical changes during a short triathlon competition in novice triathletes. *Eur J Appl Physiol* 1990; 61: 93–99.
128. Mena P, Maynar M, Campillo JE. Changes in plasma enzyme activities in professional racing cyclists. *Br J Sports Med* 1996; 30: 122–124.
129. Nagel D, Seiler D, Franz H, et al. Ultra-long distance running and the liver. *Int J Sports Med* 1990; 11: 441–445.
130. Noakes TD, Carter JW. Biochemical parameters in athletes before and having run 160 kilometres. *S Afr Med J* 1976; 50: 1562–1566.
131. Noakes TD, Carter JW. The responses of plama biochemical parameters to a 56 km race in novice and experienced ultramarathoners. *Eur J Appl Physiol* 1982; 49: 179–86.
132. Rama R, Ibáñez J, Riera M, et al. Hematological, electrolyte, and biochemical alterations after a 100-km run. *Can J Appl Physiol* 1994; 19: 411–420.
133. Richards D, Richards R, Schofield PJ, et al. Biochemical and haematological changes in Sydney's the Sun City-to-Surf fun runners. *Med J Aust* 1979; 2(9): 449–453.
134. Shapiro Y, Magazanik A, Sohar E, et al. Serum enzyme changes in untrained subjects following a prolonged march. *Can J Physiol Pharmacol* 1973; 51: 271–276.
135. Smith JE, Garbutt G, Lopes P, et al. Effects of prolonged strenuous exercise

(marathon running) on biochemical and haematological markers used in the investigation of patients in the emergency department. *Br J Sports Med* 2004; 38: 292–294.

136. Suzuki K, Peake J, Nosaka K, et al. Changes in markers of muscle damage, inflammation and HSP70 after an Ironman triathlon race. *Eur J Appl Physiol* 2006; 98: 525–534.

137. Van Rensburg JP, Kielblock AJ, van der Linde A. Physiologic and biochemical changes during a triathlon competition. *Int J Sports Med* 1986; 7: 30–35.

138. Waskiewicz Z, Klapcinska B, Sadowska-Krepa E, et al. Acute metabolic responses to a 24-h ultra-marathon race in male amateur runners. *Eur J Appl Physiol* 2012; 112: 1679–1688.

139. Wu H-J, Chen K-T, Shee B-W, et al. Effects of 24 h ultra-marathon on biochemical and hematological parameters. *World J Gastroenterol* 2004; 10: 2711–2714.

140. Apple FS, McGue MK. Serum enzyme changes during marathon training. *Am J Clin Pathol* 1983; 79: 716–719.

141. Beard ME, Hamer JW, Hamilton G, et al. Jogger's heat stroke. *NZ Med J* 1979; 89(631): 159–161.

142. Bunch TW. Blood test abnormalities in runners. *Mayo Clin Proc* 1980; 55: 113–117.

143. Hammouda O, Chtouru H, Chaouchi A, et al. Effect of short-term maximal exercise on biochemical markers of muscle damage, total antioxidant status and homocysteine levels in football players. *Asian J Sports Med* 2012; 3: 239–46.

144. Malinoski FJ. Strenuous exercise simulating hepatic injury during vaccine trials. *Vaccine* 1992; 10: 39–42.

145. Nathwani RA, Pais S, Reynolds TB, et al. Serum alanine aminotransferase in skeletal muscle diseases. *Hepatology* 2005; 41: 380–382.

146. Ohno H, Yahata T, Yamashita K, et al. Effect of physical training on immunoreactive gamma-glutamyltransferase in human plasma. *Enzyme* 1988; 39: 110–114.

147. Pettersson J, Hindorf U, Persson P, et al. Muscular exercise can cause highly pathological liver function tests in healthy men. *Br J Clin Pharmacol* 2008; 65: 253–259.

148. Takahashi I, Umeda T, Mashiko T, et al. Effects of rugby sevens matches on human neutrophil-related nonspecific immunity. *Br J Sports Med* 2007; 41: 13–18.

149. Litvinova L, Viru A. Effect of exercise and adrenal insufficiency on urea production in rats. *Eur J Appl Physiol* 1995; 70: 536–540.

150. Kayatekin BM, Gonenc S, Acikgoz O, et al. Effects of sprint exercise on oxidative stress in skeletal muscle and liver. *Eur J Appl Physiol* 2002; 87: 141–144.

151. Huang C-C, Tsai S-C, Lin W-T. Potential ergogenic effects of L-arginine against oxidative and inflammatory stress induced by acute exercise in aging rats. *Exp Gerontol* 2008; 43: 571–577.

152. Turgut G, Demir S, Genc O, et al. The effect of swimming exercise on lipid peroxidation in the rat brain, liver and heart. *Acta Physiol Pharmacol Bulg* 2003; 27: 43–45.

153. Aydin C, Ince E, Koiparan S, et al. Protective effects of long term dietary restriction on swimming exercise-induced oxidative stress in the liver, heart and kidney of rat. *Cell Biochem Funct* 2005; 25: 129–137.

154. Murakami T, Shimomura Y, Fujitsuka N, et al. Enlargement glycogen store in rat liver and muscle by fructose-diet intake and exercise training. *J Appl Physiol* 1997; 82: 772–775.

155. Coggan AR, Swanson SC, Mendenhall LA, et al. Effect of endurance training on hepatic glycogenolysis and gluconeogenesis during prolonged exercise in men. *Am J Physiol* 1995; 268: E375–E83.

156. Galbo H, Richter EA, Holst JJ, et al. Diminished hormonal responses to exercise in trained rats. *J Appl Physiol* 1977; 43: 953–958.
157. James DE, Kraegen EW. The effect of exercise training on glycogen, glycogen synthase and phosphorylase in muscle and liver. *Eur J Appl Physiol* 1984; 52: 276–281.
158. Aoi W, Naito Y, Hang LP, et al. Regular exercise prevents high-sucrose diet-induced fatty liver via improvement of hepatic lipid metabolism. *Biochem Biophys Res Comm* 2011; 413: 330–335.
159. Colombo M, Gregersen S, Kruhoeffer M, et al. Prevention of hyperglycemia in Zucker diabetic fatty rats by exercise training: effects on gene expression in insulin-sensitive tissues determined by high-density oligonucleotide microarray analysis. *Metabolism* 2005; 54: 1571–1581.
160. Bae JC, Suh S, Park SE, et al. Regular exercise is associated with a reduction in the risk of NAFLD and decreased liver enzymes in individuals with NAFLD independent of obesity in Korean adults. *PLoS ONE* 2012; 7(10): e46819.
161. Fintini D, Pietrobattista A, Morino G, et al. Energy expenditure and insulin sensitivity evaluation in obese children affected by hepatosteatosis. *Pediatr Obesity* 2012; 7(2): e4–7.
162. Gerber L, Otgonsuren M, Mishra A, et al. Non-alcoholic fatty liver disease (NAFLD) is associated with low level of physical activity: a population-based study. *Aliment Pharmacol Therap* 2012; 36: 772–781.
163. Hattar LN, Wilson TA, Tabotabo LA, et al. Physical activity and nutrition attitudes in obese Hispanic children with non-alcoholic steatohepatitis. *World J Gastroenterol* 2011; 17(39): 4396–4403.
164. Hsieh SD, Yoshinaga H, Muto T, et al. Regular physical activity and coronary risk factors in Japanese men. *Circulation* 1998; 97: 661–665.
165. Kang JH, Greenson JK, Omo JT, et al. Metabolic syndrome is associated with greater histologic severity, higher carbohydrate, and lower fat diet in patients with NAFLD. *Am J Gastroenterol* 2006; 101: 2247–2253.
166. Kistler KD, Brunt EM, Clark JM, et al. Physical activity recommendations, exercise intensity, and histological severity of nonalcoholic fatty liver disease. *Am J Gastroeneterol* 2011; 106: 470–475.
167. Leskinen T, Sipilä S, Alen M, et al. Leisure-time physical activity and high-risk fat: a longitudinal population-based twin study. *Int J Obesity* 2009; 33: 1211–1218.
168. Newton JL, Jones DEJ, Henderson E, et al. Fatigue in non-alcoholic fatty liver disease (NAFLD) is significant and associates with inactivity and excessive daytime sleepiness but not with liver disease severity or insulin resistance. *Gut* 2008; 57: 807–813.
169. Perseghin G, Lattuada G, De Cobelli F, et al. Habitual physical activity is associated with intrahepatic fat content in humans. *Diabetes Care* 2007; 30: 683–688.
170. Tiikkainen M, Beergholm R, Hakkinen AM, et al. Liver fat accumulation and insulin resistance in obese women with previous gestational diabetes. *Obesity Res* 2002; 10: 859–867.
171. Zelber-Sagi S, Ratziu V, Oren R. Nutrition and physical activity in NAFLD: an overview of the epidemiological evidence. *World J Gastroenterol* 2011; 17: 3377–3389.
172. Podolin DA, Wills BK, Wood IO, et al. Attenuation of age-related declines in glucagon-mediated signal transduction in rat liver by exercise training. *Am J Physiol* 2001; 281: E516–E23.

173. Drouin R, Robert G, Milot M, et al. Swim training increases glucose output from liver perfused in situ with glucagon in fed and fasted rats. *Metabolism* 2004; 53: 1027–1031.
174. Donovan CM, Sumida KD. Training improves glucose homeostasis in rats during exercise via glucose production. *Am J Physiol* 1990; 258: R770–R8.
175. Donovan CM, Pagliassotti MJ. Enhanced efficiency of lactate removal after endurance training. *J Appl Physiol* 1990; 68: 1053–1058.
176. Sumida KD, Donovan CM. Enhanced hepatic gluconeogenic capacity for selected precursors after endurance training. *J Appl Physiol* 1995; 79: 1883–1888.
177. Sumida KD, Donovan CM. Enhanced gluconeogenesis from lactate in perfused livers after endurance training. *J Appl Physiol* 1993; 74: 782–787.
178. Prior SJ, Jenkins NT, Brandauer J, et al. Aerobic exercise training increases circulating insulin-like growth factor binding protein-1 concentration, but does not attenuate the reduction in circulating insulin-like growth factor binding protein-1 after a high-fat meal. *Metabolism* 2012; 61: 310–316.
179. Church TS, Kuk JL, Ross R, et al. Association of cardiorespiratory fitness, body mass index, and waist circumference to nonalcoholic fatty liver disease. *Gastroenterology* 2006; 130: 2023–2030.
180. Hannukainen JC, Nuutila P, Borra R, et al. Increased physical activity decreases hepatic free fatty acid uptake: a study in human monozygotic twins. *J Physiol* 2007; 578: 347–358.
181. Haufe S, Engeli S, Budziarek P, et al. Cardiorespiratory fitness and insulin sensitivity in overweight or obese subjects may be linked through intrahepatic lipid content. *Diabetes* 2010; 59: 1640–1647.
182. Kantartzis K, Thamer C, Peter A, et al. High cardiorespiratory fitness is an independent predictor of the reduction in liver fat during a lifestyle intervention in non-alcoholic fatty liver disease. *Gut* 2009; 58: 1281–1288.
183. Krasnoff JB, Painter PL, Wallace JP, et al. Health-related fitness and physical activity in patients with nonalcoholic fatty liver disease. *Hepatology* 2008; 47: 1158–1166.
184. Kuk JL, Nichaman MZ, Church TS, et al Liver fat is not a marker of metabolic risk in lean premenopausal women. *Metabolism* 2004; 53: 1066–1071.
185. McMillan KP, Kuk JL, Church TS, et al. Independent associations between liver fat, visceral adipose tissue, and metabolic risk factors in men. *Appl Physiol Nutr Metab* 2007; 32: 265–272.
186. Nguyen-Duy TB, Nichaman MZ, Church TS, et al. Visceral fat and liver fat are independent predictors of metabolic risk factors in men. *Am J Physiol* 2003; 284: E1065–E1071.
187. O'Donovan G, Thomas EL, McCarthy JP, et al. Fat distribution in men of different waist girth, fitness level and exercise habit. *Int J Obesity* 2009; 33: 1356–1362.
188. Seppala-Lindroos A, Vehkavaara S, Hakkinen AM, et al. Fat accumulation in the liver is associated with defects in insulin suppression of glucose production and serum free fatty acids independent of obesity in normal men. *J Clin Endocrinol Metab* 2007; 87: 3023–3028.
189. Albu JB, Hellbronn LK, Kelley D, et al. Metabolic changes following a 1-year diet and exercise intervention in patients with type 2 diabetes. *Diabetes* 2010; 59: 627–633.
190. Bacchi N, Moghetti P. Exercise for hepatic fat accumulation in type 2 diabetic subjects. *Int J Endocrinobiol ID 309191* 2013: 1–5

191. Bacchi E, Negri C, Targher G, et al. Both resistance training and aerobic training reduce hepatic fat content in type 2 diabetic subjects with nonalcoholic fatty liver disease (the RAED2 randomized trial). *Hepatology* 2013; 58(4): 1287–1295.
192. Bonekamp S, Barone B, Clark JM, et al. The effect of exercise training intervention on hepatic steatosis. *Hepatology* 2008; 48 (S1): 806A.
193. Chen S-M, Liu C-Y, Li S-R, et al. Effects of therapeutic lifestyle program on ultrasound-diagnosed nonalcoholic fatty liver disease. *J Chinese Med Assoc* 2008; 71: 551–558.
194. de Piano A, de Mello M, Sanches PL, et al. Long-term effects of aerobic plus resistance training on the adipokines and neuropeptides in nonalcoholic fatty liver disease obese adolescents. *Eur J Gastroenterol Hepatol* 2012; 24: 1313–1324.
195. Devries MC, Samjoo IA, Hamadeh MJ, et al. Effect of endurance exercise on hepatic lipid content, enzymes, and adiposity in men and women. *Obesity* 2008; 16: 2281–2288.
196. Eckard C, Cole R, Lockwood J, et al. Prospective histopathologic evaluation of lifestyle modification in nonalcoholic fatty liver disease: a randomized trial. *Ther Adv Gastroenterol* 2013; 6: 249–259.
197. Fealy CE, Haus JM, Solomon TP, et al. Short-term exercise reduces markers of hepatocyte apoptosis in nonalcoholic fatty liver disease. *J Appl Physiol* 2012; 113: 1–6.
198. Finucane FM, Sharp SJ, Purslow LR, et al. The effects of aerobic exercise on metabolic risk, insulin sensitivity and intrahepatic lipid in healthy older people from the Hertfordshire Cohort Study: a randomised controlled trial. *Diabetalogia* 2010; 53: 624–631.
199. Franzese A, Vajro P, Arngeniziano A, et al. Liver involvement in obese children. Ultrasonography and liver enzyme levels at diagnosis and during follow-up in an Italian population. *Dig Dis Sci* 1997; 42: 1428–1432.
200. Goodpaster BH, Delany JP, Otto AD, et al. Effects of diet and physical activity interventions on weight loss and cardiometabolic risk factors in severely obese adults: a randomized trial. *JAMA* 2010; 304: 1795–1802.
201. Grønbæk H, Lange A, Birkebaek NH, et al. Effect of a 10-week weight loss camp on fatty liver disease and insulin sensitivity in obese Danish children. *J Pediatr Gastroenterol Nutr* 2012; 54: 223–228.
202. Hallsworth K, Fattakhova G, Hollingsworth K, et al. Resistance exercise reduces liver fat and its mediators in non-alcoholic fatty liver disease independent of weight loss. *Gut* 2011; 60: 1278–1283.
203. Hickman IJ, Jonsson JR, Prins JB, et al. Modest weight loss and physical activity in overweight patients with chronic liver disease results in sustained improvements in alanine aminotransferase, fasting insulin, and quality of life. *Gut* 2004; 53: 413–419.
204. Jin Y-J, Kim KM, Hwang S, et al. Exercise and diet modification in non-obese non-alcoholic fatty liver disease: analysis of biopsies of living liver donors. *J Gastroenterol Hepatol* 2012; 27: 1341–1347.
205. Johnson NA, Sachinwalla T, Walton DW, et al. Aerobic exercise training reduces hepatic and visceral lipids in obese individuals without weight loss. *Hepatology* 2009; 50: 1105–1112.
206. Kawaguchi T, Shiba N, Maeda T, et al. Hybrid training of voluntary and electrical muscle contractions reduces steatosis, insulin resistance, and IL-6 levels in patients with NAFLD: a pilot study. *J Gastroenterol* 2011; 46: 746–757.
207. Koot BGP, van der Baan-Slootweg OH, Tamminga-Smeulders CLJ, et al. Lifestyle intervention for non-alcoholic fatty liver disease: prospective cohort study

of its efficacy and factors related to improvement. *Arch Dis Childh* 2011; 96: 669–674.

208. Larson-Meyer DE, Newcomer BR, Heilbrunn LK, et al. Effect of 6-month calorie restriction and exercise on serum and liver lipids and markers of liver function. *Obesity* 2008; 16: 1355–1362.

209. Lazo M, Solga SF, Horska A, et al. The effect of one year of intensive lifestyle intervention on hepatic steatosis. *Hepatology* 2008; 48 (Suppl): 813A.

210. Lee S, Bacha F, Hannon T, et al. Effects of aerobic versus resistance exercise without caloric restriction on abdominal fat, intrahepatic lipid, and insulin sensitivity in obese adolescent boys: a randomized, controlled trial. *Diabetes* 2012; 61: 2787–2795.

211. Nobili V, Manco M, Devito R, et al. Lifestyle intervention and antioxidant therapy in children with nonalcoholic fatty liver disease: A randomized, controlled trial. *Hepatology* 2008; 48:119–1128.

212. Oza N, Eguchi Y, Mizuta T, et al. A pilot trial of body weight reduction for nonalcoholic fatty liver disease with a home-based lifestyle modification intervention delivered in collaboration with interdisciplinary medical staff. *J Gastroenterol* 2009; 44: 1203–1208.

213. Promrat K, Kleiner DE, Niemeier HM, et al. Randomized controlled trial testing the effect of weight loss on nonalcoholic steatohepatitis (NASSH). *Hepatology* 2010; 51: 121–129.

214. Santomauro M, Paoli-Valeri M, Fernandez M, et al. Enfermedad del hígado graso no alcohólico y su asociación con variables clínicas y bioquímicas en los niños y adolescentes obesos: efecto de una intervención de un año en el estilo de vida [Non-alcoholic fatty liver disease and its association with clinical and biochemical variables in obese children and adolescents: effect of a one-year intervention on lifestyle]. *Endocrinol Nutric* 2012; 59: 346–353.

215. Schäfer S, Kantartzis K, Machann J, et al. Lifestyle intervention in individuals with normal versus impaired glucose tolerance. *Eur J Clin Invest* 2007; 37: 535–543.

216. Shah K, Stufflebam A, Hilton TN, et al. Diet and exercise interventions reduce intrahepatic fat content and improve insulin sensitivity in obese older adults. *Obesity* 2009; 17: 2162–2168.

217. Shojaee-Moradie F, Baynes KC, Pentecost C, et al. Exercise training reduces fatty acid availability and improves the insulin sensitivity of glucose metabolism. *Diabetologia* 2007; 50: 404–413.

218. Slentz CA, Bateman LA, Willis LH, et al. Effects of aerobic vs. resistance training on visceral and liver fat stores, liver enzymes, and insulin resistance by HOMA in overweight adults from STRRIDE AT/RT. *Am J Physiol* 2012; 301: E1033–E1039.

219. Sullivan S, Kirk E, Mittendorfer B, et al. Randomized trial of exercise effect on intrahepatic triglyceride content and lipid kinetics in nonalcoholic fatty liver disease. *Hepatology* 2012; 55: 1738–1745.

220. Tamura Y, Tanaka Y, Sato F, et al. Effects of diet and exercise on muscle and liver intracellular lipid contents and insulin sensitivity in type 2 diabetic patients. *J Clin Endocrinol Metab* 2005; 90: 3191–3196.

221. Thamer C, Jürgen M, Stefan N, et al. Variations in PPARD determine the change in body composition during lifestyle intervention: A whole body magnetic resonance study. *J Clin Endocrinol Metab* 2008; 93: 1497–1500.

222. Thamer C, Machann J, Bachman OP, et al. Intramyocellular lipids: Anthropometric determinants and relationships with maximal aerobic capacity and insulin sensitivity. *J Clin Endocrinol Metab* 2003; 88: 1785–1791.

223. Thomas EL, Brynes AE, Hamilton G, et al. Effect of nutritional counselling on hepatic, muscle and adipose tissue fat content and distribution in non-alcoholic fatty liver disease. *World J Gasteroeneterol* 2006; 12(36): 5813–5819.
224. Ueno T, Sugawara H, Sujaku K, et al. Therapeutic effect of restricted diet and exercise in obese patients with fatty liver. *J Hepatol* 1997; 27: 103–107.
225. van der Heijden GJ, Wang ZJ, Chu ZD, et al. A 12-week aerobic exercise program reduces hepatic fat accumulation and insulin resistance in obese, Hispanic adolescents. *Obesity* (Silver Spring) 2010; 18: 384–390.
226. Botezelli JD, Mora RF, Dalia RA, et al. Exercise counteracts fatty liver disease in rats fed on fructose-rich diet. *Lipids Health Dis* 2010; 9: 116.
227. Cameron I, Alam MS, Wang J, et al. Endurance exercise in a rat model of metabolic syndrome. *Can J Physiol Pharmac* 2012; 90: 1490–1497.
228. Charbonneau A, Couturier K, Gauthier M-S, et al. Evidence of hepatic glucagon resistance associated with hepatic steatosis: reversal effect of training. *Int J Sports Med* 2005; 26: 432–441.
229. Cintra DE, Ropelle ER, Vitto MF, et al. Reversion of hepatic steatosis by exercise training in obese mice: the role of sterol regulatory element-binding protein-1c. *Life Sci* 2012; 91: 395–401.
230. Corriveau P, Paquette A, Brochu M, et al. Resistance training prevents liver fat accumulation in ovariectomized rats. *Maturitas* 2008; 59: 259–267.
231. Gauthier M-S, Couturier K, Latour J-G, et al. Concurrent exercise prevents high-fat-diet-induced macrovesicular hepatic steatosis. *J Appl Physiol* 2003; 94: 2127–2134.
232. Gauthier M-S, Couturier K, Charbonneau A, et al. Effects of introducing physical training in the course of a 16-week high-fat diet regimen on hepatic steatosis, adipose tissue fat accumulation, and plasma lipid profile. *Int J Obesity Rel Metab Dis* 2004; 28: 1064–1071.
233. Yasari S, Wang D, Prud'homme D, et al. Exercise training decreases plasma leptin levels and the expression of hepatic leptin receptor-a, -b, and, -e in rats. *Mol Cell Biochem* 2009; 324: 13–20.
234. Hao L, Wang Y, Duan Y, et al. Effects of treadmill exercise training on liver fat accumulation and estrogen receptor alpha expression in intact and ovariectomized rats with or without estrogen replacement treatment. *Eur J Appl Physiol* 2010; 109: 879–886.
235. Leite RD, Prestes J, Bernardes CF, et al. Effects of ovariectomy and resistance training on lipid content in skeletal muscle, liver, and heart; fat depots; and lipid profile. *Appl Physiol Nutr Metab* 2009; 34: 1079–1086.
236. Marques CMM, Motta VF, Torres TS, et al. Beneficial effects of exercise training (treadmill) on insulin resistance and nonalcoholic fatty liver disease in high-fat fed C57BL/6 mice. *Braz J Med Biol Res* 2010; 43: 467–475.
237. Moura LP, Puga GM, Beck WR, et al. Exercise and spirulina control non-alcoholic hepatic steatosis and lipid profile in diabetic Wistar rats. *Lipids Health Dis* 2011; 10: 77.
238. Pighon A, Gutkowska J, Jankowski M, et al. Exercise training in ovariectomized rats stimulates estrogenic-like effects on expression of genes involved in lipid accumulation and subclinical inflammation in liver. *Metabolism* 2011; 60: 629–639.
239. Pighon A, Paquette A, Barsalani R, et al. Substituting food restriction by resistance training prevents liver and body fat regain in ovariectomized rats. *Climacteric* 2009; 12: 153–164.

240. Rector RS, Uptergrove GM, Morris EM, et al. Daily exercise vs. caloric restriction for prevention of nonalcoholic fatty liver disease in the OLETF rat model. *Am J Physiol* 2011; 300: G874–G83.
241. Schultz A, Mendonca LS, Aguila MB, et al. Swimming training beneficial effects in a mice model of nonalcoholic fatty liver disease. *Exp Toxicol Pathol* 2012; 64: 273–282.
242. Sene-Fiorese M, Duarte FO, Scarmagnani FRR, et al. Efficiency of intermittent exercise on adiposity and fatty liver in rats fed with high-fat diet. *Obesity* (Silver Spring) 2009; 16: 2217–2222.
243. Takeshita H, Horiuchi M, Izumo K, et al. Long-term voluntary exercise, representing habitual exercise, lowers visceral fat and alters plasma amino acid levels in mice. *Environ Health Prev Med* 2012; 17: 275–284.
244. Thyfault JP, Rector RS, Uptergrove G, et al. Rats selectively bred for low aerobic capacity have reduced hepatic mitochondrial capacity and susceptibility to hepatic steatosis and injury. *J Physiol* 2009; 587: 1805–1816.
245. Yasari S, Prud'homme D, Wang D, et al. Exercise training decreases hepatic SCD-1 gene expression and protein content in rats. *Mol Cell Biochem* 2010; 335: 291–299.
246. Martin CK, Church TS, Thompson AM, et al. Exercise dose and quality of life. A randomized controlled trial. *Arch Int Med* 2009; 169: 269–278.
247. Yiamouyiannis CA, Sanders RA, Watkins JB, et al. Chronic physical activity: hepatic hypertrophy and increased total biotransformation enzyme activity. *Biochem Pharmacol* 1992; 44: 121–127.
248. Cullinane E, Siconolfi S, Saritelli A, et al. Acute decrease in serum triglycerides with exercise – is there a threshold for an exercise effect? *Metabolism* 1982; 31: 844–847.
249. Magkos F, Patterson BW, Mohammed BS, et al. A single 1-h bout of evening exercise increases basal FFA flux without affecting VLDL-triglyceride and VLDL-apolipoprotein B-100 kinetics in untrained lean men. *Am J Physiol* 2007; 292: E1568–E1574.
250. Williams P, Wood P, Haskell W, et al. EFfect of exercise intensity and duration on plasma-lipoprotein cholesterol levels. *Circulation* 1981; 64: 185.
251. Kelley GA, Kelley KS, Franklin B. Aerobic exercise and lipids and lipoproteins in patients with cardiovascular disease: a meta-analysis of randomized controlled trials. *J Cardiopulm Rehabil* 2006; 26: 131–139.
252. Kelley GA, Kelley KS, Tran ZV. Aerobic exercise, lipids and lipoproteins in overweight and obese adults: a meta-analysis of randomized controlled trials. *Int J Obseity* 2005; 29: 881–893.
253. Tsekouras YE, Magkos F, Kellas Y, et al. High-intensity interval aerobic training reduces hepatic very low-density lipoprotein-triglyceride secretion rate in men. *Am J Physiol* 2008; 295: E851–E8.
254. Thompson PD, Cullinane EM, Sady SP, et al. High-density-lipoprotein metabolism in endurance athletes and sedentary men. *Circulation* 1991; 84: 140–152.
255. Halverstadt A, Phares DA, Wilund KR, et al. Endurance exercise training raises high-density lipoprotein cholesterol and lowers small low-density lipoprotein and very low-density lipoprotein independent of body fat phenotypes in older men and women. *Metabolism* 2007; 56: 444–450.
256. Kraus WE, Houmard JA, Duscha BD, et al. Effects of the amount and intensity of exercise on plasma lipoproteins. *N Engl J Med* 2002; 347: 1483–1492.
257. Brinkley TE, Halverstadt A, Phares DA, et al. Hepatic lipase gene –514CT variant is

associated with exercise training-induced changes in VLDL and HDL by lipoprotein lipase. *J Appl Physiol* 2011; 111: 1871–1876.

258. Askew EW, Barakat H, Kuhl GL, et al. Response of lipogenesis and fatty acid synthetase to physical training and exhaustive exercise in rats. *Lipids Health Dis* 1975; 10: 491–496.

259. Fiebig R, Griffiths MA, Gore MT, et al. Exercise training down-regulates hepatic lipogenic enzymes in meal-fed rats: fructose versus complex-carbohydrate diets. *J Nutr* 1998; 128: 810–817.

260. Fiebig RG, Hollander JM, Ney D, et al. Training down-regulates fatty acid synthase and body fat in obese Zucker rats. *Med Sci Sports Exerc* 2002; 34: 1106–1114.

261. Chapados NA, Seelaender M, Levy E, et al. Effects of exercise training on hepatic microsomal triglyceride transfer protein content in rats. *Hormone Metab Res* 2009; 41: 287–293.

262. Ghanbari-Niaki A, Khabazian BM, Hossaini-Kakhak SA, et al. Treadmill exercise enhances ABCA1 expression in rat liver. *Biochem Biophys Res Comm* 2007; 36: 841–846.

263. Petridou A, Nikolaidis MG, Matsakas A, et al. Effect of exercise training on the fatty acid composition of lipid classes in rat liver, skeletal muscle, and adipose tissue. *Eur J Appl Physiol* 2005; 94: 84–92.

264. Bexfield NA, Parcell AC, Nelson WB, et al. Adaptations to high-intensity inter-mittent exercise in rodents. *J Appl Physiol* 2009; 107: 749–754.

265. Mikami T, Sumida S, Ishibashi Y, et al. Endurance exercise training inhibits activity of plasma GOT and liver caspase-3 of mice [correction of rats] exposed to stress by induction of heat shock protein 70. *J Appl Physiol* 2004; 96: 1776–1781.

266. Atalay M, Oksala NKJ, Laaksonen DE, et al. Exercise training modulates heat shock protein response in diabetic rats. *J Appl Physiol* 2004; 97: 805–811.

267. Ghanbari-Niaki A, Fathi R, Kakhak SAH, et al. Treadmill exercise's reduction of Agouti-related protein expression in rat liver. *Int J Sport Nutr Exerc Metab* 2009; 19: 473–484.

268. Velloso CP. Regulation of muscle mass by growth hormone and IGF-1. *Br J Pharmacol* 2008; 154(3): 557–568.

269. Chang S-P, Chen Y-H, Chang W-C, et al. Merit of physical exercise to reverse the higher gene expression of hepatic phosphoenolpyruvate carboxykinase in obese Zucker rats. *Life Sci* 2006; 79: 240–246.

270. Shehab M, El-Kader A. Aerobic versus resistance exercise training in modulation of insulin resistance, adipocytokines and inflammatory cytokine levels in obese type 2 diabetic patients. *J Adv Res* 2011; 2: 179–183.

271. Shaibi GQ, Cruz ML, Weigensberg MJ, et al. Effects of resistance training on insulin sensitivity in overweight Latino adolescent males. *Med Sci Sports Exerc* 2006; 38(7): 1208–1215.

272. Ibañez J, Izquierdo M, Argüelles I, et al. Twice-weekly progressive resistance training decreases abdominal fat and improves insulin sensitivity in older men with type 2 diabetes. *Diabetes Care* 2005; 28(3): 662–667.

273. van der Heijden GJ, Wang ZJ, Chu Z, et al. Strength exercise improves muscle mass and hepatic insulin sensitivity in obese youth. *Med Sci Sports Exerc* 2010; 42(11): 1973–1980.

274. Marcinko K, Sikkema SR, Constantine Samaan M, et al. High intensity interval training improves liver and adipose tissue insulin sensitivity. *Molec Metab* 2015; 4(12): 903–915.

275. Légaré A, Drouin R, Milot M, et al. Increased density of glucagon receptors in liver from endurance-trained rats. *Am J Physiol* 2001; 280: E193–E6.

276. Berglund ED, Lustig DG, Baheza RA, et al. Hepatic glucagon action is essential for exercise-induced reversal of mouse fatty liver. *Diabetes* 2011; 60: 2720–2729.

277. Paquette AW, Wang D, Gauthier M-S, et al. Specific adaptations of estrogen receptor alpha and beta transcripts in liver and heart after endurance training in rats. *Mol Cell Biochem* 2007; 306: 179–187.

278. Jackson KC, Wohlers LM, Valencia AP, et al. Wheel running prevents the accumulation of monounsaturated fatty acids in the liver of ovariectomized mice by attenuating changes in SCD-1 content. *Appl Physiol Nutr Metab* 2011; 36: 798–810.

279. Domingos MM, Rodrigues MFC, Stotzer US, et al. Resistance training restores the gene expression of molecules related to fat oxidation and lipogenesis in the liver of ovariectomized rats. *Eur J Appl Physiol* 2012; 112: 1437–1444.

280. Cha Y-S, Kim H-Y, Daily J. Exercise-trained but not untrained rats maintain free carnitine reserves during acute exercise. *Asia Pacific J Clin Nutr* 2003; 12: 120–126.

281. Ringseis R, Mooren FC, Keller J, et al. Regular endurance exercise improves the diminished hepatic carnitine status in mice fed a high-fat diet. *Mol Nutr Food Res* 2011; 55 (Suppl. 2): S193–S202.

282. Barsalani R, Chapados NA, Lavoie J-M. Hepatic VLDL-TG production and MTP gene expression are decreased in ovariectomized rats: effects of exercise training. *Hormone Metab Res* 2010; 42: 860–867.

283. Schwarz AJ, Brasel JA, Hintz RL, et al. Acute effect of brief low- and high-intensity exercise on circulating insulin-like growth factor (IGF)I, II, and IGF-binding protein-3 and its proteolysis in young healthy men. *J Clin Endocrinol Metab* 1996; 81: 3492–3497.

284. Bermon S, Ferrari P, Bernard P, et al. Responses of total and free insulin-like growth factor-I and insulin-like growth factor binding protein-3 after resistance exercise and training in elderly subjects. *Acta Physiol Scand* 1999; 165: 51–56.

285. Nishida Y, Matsubara T, Tobina T, et al. Effect of low-intensity aerobic exercise on insulin-like growth factor-I and insulin-like growth factor-binding proteins in healthy men. *Int J Endocrinol 2010*; pii: 452820. Epub 2010 Sep 22.

286. Wieczorek-Baranowska A, Nowak A, Michalak E, et al. Effect of aerobic exercise on insulin, insulin-like growth factor-1 and insulin-like growth factor binding protein-3 in overweight and obese postmenopausal women. *J Sports Med Phys Fitness* 2011; 51: 525–532.

287. Moon MK, Cho BJ, Lee YJ, et al. The effects of chronic exercise on the inflammatory cytokines interleukin-6 and tumor necrosis factor-α are different with age. *Appl Physiol Nutr Metab* 2012; 37: 631–636.

288. de Araújo CC, Silva JD, Samary CS, et al. Regular and moderate exercise before experimental sepsis reduces the risk of lung and distal organ injury. *J Appl Physiol* 2012; 112: 1206–1214.

289. Navarro A, Gomez C, Lòpez-Cepero JM, et al. Beneficial effects of moderate exercise on mice aging: Survival, behavior, oxidative stress, and mitochondrial electron transfer. *Am J Physiol* 2003; 286: R505–R511.

290. Radak Z, Chung HY, Naito H, et al. Age-associated increase in oxidative stress and nuclear factor B activation are attenuated in rat liver by regular exercise. *FASEB J* 2004; 18: 749–750.

291. Chapados NA, Lavoie J-M. Exercise training increases hepatic endoplasmic reticulum (er) stress protein expression in MTP-inhibited high-fat fed rats. *Cell Biochem Funct* 2010; 28: 202–210.
292. Burneiko RC, Diniz YS, Galhardi CM, et al. Interaction of hypercaloric diet and physical exercise on lipid profile, oxidative stress and antioxidant defenses. *Food Chem Toxicol* 2006; 44: 1167–1172.
293. da Silva LA, Pinho CA, Rocha LG, et al. Effect of different models of physical exercise on oxidative stress markers in mouse liver. *Appl Physiol Nutr Metab* 2009; 34: 60–65.
294. Gore M, Fiebig R, Hollander J, et al. Endurance training alters antioxidant enzyme gene expression in rat skeletal muscle. *Can J Physiol Pharmacol* 1998; 76: 1139–1145.
295. Huang C-C, Lin W-T, Hsu F-L, et al. Metabolomics investigation of exercise-modulated changes in metabolism in rat liver after exhaustive exercise. *Eur J Appl Physiol* 2010; 108: 557–566.
296. Hong H, Johnson P. Antioxidant enzyme activities and lipid peroxidation levels in exercised and hypertensive rat tissues. *Int J Biochem Cell Biol* 1995; 27: 923–931.
297. Eklöw L, Moldéus P, Orrenius S. Oxidation of glutathione during hydroperoxide metabolism: a study using isolated hepatocytes and the glutathione inhibitor 1,3-bis(2 chloroethyl)-1-nitrosourea. *Eur J Biochem* 1984; 138: 459–463.
298. Godin DV, Garnett ME. Species related variations in anti-oxidant status-II. Differences in susceptibility to oxidative challenge. *Comp Biochem Physiol* 1992; 103B: 743–748.
299. Ji LL, Dillon D, Wu E. Alteration of antioxidant enzymes with aging in skeletal muscle and liver. *Am J Physiol* 1990; 258: R918–R923.
300. Ho KP, Xiao DS, Ke Y, et al. Exercise decreases cytosolic aconitase activity in the liver, spleen and bone marrow in rats. *Biochem Biophys Res Comm* 2001; 282: 264–267.
301. Wilson PO, Johnson P. Exercise modulates antioxidant enzyme gene expression in rat myocardium and liver. *J Appl Physiol* 2000; 88: 1791–1796.
302. Ferreira MA. Exercise training and liver cellular turnover. Doctoral thesis, Faculty of Sport. Porto, Portugal; University of Porto, 2012.
303. Nilssen O, Forde OH, Brenn T. The Tromso Study. Distribution and population determinants of gamma-glutamyl transferase. *Am J Epidemiol* 1990; 132: 318–326.
304. Pintus F, Mascia P. Distribution and population determinants of gamma-glutamyl-transferase in a random sample of Sardinian inhabitants. 'ATS-SARDEGNA' Research Group. *Eur J Epidemiol* 1996; 12: 71–76.
305. Robinson D, Whitehead TP. Effect of body mass and other factors on serum liver enzyme levels in men attending for well population screening. *Ann Clin Biochem* 1989; 26: 393–400.
306. Whitfield JB. Gamma glutamyl transferase. *Crit Rev Clin Lab Sci* 2001; 38: 263–355.
307. Saengsirisuwan V, Phadungkij S, Pholpramool C. Renal and liver functions and muscle injuries in Thai boxers during training and after competition. *Br J Sports Med* 1998; 32: 304–308.
308. Frank S, Somani SM, Konle M. Effect of exercise on propranolol pharmacokinetics. *Eur J Clin Pharmacol* 1990; 39: 391–394.
309. Panton LB, Guillen GJ, Williams L, et al. The lack of effect of aerobic exercise training on propranolol pharmacokinetics in young and elderly adults. *J Clin Pharmacol* 1995; 35: 885–894.

310. Ducry JJ, Howald H, Zysset T, et al. Liver function in physically trained subjects. Galactose elimination capacity, plasma disappearance of ICG, and aminopyrine metabolism in long distance runners. *Dig Dis Sci* 1979; 24: 192–196.
311. Orioli S, Bandinelli I, Birardi A, et al. Hepatic antipyrine metabolism in athletes. *J Sports Med Phys Fitness* 1990; 30: 261–263.
312. Villa JG, Cuadrado G, Bayón JE, et al. The effect of physical conditioning on antipyrine clearance. *Eur J Appl Physiol* 1998; 77: 106–111.
313. Boel J, Andersen LB, Hansen SH, et al. Hepatic drug metabolism and physical fitness. *Clin Pharmacol Therap* 1984; 36: 121–126.
314. Mauriz JL, Tabernero B, Garcia-Lopez J, et al. Physical exercise and improvement of liver oxidative metabolism in the elderly. *Eur J Appl Physiol* 2000; 81: 62–66.
315. Dyke TM, Sams RA, Hinchcliff KW. Intensity-dependent effects of acute submaximal exercise on the pharmacokinetics of bromsulphalein in horses. *Am J Vet Res* 1998; 59: 1481–1487.
316. Daggan RN, Zafeiridis A, Dipla K, et al. The effects of chronic exercise on anaethesia-induced hepatotoxicity. *Med Sci Sports Exerc* 2000; 32: 2024–2028.
317. Frenkl R, Gyore A, Szeberenyi S. The effect of muscular exercise on the microsomal enzyme system of the rat liver. *Eur J Appl Physiol* 1980; 44: 135–140.
318. Yiamouyiannis CA, Martin BJ, Walkins JB. Chronic physical activity alters excretory function in rats. *J Pharmacol Exp Therap* 1993; 265: 321–327.

2 Physical activity and hepatic pathologies

Introduction

The effects of physical activity upon the metabolism of the health liver were examined in Chapter 1. We here examine interactions between physical activity and some clinically important chronic hepatic disorders, including the metabolic syndrome, non-alcoholic fatty liver disease (NAFLD), various types of hepatic inflammation and resulting fibrosis, cirrhosis and hepatic carcinoma, as well as issues of liver transplantation. We look specifically at the role of inadequate habitual physical activity in the genesis and progression of these various syndromes, and will consider appropriate exercise recommendations for the prevention and treatment of such disorders.

Physical activity and the metabolic syndrome

The metabolic syndrome is a relatively new diagnosis. It is now perhaps the commonest of the clinical disorders associated with hepatic dysfunction, and it has played a prominent role in stimulating the development of exercise-related wellness programmes. But as long as 250 years ago, the Italian physician and anatomist Giovanni Battista Morgagni (1682–1771) identified an association between visceral obesity, a high blood pressure, atherosclerosis, high levels of uric acid in the blood and frequent episodes of obstructed breathing during sleep.[1] The distinct characteristics of male-type (android) obesity were described by the French physician Jean Vague,[2] and he noted its association with various metabolic disorders, including diabetes mellitus and a premature onset of atherosclerosis. Another historical landmark was Reaven's 1988 Banting lecture, where he coined the term "Syndrome X" for a clustering of glucose intolerance, hypertension, low concentrations of high density lipoprotein (HDL) cholesterol, raised serum triglycerides and hyperinsulinaemia.[3] The term "Syndrome X" did not gain wide acceptance, but the idea of this particular clustering of risk factors persisted and soon became identified as the metabolic syndrome.

The metabolic syndrome is now found widely in most developed societies, with a prevalence ranging from 16–33%.[4] It has been associated with an "obesity epidemic" that probably reflects, among other possible causes, a progressive reduction of habitual physical activity and an increased consumption of refined carbohydrates.[5] There is a strong association between the metabolic syndrome and non-alcoholic fatty liver disease,[6, 7] although it is less clear which of these conditions is cause and which is effect.

Diagnostic criteria for the metabolic syndrome

The World Health Organization[8] has defined the metabolic syndrome by the presence of insulin resistance (type 2 diabetes, impaired fasting glucose, impaired glucose tolerance or impaired glucose uptake when insulin levels are increased), plus two of four other factors: a blood pressure >140/90 mm Hg (or use of hypotensive medication), triglycerides >150 mg/dL, HDL cholesterol <35 mg/dl (men) or 39 mg/dL (women) and obesity (a body mass index >30 kg/m2 or a waist/hip circumference ratio >0.9 [men] or >0.85 [women]), with traces of protein in the urine.

A joint committee of the US National Heart, Lung and Blood Institute and the American Heart Association[9] advanced slightly different criteria: abdominal obesity, atherogenic dyslipidaemia (raised triglycerides and reduced HDL cholesterol), a raised resting blood pressure, insulin resistance, a pro-inflammatory state and a prothrombotic state. Specific criteria included a waist circumference >1.02 m (men) or 0.88 m (women), triglycerides >150 mg/dL, HDL cholesterol <40 mg/dL (men) or <50 mg/dL (women), a blood pressure >130/85 mm Hg and a fasting blood glucose >110 mg/dL.

Another set of identifiers adopted in our study of a Japanese population[10] was the presence of three or more of the following: (1) a body mass index >25 kg/m², (2) fasting triglycerides >150 mg/dL, (3) a fasting serum HDL cholesterol <40 mg/dL(men) or 50 mg/dL (women), (4) a blood pressure >130/85 mmHg, and (5) a fasting plasma glucose >110 mg/dL) and/or a haemoglobin A1c >5.5%.

Role of physical activity in prevention and treatment

Many of the characteristics of the metabolic syndrome reflect a malfunction of the liver, and most can be reversed by regular physical activity. A number of investigations based upon physical activity questionnaires have demonstrated associations between development of the metabolic syndrome, a low level of habitual physical activity[11, 12] and a high proportion of sedentary time.[13, 14]

Thus, a study of 1144 elderly people in Northern Italy found a highly significant inverse relationship of reported leisure activity with triglycerides, waist circumference and insulin resistance.[11] Likewise, a four-year follow-up of 612 Finnish middle-aged men found 107 developing the metabolic syndrome;[12] this risk was halved in those who took >3 hours/week of moderate leisure-time physical activity, and men in the upper third of the maximal oxygen intake distribution were 75% less likely to be affected by the metabolic syndrome than those who were sedentary. An analysis of data for 1626 adults from the NHANES survey of 1999–2000 found that those who engaged in >150 minutes/week of moderate or vigorous physical activity had approximately half the risk of the metabolic syndrome relative to those who were sedentary (odds ratio 1.90 [1.22-2.97]), although data adjustments for age, sex, ethnicity, smoking and alcohol use attenuated the odds ratio to 1.46.[13] Frequent use of a computer or TV watching was also associated with an increased prevalence of the condition; risk ratios were for 1 hour, 1.41; 2 hours, 1.37; 3 hours, 1.70 and >4 hours, 2.10.[13] Likewise, in Europe, a study of 992 adults found that the risk of the metabolic syndrome was positively associated with the number of hours per day spent watching television or working at a computer screen.[14]

The Nakanojo study provided objective evidence of the inverse association between habitual physical activity (as measured by a pedometer/accelerometer over an entire year) and incidence of the metabolic syndrome in a sample of 220 Japanese aged 65–84 years.[10] The risk was 4.3 times greater in the least active quartile of this population (those taking <4700 steps/day and spending <9 min/d at an exercise intensity >3 METs) than in the most active quartile (those taking >8500 steps/day and spending >24 min/d at an intensity >3 METs).

Bankoski and associates[15] focused specifically on sedentary time, as monitored by an accelerometer. Their subjects were 1367 adults aged >60 years, participants in the 2003–2006 NHANES survey, and they noted small differences pointing to an association between sedentary time and the risk of developing the metabolic syndrome. In affected individuals, the sedentary portion of the day was greater (67.3 vs. 62.2%), sedentary bouts were longer in duration (17.7 vs. 16.7 minutes) and accelerometer counts were lower during sedentary periods (14.8 vs. 15.8 counts/minute); further, these differences in risk persisted after adjusting statistically for differences in physical activity levels, showing that sedentary time was an independent risk factor. Healy et al.[16, 17] also used accelerometers to categorize sedentary time in 169 Australians. They found that independently of moderate to vigorous physical activity, there were significant associations of sedentary time, light-intensity time and mean activity intensity with waist circumference and clustered metabolic risk. Moreover, breaks in sedentary time were associated with reductions in waist circumference and triglyceride levels and enhanced glucose tolerance, independently of total sedentary time and moderate to vigorous physical activity.[16]

There remains a need for additional longitudinal studies, but whether based on subjective or objective measures of physical activity patterns, cross-sectional investigations provide convincing evidence of an association between both an active lifestyle and a minimization of sedentary time and a reduced risk of the metabolic syndrome.

Non-alcoholic fatty liver disease

Non-alcoholic fatty liver disease (NAFLD) was first described in 1980.[18] It is characterized by the accumulation of fat in hepatocytes, much as seen with an excessive alcohol consumption, and it is often discovered accidentally as a rise in the serum enzymes that are used as markers of hepatic dysfunction. The healthy liver contains some fat (triglycerides that are stored in the hepatocytes), but NAFLD is commonly diagnosed when fat stores exceed 5% of hepatic mass. NAFLD accounts for the majority of liver disease worldwide. It affects 25 to 45% of adults[18–21] including most individuals who are obese.[22] Moreover, its prevalence appears to be increasing.[23] NAFLD even affects 2.6 to 9.6% of children, depending upon age, sex, ethnic group and habitual activity.[24, 25]

Diagnosis and patho-physiology of NAFLD

Liver biopsy and histological assessment provide gold standards for the diagnosis of NAFLD, but in human research the liver fat content is more commonly inferred from proton magnetic resonance spectroscopy or computed tomography. In animals, the usual approach has been chemical or histological analysis of hepatic tissue at sacrifice.

Hepatic fat accumulation is an important form of liver dysfunction, and is commonly associated with obesity, cardiovascular disease and diabetes mellitus. The build-up of triglycerides could reflect an increased delivery of fatty acids to the liver, either from adipose tissue or directly from the diet, increased *de novo* hepatic lipogenesis, decreased hepatic fatty acid oxidation or a decreased exit of fatty acids from the liver in the form of VLDL triglycerides (Chapter 1). The first of these mechanisms is probably the most important.[26] Studies using radioactive markers found that 59% of the fat was derived from non-esterified fatty acids, 26% from *de novo* lipogenesis and 15% from the diet.[27] The increase in hepatic fat impairs insulin sensitivity by suppressing the activity of phosphatidyl-linositol-3-kinase, a key enzyme mediating the action of insulin on the liver.[26] Adipose tissue also manifests insulin resistance in NAFLD.[28] Any given secretion of insulin becomes less effective in increasing muscle glucose uptake and in suppressing the release of fatty acids from fat.[29]

NAFLD can progress from a simple accumulation of fat in the hepatocytes (the condition of steatosis) through inflammation of the liver tissue (steato-hepatitis) to fibrosis, cirrhosis, liver failure and even hepatic carcinoma.[30] It is not entirely clear why the condition remains a simple steatosis in some individuals but progresses to more serious complications in others. Inter-individual differences in reactions to reactive oxygen species, cytotoxic dicarboxylic acids, and hormonal balance as well as mitochondrial abnormalities may be involved.[30] Progression to steatohepatitis probably reflects the combined effects of hepatic fat accumulation and oxidant stress, possibly supplemented by a fatty acid mediated apoptosis of liver cells,[31] and gut barrier dysfunction with entry of endotoxins into the hepatic circulation.[32] However, anti-oxidant therapy is not necessarily helpful in preventing disease progression. In one study of children, Nobili et al.[33] found that provision of anti-oxidants such as alpha-tocopherol and ascorbic acid did not enhance the benefits gained from treatment with a simple combination of exercise and weight loss.

NAFLD is commonly associated with other markers of inadequate physical activity, including cardiovascular disease, metabolic syndrome and type 2 diabetes mellitus. Although body fatness is a prime determinant of whole-body insulin sensitivity, the main factor influencing hepatic insulin sensitivity seems to be the individual's active energy expenditure.[34] A follow-up of 6003 patients with NAFLD found that 411 developed type 2 diabetes over 4.9 years. Less than 60 minutes of exercise per week and a gamma glutamyl transferase (GGT) level >109 IU/L were significant predictors of a risk of developing diabetes; for both indicators, hazard ratios averaged 1.60.[35] GGT facilitates the intracellular transport of glutathione; increases in GGT levels are thus a possible indicator of attempts to counter the oxidant stress which can predispose to diabetes.[36]

Low levels of habitual physical activity predispose to obesity, dyslipidaemia, impaired glucose tolerance and high blood pressure, and physical activity is effective in the clinical management of these problems. However, a reduction in liver fat content is also an important component of both prevention and treatment. A decrease of hepatic fat content can avert type 2 diabetes mellitus, particularly in older individuals.[37, 38] Similarly, a normalizing of liver fat content improves the insulin-induced suppression of hepatic glucose output and restores normal fasting blood glucose concentration in patients with type 2 diabetes.[39]

Habitual physical activity, attained fitness and liver fat content

Many reviews have pointed to the possible role of physical activity in the prevention and management of NAFLD (Table 2.1). There is general agreement on the benefits obtained from a combination of regular exercise and dieting. Some authors have suggested that these two treatment options act independently of each other, but others have found the benefits of exercise are linked rather closely to resulting reductions in body mass. The optimal intensity, duration and frequency of exercise sessions remain unclear, and in many studies poor compliance with exercise and/or dietary regimens has been a major problem with both therapy and data analysis. Some reviewers have pointed to adjuvant benefits from certain drugs and behavioural counselling, but others maintain that no drugs are useful in treating NAFLD. Despite these various uncertainties, there is good evidence, drawn from cross-sectional and longitudinal human studies as well as animal research, that regular physical activity can reduce the accumulation of fat in the liver (see also Chapter 1), and some (but not all) studies of physical activity programmes have demonstrated a reversal of the increased levels of enzymes such as alanine transaminase that were signalling hepatic dysfunction.

Cross-sectional studies in humans

Many cross-sectional investigations have shown associations between low levels of habitual physical activity and/or aerobic fitness and the prevalence of excessive amounts of fat in the liver (Table 1.3), usually with evidence of liver dysfunction in the form of increased hepatic enzyme levels. Most authors have used questionnaires to assess habitual physical activity, but three studies used objective activity monitors,[64–66] and one report classified subjects based upon

Table 2.1 Conclusions of published reviews concerning the role of physical activity in the prevention and treatment of NAFLD

Author	Number of references	Conclusions	Comments
Systematic reviews			
Eslami et al.[40]	70	No effective treatment for steatosis but increased physical activity and weight loss can improve enzymes and hepatic histology	
Keating et al.[41]	47	Beneficial effect of exercise on liver fat seen with little or no weight loss. Exercise has no effect on ALT	12 studies included in meta-analysis
Musso et al.[42]	140	Lifestyle weight loss >7% safe, improved hepatic risk profile, but achieved by <50% of patients	Statins and polyunsaturated fats improved steatosis, but effects on liver histology unclear
Rodriguez et al.[43]	25	Optimal exercise regimen in terms of effectiveness and compliance has yet to be determined; reduction in sedentary time might also help	Semi-structured review
Socha et al.[44]	57	Benefit from enhanced lifestyle; data insufficient to determine value of alternatives	Main focus on patients unable or unwilling to change lifestyle
Thoma et al.[45]	49	Consistent reductions in liver fat and ALT with exercise, correlated most strongly with decrease in body mass. Usually reduced insulin resistance, but changes of fibrosis less consistent	
Unstructured reviews			
Alisi et al.[46]	54	Combination of diet and exercise can modify course of simple steatosis	Drugs might enhance response
Bacchi and Moghetti[47]	18	Exercise may reduce hepatic fat and hepatic enzyme concentrations, independent of dietary modifications	
Caldwell and Lazo[48]	48	More exercise seems better, but optimal intensity not known	
Centis et al.[49]	65	Weight loss and physical activity have specific therapeutic roles	Drugs should remain a second line of treatment
Cheung and Sanyal[50]	101	Weight loss and increased exercise consistently associated with improved liver histology	Some discussion of cellular mechanisms

Table 2.1 continued

Author	Number of references	Conclusions	Comments
Conjeevaram and Tiniakos[51]	26	Physical activity recommended, but lack of criteria for intensity, volume and duration of exercise	
Della Corte et al.[52]	96	Weight loss diet and exercise are first line therapeutic measures	Drugs may serve as adjuvants
Dowman et al.[53]	167	Need for multifaceted treatment: diet, exercise and behavioural counselling	No highly effective drug treatment
Duvnjak et al.[54]	151	Diet and exercise first line interventions, but problems of poor compliance. Lack of specific exercise guidelines	Value of pharmacologic adjuvants not proven
Johnson and George[55]	57	Enzyme levels reduced and steatosis improved with exercise independent of weight loss	Weight loss needs to be 3–10% of body mass to reduce steatosis
Mencin and Lavine[56]	95	Main treatment remains diet and exercise	Vitamin E may be a helpful adjunct
Nobili et al.[57]	40	Improved physical activity and nutrition needed to manage and treat condition	
Nobili and Sanyal[58]	72	Best approach is exercise + diet, but motivation is difficult	No drugs yet of proven value
Rector and Thyfault[59]	93	Condition due to physical inactivity, low aerobic fitness and over-nutrition singly or in combination	
Reynoso and Lavine[60]	12	Exercise (unspecified) may reduce steatosis, but effects on other aspects of histology unknown	Based on consensus guidelines
Spassiani and Kuk[61]	28	Independent effect of exercise upon liver fat content unclear	Most studies to date have included multiple therapies
Targher et al.[62]	125	Team of experts including exercise specialist needed to correct "unhealthy" lifestyle	Drugs a questionable option
Zelber-Sagi et al.[63]	151	Lifestyle modification with increased physical activity first line, aim of 5–10% weight reduction	Two-year compliance with physical activity as low as 20%

their obesity.[67] The sample size of study populations has ranged from small groups to >30,000 people, and one analysis was based upon twins with dissimilar activity patterns, allowing an examination of possible genetic contributions to the disorder.[68] In one instance, the data obtained by objective monitoring suggested an effect of physical activity, but (probably because of a lesser reliability and validity of the test instruments) classifications of the same individuals based upon subjective questionnaires did not.[64] Collectively, cross-sectional studies have shown that habitual physical activity is an important correlate of hepatic fat content, with a possible dose-response relationship.[69] However, two reports found no relationship between the severity of histological abnormalities in the liver and the volume of habitual physical activity.[70, 71] Other analyses (including the twin study of Leskinen et al.[68]) related hepatic fat accumulation to aerobic fitness (Table 1.4). With two exceptions,[72, 73] hepatic fat levels were inversely associated with aerobic fitness, although in some studies the association was relatively weak,[74, 75] particularly when data were co-varied for inter-individual differences in obesity.

Longitudinal studies in humans

Longitudinal trials in humans have usually had only a small sample size (Table 1.5), with "usual treatment" or a dietary regimen serving as the control treatment. Interventions have ranged widely from general lifestyle recommendations to closely supervised interventions with careful control of both exercise and diet. Typically, liver fat content has decreased, often with increases in insulin sensitivity, as activity levels have been augmented. One report noted an associated improvement of histopathology in response to an exercise and weight loss programme,[76] but there is as yet little evidence to support the idea that increased exercise can reverse cell damage. Beneficial effects of exercise upon serum aminotransferase levels have also been unclear, possibly because in some studies levels of this enzyme were close to normal prior to the initiation of treatment.[41, 77]

Moat studies have pointed to a maximization of reductions in hepatic fat content and a possible normalization of serum amino-transferases from program-mes that induced a significant weight loss through a combination of physical activity and dieting, but the respective contributions of regular physical activity, dietary change and weight loss to improvements in hepatic function remain to be clarified.[77] Exercise has traditionally been employed with the goal of facilitating weight loss, but some investigators have found benefits from exercise in the absence of either dieting[78] or any change in body mass.[79] Furthermore, in some reports benefits have persisted after statistical adjustment of data for changes in body mass,[80] and at least one study found that dietary manipulation did not enhance the effects of exercise alone.[81]

Nevertheless, much of the current evidence suggests that physical activity benefits the liver primarily by enhancing the effects of dieting;[76] it may[82] or may not[37, 83] increase the insulin sensitization induced by dieting alone. A weight loss of 10% or more seems the most effective means to lower liver fat content and normalize amino-transferase levels; effects are smaller if the decrease in body mass is 5% or less.[84] Several reports have suggested that although exercise brings other health benefits, including a sensitization to insulin, it does not enhance the hepatic response to dieting alone.[37, 83, 85]

Although most investigators have looked at the benefits of aerobic training programmes, a few reports have examined hepatic responses to resistance training. Unfortunately, the findings have been inconsistent. A controlled three-month trial in obese adolescent boys reported that thrice weekly 60-min sessions of either aerobic or resistance exercise reduced liver fat, but only resistance exercise was effective in increasing insulin sensitivity.[86] Two of three comparisons between aerobic and resistance training[47, 86] found similar decreases of hepatic fat with both types of exercise. However, the third and largest study found no benefit from resistance training alone, and the response to aerobic training was not augmented by adding a resistance training component.[87] Another study of a resistance exercise found no reduction of inflammatory markers with this type of treatment,[88] and a 12-week trial of resistance exercise found a decrease of insulin resistance without a change of hepatic fat content.[89] Thus, although resistance exercise helps to correct the muscular weakness and autonomic dysfunction that is often associated with NAFLD,[90] it remains unclear whether it is effective in decreasing steatosis; for the present, it seems best to advocate aerobic exercise.

Longitudinal studies in animals

Animal studies of exercise and hepatic steatosis generally confirm the findings from human investigations (Table 1.6). The animal data provide growing empirical evidence that fat accumulation has adverse effects upon hepatic function, and that these changes can be reversed by a programme of sustained exercise. Further, the animal research adds helpful information on underlying cellular mechanisms.

In mice that were fed a high-fat diet, regular physical activity reduced hepatic fat accumulation, improved insulin resistance and reduced circulating levels of cholesterol, triglycerides, and aspartate transaminase and alanine transaminase.[91] Regimens based on dietary restriction, voluntary wheel running and imposed swimming or treadmill running have all seemed effective in preventing steatosis (Table 1.6), and in one report beneficial changes were elicited more readily by intermittent than by continuous bouts of swimming.[92] Yasari et al.[93] commented that after six weeks of detraining, rats that had run on a treadmill for four weeks had regained a similar body fat to their sedentary peers, but liver lipid infiltration had not yet increased. In contrast, Linden et al.[94] found that four weeks of inactivity following 16 weeks of wheel-running caused the development of hepatic steatosis in obese rats, although liver triglycerides were still 60% lower than in animals that had remained sedentary throughout.

Underlying mechanisms

Details of the mechanisms underlying the adverse effects of hepatic fat are discussed in a recent review.[95] Lipid accumulation appears to down-regulate phosphatidylinositol 3-kinase, a key enzyme mediating the action of insulin in hepatocytes.[26] Rats fed an obesity-inducing diet not only developed peripheral insulin resistance, but also showed activation of the pro-inflammatory molecules c-jun N-terminal kinase (JNK) and nuclear factor kappa-B (NF-kB).

Cellular adaptations seen with enhanced physical activity have included increased hepatic mitochondrial fatty acid oxidation, enhanced oxidative enzyme function and protein content, and suppression of *de novo* hepatic lipogenesis.[96] Specific molecular mechanisms include increased hepatic mitochondrial activity and subsequent beta-oxidation of fats,[96] a decreased level of transcription factors regulating the genes involved in cholesterol and fatty acid synthesis,[97] down-regulation of a rate-limiting enzyme in the biosynthesis of monounsaturated fats[98] and a decrease of hepatic ketone synthesis.[99] Regular exercise also normalizes the catabolism of branched-chain amino acids[100] and attenuates the reduced levels of hepatic IGF-1 seen in alloxan-diabetic rats.[101]

Further, exercise training lessens endoplasmic reticular stress in the liver, as shown by decreased phosphorylation of the two major metabolic markers of this condition.[102] Moreover, the glucose stimulation of insulin secretion is decreased in rats with access to an exercise-wheel, without any deterioration in their capacity for glucose homeostasis.[103] Seven days of voluntary wheel running increased release of the hormone-like hepatic insulin sensitizing substance (HISS), thus decreasing insulin resistance.[104, 105] Finally, exercise partially reversed attenuated insulin and leptin signalling in rats with chlorpromazine-induced diabetes.[106]

One way in which aerobic exercise appears to exert a beneficial influence on hepatic function is by decreasing myostatin output.[107] This substance inhibits muscle growth, thus predisposing to obesity, hepatic insulin resistance and diabetes.[107] It may also have more direct effects upon hepatocytes.[108] Inactivation of the gene for myostatin binding increased myostatin levels, causing hepatic steatosis in mice in the absence of any change in muscle mass.[109] Moreover, injection of recombinant myostatin slowed overall growth, again without change of muscle mass.[107] Finally, normal liver function depends on an appropriate balance between cell proliferation and apoptosis; however, both mouse and human liver cell cultures have shown increased apoptosis when incubated with recombinant activin, which binds to the same receptors as myostatin.[110, 111]

Exercise training also has beneficial effects that arise outside the liver. Positive influences on insulin sensitivity include an increase in muscle mass, an alteration in muscle quality, an increase in the energy demands of skeletal muscle and a reduction of fat stores in other viscera.

Following a sudden one-week cessation of exercise, several metabolic precursors of steatosis were seen in obese rats, along with an increased appetite. Other changes included a decrease in hepatic mitochondrial oxidative capacity, an increased hepatic expression of lipogenetic proteins and increased levels of hepatic malonyl CoA, a key factor in lipid synthesis.[112]

Hepatic inflammation, fibrosis and cirrhosis

Chronic liver inflammation, whether from NAFLD, alcohol abuse or viral infection, drives hepatic fibrosis, but the pathological process can be prevented, stabilized or reversed by immuno-suppressive, anti-inflammatory, anti-oxidant and antiviral agents.[113] Cirrhosis is a late stage in the process, where there is severe fibrotic scarring of the liver and a gross hepatic malfunction that leads to jaundice, fatigue, weakness, loss of appetite, itching and easy bruising.

Responses to exercise therapy seem relatively independent of the cause of liver inflammation. Positive influences include an increase in muscle mass, an alteration in muscle quality, an increase in the energy demands of skeletal muscle and a reduction of visceral fat stores (leading to a reduced incorporation of fatty acids into the liver). Exercise also seems to exert a direct beneficial influence on hepatic pathology beyond any reduction in liver fat content. As fibrosis develops, markers of hepatic apoptosis increase,[114] but the prevalence of these changes is inversely associated with the individual's level of habitual physical activity.[115]

Hepatitis

About a tenth of those who have developed steatosis progress to the inflammatory stage of steato-hepatitis. Regular physical activity reduces the likelihood of developing a NAFLD hepatitis because it reduces the fat content of the liver (above). The shift from NAFLD fibrosis to cirrhosis is usually seen only in those individuals who are over the age of 50 years, and it is thought to reflect a progressive dysfunction of the hepatic mitochondria.[116]

Alcoholic hepatitis

Alcoholic hepatitis is seen following an excessive intake of alcohol, usually repeated over the course of many years. In one biopsy survey, 20% of alcoholics showed hepatitis.[117] As with NAFLD, alcoholic hepatitis is commonly marked by an accumulation of fat in the liver and increases of serum enzymes that indicate liver damage.[118] The 28-day mortality of acute alcoholic hepatitis can be as high as 30–50%.[119] It has sometimes been hypothesized that regular physical activity can play a preventive role, reducing the risk to the liver from an excessive alcohol consumption, but this view is not supported by current research.[120, 121] There seems to have been no systematic study of physical activity in the treatment of alcoholic hepatitis, once this is established.

Steato-hepatitis

Baba et al.[122] had a group of 65 patients with steato-hepatitis participate in a moderate intensity exercise programme (30 minutes at 60–70% of maximal heart rate five days/week) for three months. This regimen apparently contributed to a functional reversal of the pathology in the 44 individuals who complied with the prescribed exercise; serum amino-transferase levels were reduced in the compliant group, and there was complete normalization of hepatic enzyme levels in 20 of the 44 compliant individuals. Hickman et al.[123, 124] also noted a 17% improvement of aerobic fitness and decreased hepatic enzyme levels, but no reversal of histological changes after six months of a progressive 15-item circuit training routine. In contrast, some studies in rats have suggested that endurance training can reverse structural damage in the liver, including mitochondrial abnormalities.[125] He et al.[126] fed rats a high-fat diet, and they noted less severe histological changes in animals that undertook vigorous swimming exercise relative to control animals.

Viral hepatitis

Viral hepatitis develops in about 15% of those infected with the hepatitis B virus, but is more commonly a consequence of hepatitis C infections. Prevalence of the disease is high among athletes, perhaps because of exposures through international travel and/or the sharing of water bottles. During the acute phase, there is commonly enlargement of the liver and spleen, with complaints of nausea, abdominal pain and fatigue. Some clinicians have recommended prohibiting sports participation until such findings are resolved.[127] However, there have been very few reported cases of exercise-induced hepatic rupture even during the acute phase of the disease, and such guidelines may be overly restrictive.[128]

Viral hepatitis is regarded as chronic if the disease has persisted for siz months. At this stage, affected individuals are still less active than their peers.[129] Complaints of fatigue may persist, but those with mild disease tolerate exercise programmes quite well.[127, 130] Ritland et al.[131] examined nine patients with chronic active hepatitis who were receiving immuno-suppressive therapy, and they found that 12 weeks of interval training (30 minute sessions, three to four times per week, with the active component rising to 75% of maximal heart rate) yielded improvements of aerobic function (a 20% gain in Åstrand predictions of maximal oxygen intake), without any worsening of enzyme markers of liver dysfunction.

Fibrosis

Unfortunately, physical inactivity causes a worsening of NAFLD, and this can create a vicious cycle of fatigue that further discourages physical activity. A sedentary lifestyle is particularly likely in those who have become obese. An adequate intensity of physical activity is important in preventing disease progression. Neither the risk of steato-hepatitis nor the histological stage of fibrosis were associated with either the total volume of physical activity or the duration of moderate physical activity,[71] but in individuals who met the currently recommended weekly amount of *vigorous* physical activity, the odds of finding steato-hepatitis was 0.65, and in those who reported undertaking twice the recommended amount of *vigorous* physical activity, the odds were reduced to 0.53.[71] Others have noted little cellular repair response to modest doses of physical activity. Ueno et al.[132] found that a three-month programme of walking and jogging reduced liver fat content, but did not change the extent of hepatic fibrosis. Likewise, Krasnoff and associates[72] found no association between currently reported physical activity and the histological severity of NAFLD, although a possible effect of exercise intensity was signalled by milder disease in those with a higher peak oxygen intake.

However, Oh et al.[133] examined the response to a 12-week exercise programme (fast walking and mild jogging for 40–60 minutes, three times/week) in 42 NAFLD patients where liver fibrosis was suspected, and they found a favourable response matching that seen with dietary restriction. There were equivalent reductions in serum alanine aminotransferase and gamma glutamyl transpeptidase levels (–20.6% vs. –16.1% and –25.7% vs –34.0%), and similar improvements of insulin resistance (–29.7% vs. –26.9%), and increases in serum adiponectin levels (+33.4% vs. +15.1%). Moreover, exercise training reduced serum levels of the markers of inflammation and oxidative stress usually associated with fibrosis: ferritin and thiobarbituric acid reactive substances (–25.0% vs. +1.1% and –33.5% vs. –10.5%). Other reports also found substantial benefits from vigorous exercise. A group of 13 obese individuals (body mass index 35 kg.m²) with NAFLD undertook one week of vigorous exercise (60 minutes/day at 80–85% of maximal heart rate);[114] despite the short duration of this trial, the intervention reduced circulating levels not only of alanine transaminase, but also of a marker of hepatic cell apoptosis (CK18 fragments), thus increasing the potential for regeneration of healthy liver tissue. We may thus conclude that vigorous exercise can attenuate the stimuli leading to hepatic fibrosis in NAFLD, and correct some metabolic markers of hepatic dysfunction, although it is less likely it will reverse fibrotic changes that have already occurred.

These conclusions are reinforced by animal experimentation. In some animal studies, not only enzyme markers, but also histological appearances have improved. In mice where hepatic fibrosis was induced by feeding a high fat diet and large amounts of fructose,[134] vigorous exercise (16 weeks of treadmill running, 60 minutes per day at speeds increasing from 15–20 m/minute) reduced histological evidence of fibrosis relative to control animals. A second animal study noted histological evidence of inflammation and steatohepatitis (macro-vesicular steatosis and lymphocytosis) in sedentary rats that were fed a high-fat diet, but such findings were greatly attenuated in their peers who undertook vigorous daily physical activity (swimming for 30 rising to 90 minutes per day); alanine transaminase but not aspartase transaminase levels were also reduced in the exercised animals.[126]

Cirrhosis

Although regular physical activity can prevent the progression of NAFLD to cirrhosis, exercise programmes seem unlikely to reverse the advanced pathological changes associated with this diagnosis. The primary clinical rationale for advocating exercise therapy in hepatic cirrhosis is rather to reduce associated physical weakness and co-morbidities,[147] and to enhance survival prospects if the patient receives a liver transplant.[138, 140] Lemyze et al.[148] have pointed to multiple factors that impair physical performance in advanced hepatic cirrhosis, including deconditioning, malnutrition, anaemia, cirrhotic cardiomyopathy and the hepato-pulmonary syndrome.

The impairment of physical capacity seems proportional to disease severity as measured by the Pugh index of liver failure, but is independent of aetiology (NAFLD, alcoholism or viral hepatitis).[135, 142, 143] Even moderate physical activity (30% of peak work rate) increases pressures in the hepatic portal vein, with a danger of precipitating oesophageal bleeding,[149] particularly if varices have developed in the lower part of the oesophagus.

Clinical concerns over possible oesophageal haemorrhage have led many investigators to report the anaerobic threshold, or to predict maximal oxygen intake from submaximal data rather than to assess aerobic capacity by direct measurements of peak treadmill or cycle ergometer effort (Table 2.2). Levels of anaerobic threshold, aerobic fitness and exercise tolerance are all low,[77, 131, 135–138, 141–144] particularly if there is an associated accumulation of ascitic fluid in the peritoneal cavity.[135, 144]

Patients with cirrhosis usually show muscular weakness,[141, 143, 145, 146] probably in part because of a decrease in protein synthesis.[150] Thus, Campillo et al.[135] noted that individuals with cirrhosis had low levels of prealbumin (0.10 g/L, vs. norms of 0.28–0.32 g/L) and albumin (30 g/L, vs. norms of 40–435 g/L), and Wong et al. also found low albumin levels, particularly in patients who had developed ascites.[144]

When exercising at three to four times resting oxygen consumption, the respiratory quotient of sedentary individuals normally indicates a roughly equal usage of fat and carbohydrate; however, Camillo et al.[136] saw an almost exclusive use of carbohydrate in patients with cirrhosis who were exercising. This could reflect in part a low maximal oxygen intake-even exercise demanding four times resting oxygen consumption approaches maximal effort for some patients with cirrhosis. Over 32 minutes of moderate physical activity, Campillo et al.[136] found that the patients also showed a progressive decrease of blood glucose and an accumulation of blood lactate, likely reflecting defective hepatic gluconeogenesis. DeLissio et al.[137] also commented on a defective endogenous production of glucose in those with cirrhosis, although in their four subjects blood glucose levels did not fall during exercise, because (in contrast to Campillo et al.) fat usage was greater than in controls.

There have been few investigations of the effect of aerobic training in patients with cirrhosis. One investigation reported a 29% gain of predicted $\dot{V}O_{2max}$ over 10–12 weeks of conditioning,[131] and a second trial with only four subjects found an increase of $\dot{V}O_{2max}$ in two of the four individuals following training, with an 18–20% improvement of muscle strength in these two individuals.[135] Exercise that includes an element of resistance training is arguably a useful therapy for restoring muscle mass and improving fitness, strength and functional capacity, but it remains unclear whether an increase of habitual physical activity can restore liver health (and if so, the dose of activity that is needed). One major obstacle to implementing and sustaining exercise training in advanced liver disease is the initial fatigue of the patient. This has an adverse effect upon the individual's quality of life[151] and by discouraging physical activity, it progressively

Table 2.2 Aerobic power and muscle strength of individuals with hepatic cirrhosis

Author	Sample	Measurement technique	Findings	Comments
Aerobic power				
Campillo et al.[135]	24 cases of liver cirrhosis (? cause) in good clinical condition	Incremental treadmill exercise (3 min/stage) to subjective exhaustion	$\dot{V}O_{2peak}$ 19.6 ml/[kg.min]	$\dot{V}O_{2peak}$ inversely related to Pugh score for liver failure (r = –0.57), may reflect loss of muscle mass
Campillo et al.[136]	10 cases of alcoholic liver cirrhosis, 6 sedentary controls	32 minutes exercise at 3–4 times resting oxygen consumption	Patients metabolized exclusively carbohydrates, whereas controls used equal parts of fat and carbohydrate	Patients showed decreased blood glucose and increased lactate levels, indicating impaired gluconeogenesis
DeLissio et al.[137]	4 cases of hepatic cirrhosis	Prediction of $\dot{V}O_{2peak}$ from treadmill exercise at 50% of maximal effort	$\dot{V}O_{2peak}$ 29.9 ml/[kg.min] vs. 49.0 ml/[kg.min] in controls	Lack of normal endogenous gluconeogenesis in patients, as seen from infusions of isotopically marked glucose
Dharancy et al.[138]	135 cases of hepatic cirrhosis	Progressive cycle ergometer test with 10W/min increments of loading to exhaustion	$\dot{V}O_{2peak}$ 17.2 ml/[kg.min], 61% of predicted; 54% of patients had $\dot{V}O_{2peak}$ 60% of predicted $\dot{V}O_2$-AT also low	Patients with $\dot{V}O_{2peak}$ <60% of normal had decreased 1 yr survival following transplant operation (64.7% vs. 96.4%. p = 0.0003). MELD score of disease severity inversely related to $\dot{V}O_{2peak}$
Epstein et al.[140]	156 patients on transplant waiting list, 59 received transplants	Cycle ergometer test, ramp protocol to $\dot{V}O_{2peak}$	6 died within 100 days of transplant had $\dot{V}O_{2peak}$ <50% predicted and $\dot{V}O_2$-AT also reduced	
Pieber et al.[141]	15 patients on transplant waiting list	Cycle ergometer test, 25 W increase of loading every 2 minutes	$\dot{V}O_{2max}$-AT 10.3 mL/[kg/min]	Associated decreases in health-related quality of life

Table 2.2 continued

Author	Sample	Measurement technique	Findings	Comments
Ritland et al.[131]	9 cases of hepatitis receiving immuno-suppressive therapy, 5 with cirrhosis	Prediction of $\dot{V}O_{2max}$ from submaximal test, using Åstrand nomogram	Predicted $\dot{V}O_{2max}$ 31 ml/[kg.min]	$\dot{V}O_{2max}$-increased by interval training, 19% at 4–5 wk, 29% at 10–12 wk
Terziyski et al.[142]	19 cases of hepatic cirrhosis	Treadmill test, Bruce protocol	$\dot{V}O_{2peak}$ 23.9 ml/[kg.min] 72.1% of predicted	Patients with mild and moderate hepatic cirrhosis have reduced exercise capacity, which correlates with Child-Pugh score ($p = 0.031$)
Wiesinger et al.[143]	12 alcoholic cirrhosis, 8 post viral hepatitis, 6 other causes of cirrhosis	Cycle ergometer, loading increased 25 W every 2 minutes	19 pts completed cycle ergometer test. $\dot{V}O_2$AT Child-Pugh class: A = 11.6 ml/[kg.min] (54% pred $\dot{V}O_{2-max}$) B = 10.3 ml/[kg.min] (37% pred $\dot{V}O_{2-max}$) C = 8.7 ml/[kg.min] (32% pred $\dot{V}O_{2-max}$)	Patients with advanced stage liver disease are stage dependently impaired in their physical capacity
Wong et al.[144]	39 cases of hepatic cirrhosis	Exercise capacity – $\dot{V}O_{2peak}$ – $\dot{V}O_2$-At	$\dot{V}O_{2peak}$ (ml/kg.min) (from graph): pre-ascitic 24, ascitic 13.5 controls: 28.5	Patients had a significant reduction in exercise capacity and an early anaerobic threshold; associated myocardial thickening and ventricular stiffness

Muscle strength

Author	Sample	Measurement technique	Findings	Comments
Andersen et al.[145]	24 cases of alcoholic cirrhosis	Isokinetic strength flexion and extension of ankle, hip, knee, elbow and wrist; abduction and adduction of shoulder Anthropometry	Strength reduced 29–35% in patients compared with controls LBM 35.6kg (79% of predicted)	

Table 2.2 continued

Author	Sample	Measurement technique	Findings	Comments
Pieber et al.[141]	15 patients on liver transplant waiting list	Isokinetic dynamometer, handgrip dynamometer	Peak torque of knee extensors 97 N-m, Handgrip force 524 N	Patients with end-stage liver disease have deficits of muscle strength
Tarter et al.[146]	49 alcoholic, 42 non-alcoholic cirrhosis	Isokinetic device, concentric and eccentric contraction force in upper and lower limbs	Upper limb peak concentric peak (N): alcoholic = 50.5 nonalcoholic = 55.0 controls = 68.1 Eccentric force (N): alcoholic = 95.0 nonalcoholic = 94.6 controls = 122.2 Lower limb peak concentric force (N): alcoholic = 104.6 nonalcoholic = 108.2 controls = 140.8 Eccentric force (N): alcoholic = 187.5 nonalcoholic = 196.8 controls = 241.5	Psychomotor capacity correlates negatively with isokinetic strength in cirrhosis
Wiesinger et al.[143]	12 alcoholic cirrhosis, 8 post viral hepatitis, 6 other causes of cirrhosis	Isokinetic dynamometer and handgrip dynamometer	Knee torque depends on Child-Pugh score: Class A 149 N-m, Class B 108 N-m, Class C 89 N-m Handgrip Class A 680 N, Class B 569N, Class C 451N	Patients with advanced liver disease are stage dependently impaired in their physical capacity. Impairment unrelated to disease aetiology

exacerbates the initial loss of muscular strength.[152] Nevertheless, regular progressive exercise can counter such fatigue, even in people with advanced fibrosis.[153] Moreover, given adequate motivation and a progressive programme, patients with cirrhosis can tolerate quite vigorous exercise; they can maintain oxygenation of the brain and muscles even during incremental cycle ergometry to exhaustion[154] and they show no evidence of hypoglycemia while undertaking 90 minutes of treadmill exercise at 50% of maximal oxygen intake.[137]

We may conclude that exercise rehabilitation programmes can have favourable effects even in advanced hepatic disease, if the affected individuals can be motivated to sustain their participation in such activity.

Hepatocellular carcinoma

Hepatocellular carcinoma is usually a secondary complication of advanced NAFLD, hepatitis B or C infection, or alcoholic cirrhosis. In countries where viral hepatitis is prevalent, this is the dominant cause of hepatic cancer, but in North America alcoholism and NAFLD are more important antecedents.

Interactions between physical activity and hepato-cellular carcinoma have had little study, although given that physical activity reduces the risk of NAFLD, some preventive value would be anticipated. A ten-year follow-up of 507,897 retired Americans found a significantly reduced risk of hepatic carcinoma (odds ratio 0.64) in those who reported regular activity (>5 times a week) versus those who exercised never or rarely.[155] Likewise, a comparison between sedentary mice and those assigned to daily treadmill running for 32 weeks showed that although both groups were fed a diet that induced NAFLD, the exercisers had a lower incidence of hepatic tumours.[156]

Moderate physical activity may offer palliative therapy in those with established disease. One case report noted that six weeks of supervised aerobic exercise (cycling twice per week) produced a 20% increase in peak work capacity, along with an increase in the six minute walking distance and quality of life.[157]

Liver transplants

An increasing proportion of patients with advanced liver disease are now treated by hepatic transplantation. Maximization of physical condition is important to the success of such surgery. Patients remain at risk of NAFLD following transplants, and it is thus important to continue regular physical activity following operation. Empirical non-randomized data further suggest that those who exercise have a higher quality of life after hepatic transplantation,[158] although the direction of causality in this relationship remains debatable.

Areas for further research

Much of the research on physical activity and hepatic pathologies has been cross-sectional in type, and there remains scope for substantial prospective trials that examine the value of various patterns of physical activity in preventing and treating disorders of liver function. The respective contributions of physical activity, dietary change and weight loss to improvements in hepatic function remain to be clarified, and there is a need to clarify whether a reduction of sedentary behaviour will augment the benefit yielded simply by an increase of habitual physical activity.

Although regular physical activity improves effort tolerance and enhances the quality of life in advanced liver disease, often with a reversal of high levels of hepatic enzymes, it is less clear whether liver histopathology can be improved in response to a combined exercise and weight loss programme.[76] Methods of increasing compliance with prescribed exercise also require further study.

A few reports have noted favourable responses to resistance exercise in NAFLD, although its effectiveness in management and treatment is not yet clearly established. There also remains a need to define the minimum dose of physical activity that is required for benefit, to clarify the exercise tolerance of individuals with impaired hepatic function and to determine doses of exercise that may lead to hepatic injury. Finally, there has as yet been little systematic study of the possible role of exercise programmes in the treatment of patients with alcoholic hepatitis.

Practical implications and conclusions

Many features of the metabolic syndrome suggest hepatic dysfunction, and there is a close association between this syndrome and the non-alcoholic fatty infiltration of NAFLD. Risks of developing the metabolic syndrome are reduced independently by both regular physical activity and the avoidance of sedentary habits. Sedentary behaviour also predisposes to steatosis and associated disorders, including atherosclerotic disease and diabetes mellitus. If untreated, simple steatosis, NAFLD, alcoholic inflammation and exposure to hepatitis B or C can all initiate a sequence of fibrosis, cirrhosis and even cancerous change in liver tissue, particularly if habitual physical activity is inadequate.

Regular physical activity and dieting can restore insulin sensitivity, counteract diabetes and steatosis, and possibly facilitate recovery from various forms of hepatitis. Optimization of functional capacity is important to quality of life and the success of liver transplantation if such treatment is undertaken. The majority of therapeutic programmes have prescribed moderate to vigorous aerobic exercise for three to five days per week. However, further information is needed on the efficacy of resistance versus aerobic exercise, on the minimum dose of activity required for benefit, on the exercise tolerance of individuals with chronic liver disease, and on the dose of exercise that may lead to hepatic injury.

Programme compliance is a problem for the obese. Fatigue (probably centrally mediated) is frequent in hepatic steatosis,[159] and this may reduce motivation or even preclude sustained vigorous activity. The one study of NAFLD that examined predictors of exercise adoption and adherence concluded that initial confidence in the ability to exercise was often low in hepatic dysfunction, in part because of a fear of falling.[160] Supervised exercise with similarly affected individuals can often improve self-confidence and reduce fears of falling, but if such an approach is ineffective, less conventional tactics may be needed to increase daily energy expenditures. One investigation achieved a significant reduction of alanine transaminase through a combination of regular voluntary and electrical stimulation of the quadriceps and hamstring muscles.[161]

References

1. Morgagni GB. *The seats and causes of diseases invesigated by anatomy*. London, UK: A, Millar and T. Cadel, 1769
2. Vague J. The degree of masculine differentiation of obesities. A factor determining predisposition to diabetes, atherosclerosis, gout and uric calculous disease. *Am J Clin Nutr* 1956; 4: 20–34.
3. Reaven G. Role of insulin resistance in human disease. *Diabetes Care* 1988; 37: 1595–1607.
4. Cameron AJ, Shaw JE, Zimmet P. The metabolic syndrome: prevalence in worldwide populations. *Endocrinol Metab Clin N Am* 2004; 33: 351–357.
5. McAllister MJ, Dhurandhar NV, Keith SW, et al. Ten putative contributors to the obesity epidemic. *Crit Rev Food Sci Nutr* 2009; 49(10): 868–913.
6. Chen SH, He F, Zhou L, et al. Relationship between nonalcoholic fatty liver disease and metabolic syndrome. *J Dig Dis* 2011; 12(2): 125–130.
7. Patton HM, Yates K, Unalp-Arida A, et al. Association between metabolic syndrome and liver histology among children with nonalcoholic fatty liver disease. *Am J Gastroenterol* 2010; 105(9): 2093–2102.
8. Alberti KG, Zimmet PZ. Definition, diagnosis and classification of diabetes mellitus and its complications. Part 1: diagnosis and classification of diabetes mellitus: provisional report of a WHO consultation. *Diabet Med* 1998; 15: 539–553.
9. Grundy SM, Brewer HB, Cleeman JI, et al. Definition of metabolic syndrome. Report of the National Heart, Lung, and Blood Institute/American Heart Association conference on scientific issues related to definition. *Circulation* 2004; 109: 433–438.
10. Park S, Park H, Togo F, et al. Year-long physical activity and metabolic syndrome in older Japaese adults: Cross-sectional data from the Nakanojo study. J *Gerontol Med Sci* 2008; 63A(10): 1119–1123.
11. Bianchi G, Rossi V, Muscari A, et al. Physical activity is negatively associated with the metabolic syndrome in the elderly. *Quart J Med* 2008; 101: 713–721.
12. Laaksonen DE, Lakka HM, Salonen JT, et al. Low levels of leisure-time physical activity and cardiorespiratory fitness predict development of the metabolic syndrome. *Diabetes Care* 2002; 25: 1612–1618.
13. Ford ES, Kohl HW, Mokdad AH, et al. Sedentary behavior, physical activity, and the metabolic syndrome among US adults. *Obes Res* 2005; 13: 608–614.
14. Wijndaele K, Duvigneaud N, Matton L, et al. Sedentary behaviour, physical activity and a continuous metabolic syndrome risk score in adults. *Eur J Clin Nutr* 2009; 63: 421–429.
15. Bankoski A, Harris TB, McClain JJ, et al. Sedentary activity associated with metabolic syndrome independent of physical activity. *Diabetes Care* 2011; 34: 497–503.
16. Healy GN, Dunstan DW, Salmon J, et al. Breaks in sedentary time: beneficial associations with metabolic risk. *Diabetes Care* 2008; 31: 661–666.
17. Healy GN, Wijndaele K, Dunstan DW, et al. Objectively measured sedentary time, physical activity, and metabolic risk: the Australian Diabetes, Obesity and Lifestyle Study (AusDiab). *Diabetes Care* 2008; 31: 369–371.

18. Rinella ME. Non-alcoholic fatty liver disease. A systematic review. *JAMA* 2015; 313(22): 2263–2273.
19. Browning JD, Szczepaniak LS, Dobbins R, et al. Prevalence of hepatic steatosis in an urban population in the United States: impact of ethnicity. *Hepatology* 2004; 40: 1387–1395.
20. Shaker M, Tabbaa A, Albeldawi Meab KG. Liver transplantation for nonalcoholic fatty liver disease: New challenges and new opportunities. *World J Gastroenterol* 2014; 20(18): 5320–5330.
21. Szczepaniak LS, Nurenberg P, Leonard D, et al. Magnetic resonance spectroscopy to measure hepatic triglyceride content: prevalence of hepatic steatosis in the general population. *Am J Physiol* 2005; 288: E462–468.
22. Bellentani S, Saccoccio G, Masutti F, et al. Prevalence of and risk factors for hepatic steatosis in Northern Italy. *Ann Int Med* 2000; 132: 112–117.
23. Lazo M, Hernaez R, Bonekamp S, et al. Non-alcoholic fatty liver disease and mortality among US adults: prospective cohort study. *Br Med J* 2011; 343: d6891.
24. Takahashi Y, Fukusato T. Pediatric nonalcoholic fatty liver disease: overview with emphasis on histology. *World J Gastroenterol* 2010; 16: 5280–5285.
25. Tsuruta G, Tanaka N, Hongo M, et al. Nonalcoholic fatty liver disease in Japanese junior high school students: its prevalence and relationship to lifestyle habits. *J Gastroenterol* 2010; 45: 666–672.
26. Katsanos CS. Lipid-induced insulin resistance in the liver: role of exercise. *Sports Med* 2004; 34: 955–965.
27. Donnelly KL, Smith CI, Schwarzenberg SJ, et al. Sources of fatty acids stored in liver and secreted via lipoproteins in patients with nonalcoholic fatty liver disease. *J Clin Invest* 2005; 115: 1343–1351.
28. Kotronen A, Juurinen L, Tiikkainen M, et al. Increased liver fat, impaired insulin clearance, and hepatic and adipose tissue insulin resistance in type 2 diabetes. *Gastroenterology* 2008; 135(1): 122–130.
29. Korenblat KM, Fabbrini E, Mohammed BS, et al. Liver, muscle, and adipose tissue insulin action is directly related to intrahepatic triglyceride content in obese subjects. *Gastroenterology* 2008; 134(5): 1369–1375.
30. Angulo P. Non-alcoholic fatty liver disease. *New Engl J Med* 2002; 346: 1221–1231.
31. Malhi N, Kaufman RJ. Endoplasmic reticulum stress in liver disease. *J Hepatol* 2011; 54(4): 795–809.
32. Rao R. Endotoxemia and gut barrier disease in alcoholic liver disease. *Hepatology* 2009; 50: 638–644.
33. Nobili V, Manco M, Devito R, et al. Lifestyle intervention and antioxidant therapy in children with nonalcoholic fatty liver disease: A randomized, controlled trial. *Hepatology* 2008; 48: 119–128.
34. Holt HN, Wild SH, Wareham N, et al. Differential effects of fatness, fitness and physical activity energy expenditure on whole-body, liver and fat insulin sensitivity. *Diabetologia* 2007; 50: 1698–706.
35. Arase Y, Suzuki F, Ikeda K, et al. Multivariate analysis of risk factors for the development of type 2 diabetes in nonalcoholic fatty liver disease. *J Gastroenterol* 2009; 44: 1064–1070.
36. Nannipierri M, Gonzales C, Baldi S, et al. Liver enzymes, the metabolic syndrome, and incident diabetes: The Mexico City diabetes study. *Diabetes Care* 2005; 28: 1757–1762.

37. Tamura Y, Tanaka Y, Sato F, et al. Effects of diet and exercise on muscle and liver intracellular lipid contents and insulin sensitivity in type 2 diabetic patients. *J Clin Endocrinol Metab* 2005; 90: 3191–3196.

38. Thamer C, Machann J, Stefan N, et al. High visceral. fat mass and high liver fat are associated with resistance to lifestyle intervention. *Obesity* (Silver Spring) 2007; 15: 531–538.

39. Petersen KF, Dufour S, Befroy D, et al. Reversal of nonalcoholic hepatic steatosis, hepatic insulin resistance, and hyperglycemia by moderate weight reduction in patients with type 2 diabetes. *Diabetes* 2005; 54(3): 603–608.

40. Eslami L, Merat S, Nasseri-Moghaddam S. Treatment of non-alcoholic fatty liver disease (NAF LD): a systematic review. *Middle East J Dig Dis* 2009; 1: 89–99.

41. Keating SE, Hackett DA, George J, et al. Exercise and non-alcoholic fatty liver disease: a systematic review and meta-analysis. *J Hepatol* 2012; 57: 157–66.

42. Musso G, Cassader M, Rosina F, et al. Impact of current treatments on liver disease, glucose metabolism and cardiovascular risk in non-alcoholic fatty liver disease (NAFLD): a systematic review and meta-analysis of randomised trials. *Diabetalogia* 2012; 55: 885–904.

43. Rodriguez B, Torres DM, Harrison SA. Physical activity: an essential component of lifestyle modification in NAFLD. *Nature Rev Gastroenterol Hepatol* 2012; 9: 726–731.

44. Socha P, Horvath A, Vajro P, et al. Pharmacological interventions for non-alcoholic fatty liver disease in adults and in children: a systematic review. *J Pediatr Gastroenterol Nutr* 2009; 48: 587–596.

45. Thoma CD, Day CP, Trenell MI. Lifestyle interventions for the treatment of non-alcoholic fatty liver disease in adults: A systematic review. *J Hepatol* 2012; 56: 255–266.

46. Alisi A, Locatelli M, Nobili V. Nonalcoholic fatty liver disease in children. *Curr Opin Clin Nutr Metab Care* 2010; 13: 397–402.

47. Bacchi N, Moghetti P. Exercise for hepatic fat accumulation in type 2 diabetic subjects. *Int J Endocrinol* 2013: ID 309191: 1–5.

48. Caldwell S, Lazo M. Is exercise an effective treatment for NASH? Knowns and unknowns. *Ann Hepatol* 2009; 8 (Suppl. 1): S60–S66.

49. Centis E, Marzocchi R, Di Domizio S, et al. The effect of lifestyle changes in non-alcoholic fatty liver disease. *Dig Dis* 2010; 28: 267–273.

50. Cheung O, Sanyal AJ. Recent advances in nonalcoholic fatty liver disease. *Curr Opin Gastroenterol* 2009; 25: 230–237.

51. Conjeevaram HS, Tiniakos DG. Editorial: exercise for NAFLD: does intensity matter? *Am J Gastroenterol* 2011; 106: 470–475.

52. Della Corte C, Alisi A, Iorio R, et al. Expert opinion on current therapies for nonalcoholic fatty liver disease. *Expert Opin Pharmacother* 2011; 12: 1901–1911.

53. Dowman JK, Armstrong MJ, Tomlinson JW, et al. Current therapeutic strategies in non-alcoholic fatty liver disease. *Diabetes, Obes Metab* 2011; 13: 692–702.

54. Duvnjak M, Tomasic V, Gomercic M, et al. Therapy of nonalcoholic fatty liver disease: current status. *J Physiol Pharmacol* 2009; 60 (Suppl. 7): 57–66.

55. Johnson NA, George J. Fitness versus fatness: moving beyond weight loss in nonalcoholic fatty liver disease. *Hepatology* 2010; 52: 370–381.

56. Mencin AA, Lavine JE. Nonalcoholic fatty liver disease in children. *Curr Opin Clin Nutr Metab Care* 2011; 14: 151–157.

57. Nobili V, Carter-Kent C, Feldstein AE. The role of lifestyle changes in the management of chronic liver disease. *BMC Med* 2011; 9: 70.
58. Nobili V, Sanyal AJ. Treatment of nonalcoholic fatty liver disease in adults and children: a closer look at the arsenal. *J Gastroenterol* 2012; 47: 29–36.
59. Rector SR, Thyfault JP. Does physical inactivity cause nonalcoholic fatty liver disease? *J Appl Physiol* 2011; 111: 1828–1835.
60. Reynoso E, Lavine JE. NAFLD: The role of exercise in treating NAFLD. *Nature Rev Gastroenterol Hepatol* 2012; 9: 368–370.
61. Spassiani NA, Kuk JL. Exercise and the fatty liver. *Appl Physiol Nutr Metab* 2008; 33: 802–807.
62. Targher GB, Bellis A, Fornengo P, et al. Prevention and treatment of nonalcoholic fatty liver disease. *Dig Liver Dis* 2010; 42: 331–340.
63. Zelber-Sagi S, Ratziu V, Oren R. Nutrition and physical activity in NAFLD: an overview of the epidemiological evidence. *World J Gastroenterol* 2011; 17: 3377–3389.
64. Fintini D, Pietrobattista A, Morino G, et al. Energy expenditure and insulin sensitivity evaluation in obese children affected by hepatosteatosis. *Pediatr Obesity* 2012; 7: (2) e4–7.
65. Gerber L, Otgonsuren M, Mishra A, et al. Non-alcoholic fatty liver disease (NAFLD) is associated with low level of physical activity: a population-based study. *Aliment Pharmacol Therap* 2012; 36: 772–781.
66. Newton JL, Jones DEJ, Henderson E, et al. Fatigue in non-alcoholic fatty liver disease (NAFLD) is significant and associates with inactivity and excessive daytime sleepiness but not with liver disease severity or insulin resistance. *Gut 2008*; 57: 807–813.
67. Viitasalo A, Laaksonen DE, Lindi V, et al. Clustering of metabolic risk factors is associated with high-normal levels of liver enzymes among 6- to 8-year-old children: the PANIC study. *Metab Syndr Relat Disord* 2012; 10: 337–343.
68. Leskinen T, Sipilä S, Alen M, et al. Leisure-time physical activity and high-risk fat: a longitudinal population-based twin study. *Int J Obesity* 2009; 33: 1211–1208.
69. Hsieh SD, Yoshinaga H, Muto T, et al. Regular physical activity and coronary risk factors in Japanese men. *Circulation* 1998; 97: 661–665.
70. Kang JH, Greenson JK, Omo JT, et al. Metabolic syndrome is associated with greater histologic severity, higher carbohydrate, and lower fat diet in patients with NAFLD. *Am J Gastroenterol* 2006; 101: 2247–2253.
71. Kistler KD, Brunt EM, Clark JM, et al. Physical activity recommendations, exercise intensity, and histological severity of nonalcoholic fatty liver disease. *Am J Gastroenterol* 2011; 106: 470–475.
72. Krasnoff JB, Painter PL, Wallace JP, et al. Health-related fitness and physical activity in patients with nonalcoholic fatty liver disease. *Hepatology* 2008; 47: 1158–1166.
73. Seppala-Lindroos A, Vehkavaara S, Hakkinen AM, et al. Fat accumulation in the liver is associated with defects in insulin suppression of glucose production and serum free fatty acids independent of obesity in normal men. *J Clin Endocrinol Metab* 2007; 87: 3023–3028.
74. McMillan KP, Kuk JL, Church TS, et al. Independent associations between liver fat, visceral adipose tissue, and metabolic risk factors in men. *Appl Physiol Nutr Metab* 2007; 32: 265–272.
75. Nguyen-Duy TB, Nichaman MZ, Church TS, et al. Visceral fat and liver fat are independent predictors of metabolic risk factors in men. *Am J Physiol* 2003; 284: E1065–E1071.

76. Goodpaster BH, Delany JP, Otto AD, et al. Effects of diet and physical activity interventions on weight loss and cardiometabolic risk factors in severely obese adults: a randomized trial. *JAMA* 2010; 304: 1795–1802.
77. Hallsworth K, Fattakhova G, Hollingsworth K, et al. Resistance exercise reduces liver fat and its mediators in non-alcoholic fatty liver disease independent of weight loss. *Gut* 2011; 60: 1278–1283.
78. Larson-Meyer DE, Newcomer BR, Heilbrunn LK, et al. Effect of 6-month calorie restriction and exercise on serum and liver lipids and markers of liver function. *Obesity* 2008; 16: 1355–1362.
79. Johnson NA, Sachinwalla T, Walton DW, et al. Aerobic exercise training reduces hepatic and visceral lipids in obese individuals without weight loss. *Hepatology* 2009; 50: 1105–1112.
80. Bonekamp S, Barone B, Clark JM, et al. The effect of exercise training intervention on hepatic steatosis. *Hepatology* 2008; 48 (S1): 806A.
81. Eckard C, Cole R, Lockwood J, et al. Prospective histopathologic evaluation of lifestyle modification in nonalcoholic fatty liver disease: a randomized trial. *Ther Adv Gastroenterol* 2013; 6: 249–259.
82. Coker RH, Williams RH, Yeo SE, et al. The impact of exercise training compared to caloric restriction on hepatic and peripheral insulin resistance in obesity. *J Clin Endocrinol Metab* 2009; 94: 4258–4266.
83. Shah K, Stufflebam A, Hilton TN, et al. Diet and exercise interventions reduce intrahepatic fat content and improve insulin sensitivity in obese older adults. *Obesity* 2009; 17: 2162–2168.
84. Chen S-M, Liu C-Y, Li S-R, et al. Effects of therapeutic lifestyle program on ultrasound-diagnosed nonalcoholic fatty liver disease. *J Chin Med Assoc* 2008; 71: 551–558.
85. Straznicky NE, Lambert EA, Grima MT, et al. The effects of dietary weight loss with or without exercise training on liver enzymes in obese metabolic syndrome subjects. *Diabetes Obes Metab* 2012; 14: 139–148.
86. Lee S, Bacha F, Hannon T, Kuk JL, et al. Effects of aerobic versus resistance exercise without caloric restriction on abdominal fat, intrahepatic lipid, and insulin sensitivity in obese adolescent boys: a randomized, controlled trial. *Diabetes* 2012; 61: 2787–2795.
87. Slentz CA, Bateman LA, Willis LH, et al. Effects of aerobic vs. resistance training on visceral and liver fat stores, liver enzymes, and insulin resistance by HOMA in overweight adults from STRRIDE AT/RT. *Am J Physiol* 2012; 301: E1033–E9.
88. Levinger I, Goodman C, Peake J, et al. Inflammation, hepatic enzymes and resistance training in individuals with metabolic risk factors. *Diabetes Med* 2009; 26: 220–227.
89. van der Heijden GJ, Wang ZJ, Chu Z, et al. Strength exercise improves muscle mass and hepatic insulin sensitivity in obese youth. *Med Sci Sports Exerc* 2010; 42: 1973–1980.
90. Jakovljevic D, Hallsworth K, Zalewski P, et al. Resistance exercise improves autonomic regulation at rest and haemodynamic response to exercise in non-alcoholic fatty liver disease. *Clin Sci* 2013; 125: 143–149.
91. Marques CMM, Motta VF, Torres TS, et al. Beneficial effects of exercise training (treadmill) on insulin resistance and nonalcoholic fatty liver disease in high-fat fed C57BL/6 mice. *Braz J Med Biol Res* 2010; 43: 467–475.
92. Sene-Fiorese M, Duarte FO, Scarmagnani FRR, et al. Efficiency of intermittent exercise on adiposity and fatty liver in rats fed with high-fat diet. *Obesity* (Silver Spring) 2009; 16: 2217–2222.

93. Yasari S, Paquette A, Charbonneau A, et al. Effects of ingesting a high-fat diet upon exercise-training cessation on fat accretion in the liver and adipose tissue of rats. *Appl Physiol Nutr Metab* 2006; 31: 367–375.

94. Linden MA, Meers GM, Ruebel ML, et al. Hepatic steatosis development with four weeks of physical inactivity in previously active, hyperphagic OLETF rats. *Am J Physiol* 2013; 304(9): R763–R771.

95. Shephard RJ, Johnson N. Effects of physical activity upon the liver. *Eur J Appl Physiol* 2015; 115(1): 1–46.

96. Rector RS, Uptergrove GM, Morris EM, et al. Daily exercise vs. caloric restriction for prevention of nonalcoholic fatty liver disease in the OLETF rat model. *Am J Physiol* 2011; 300: G874–G883.

97. Cintra DE, Ropelle ER, Vitto MF, et al. Reversion of hepatic steatosis by exercise training in obese mice: the role of sterol regulatory element-binding protein-1c. *Life Sci* 2012; 91: 395–401.

98. Yasari S, Prud'homme D, Wang D, et al. Exercise training decreases hepatic SCD-1 gene expression and protein content in rats. *Mol Cell Biochem* 2010; 335: 291–299.

99. El Midaoui A, Chiasson JL, Tancrede G, et al. Physical training reverses the increased activity of the hepatic ketone body synthesis pathway in chronically diabetic rats. *Am J Physiol* 2006; 290: E207–E212.

100. Li Z, Murakami T, Nakai N, et al. Modification by exercise training of activity and enzyme expression of hepatic branched-chain alpha-ketoacid dehydrogenase complex in streptozotocin-induced diabetic rats. *J Nutr Sci Vitaminol* 2001; 47: 345–350.

101. Leme JACA, Silveira RF, Gomes RJ, et al. Long-term physical training increases liver IGF-I in diabetic rats. *Growth Hormone IGF Res* 2009; 19: 262–266.

102. da Luz G, Frederico MJS, da Silva S, et al. Endurance exercise training ameliorates insulin resistance and reticulum stress in adipose and hepatic tissue in obese rats. *Eur J Appl Physiol* 2011; 111: 2015–2023.

103. Zawalich W, Maturo S, Felig P. Influence of physical training on insulin release and glucose utilization by islet cells. *Am J Physiol* 1982; 243: E464–E469.

104. Chowdhury KK, Legare DJ, Lautt WW. Exercise enhancement of hepatic insulin-sensitising substance-mediated glucose uptake in diet-induced prediabetic rats. *Br J Nutr* 2013; 109: 844–852.

105. Chowdhury KK, Legare DJ, Lautt WW. Insulin sensitization by voluntary exercise in aging rats is mediated through hepatic insulin sensitizing substance (HISS). *Exp Gerontol* 2011; 46: 73–80.

106. Park S, Hong SM, Lee JE, et al. Chlorpromazine exacerbates hepatic insulin sensitivity via attenuating insulin and leptin signaling pathway, while exercise partially reverses the adverse effects. *Life Sci* 2007; 80: 2428–2435.

107. Hittel DS, Axelson M, Sarna N, et al. Myostatin decreases with aerobic exercise and associates with insulin resistance. *Med Sci Sports Exerc* 2010; 42: 2023–2029.

108. Allen DL, Hittel DS, McPherron AC. Expression and function of myostatin in obesity, diabetes, and exercise adaptation. *Med Sci Sports Exerc* 2011; 43: 1828–1835.

109. Mukherjee A, Sidis Y, Mahan A, et al. FSTL3 deletion reveals roles for TGF-beta family ligands in glucose and fat homeostasis in adults. *Proc Natl Acad Sci USA* 2007; 104: 1348–1353.

110. Chen W, Woodruff TK, Mayo KE. Activin A-induced HepG2 liver cell apoptosis: involvement of activin receptors and smad proteins. *Endocrinology* 2000; 141: 1263–1272.

111. Woodruff TK, Krummen L, Chen SA, et al. Pharmacokinetic profile of recombinant human (rh) inhibin A and activin A in the immature rat. II. Tissue distribution of [125I]rh-inhibin A and [125I]rh-activin A in immature female and male rats. *Endocrinology* 1993; 132: 725–734.

112. Rector RS, Thyfault JP, Laye MJ, et al. Cessation of daily exercise dramatically alters precursors of hepatic steatosis in Otsuka Long-Evans Tokushima Fatty (OLETF) rats. *J Physiol* 2008; 586: 4241–4249.

113. Czaja AJ. Hepatic inflammation and progressive liver fibrosis in chronic liver disease. *World J Gastroenterol* 2014; 29(10): 2515–2532.

114. Fealy CE, Haus JM, Solomon TP, et al. Short-term exercise reduces markers of hepatocyte apoptosis in nonalcoholic fatty liver disease. *J Appl Physiol* 2012; 113: 1–6.

115. Lee YS, Kek BLK, Poh LKS, et al. Association of raised liver transaminases with physical inactivity, increased waist-hip ratio, and other metabolic morbidities in severely obese children. *J Pediatr Gastroenterol Nutr* 2008; 47: 172–178.

116. Gonçalves IO, Oliveira PJ, Ascensão A, et al. Exercise as a therapeutic tool to prevent mitochondrial degeneration in nonalcoholic steatohepatitis. *Eur J Clin Invest* 2013; 43(11): 1184–1194.

117. Naveau S, Giraud V, Borotto E, et al. Excess weight as a factor for alcoholic liver disease. *Hepatology* 1997; 25: 108–111.

118. Basra S, Anand BS. Definition, epidemiology and magnitude of alcoholic hepatitis. *World J Hepatol* 2011; 3(5): 109–113.

119. Madrey WC, Boitnott JK, Bedine MS, et al. Corticoid therapy of alcoholic hepatitis. *Gastroeneterology* 1978; 75: 193–199.

120. Buscemi J, Martens MP, Murphy JG, et al. Moderators of the relationship between physical activity and alcohol consumption in college students. *J Am Coll Health* 2011; 59(6): 503–509.

121. Kendzor DE, Dubbwert PM, Olivier J, et al. The influence of physical activity on alcohol consumption among heavy drinkers participating in an alcohol treatment intervention. *Addict Behav* 2008; 33(10): 1337–1343.

122. Baba CS, Alexander G, Bikkasani K, et al. Effect of exercise and dietary modification on serum aminotransferase levels in patients with nonalcoholic steatohepatitis. *J Gastroentgerol Hepatol* 2006; 21: 191–198.

123. Hickman IJ, Jonsson JR, Prins JB, et al. Modest weight loss and physical activity in overweight patients with chronic liver disease results in sustained improvements in alanine aminotransferase, fasting insulin, and quality of life. *Gut* 2004; 53: 413–419.

124. Hickman IJ, Byrne NM, Croci I, et al. A pilot randomized study of the metabolic and histological effects of exercise in non-alcoholic steatohepatitis. *J Diabetes Metab* 2013; 4: 8.

125. Gonçalves IO, Passos E, Rocha-Rodrigues S, et al. Physical exercise prevents and mitigates non-alcoholic steatohepatitis-induced liver mitochondrial structural and bioenergetics impairments. *Mitochondrion* 2014; 15: 40–51.

126. He Y, Zhang H, Fu F. The effects of swimming exercise on high-fat-diet-induced steatohepatitis. *J Sports Med Phys Fitness* 2008; 48: 259–265.

127. Harrington DW. Viral hepatis and exercise. *Med Sci Sports Exerc* 2000; 32: S422–S430.

128. Anish EJ. Viral hepatitis: Sports-related risk. *Curr Sports Med Rep* 2004; 3: 100–106.

129. Moon J, Kallman J, Winter P, et al. Disparities in activity level and nutrition between patients with chronic hepatitis C and blood donors. *PM R* 2012; 4(6): 436–441.

130. Ritland S, Foss NE, Gjone E. Physical activity in liver disease and liver function in sportsmen. *Scand J Soc Med* 1982; 29(Suppl.): 221–226.

131. Ritland S, Petlund CF, Knudsen T, et al. Improvement of physical capacity after long-term training in patients with chronic active hepatitis. *Scand J Gastroenterol* 1983; 18: 1083–1087.

132. Ueno T, Sugawara H, Sujaku K, et al. Therapeutic effect of restricted diet and exercise in obese patients with fatty liver. *J Hepatol* 1997; 27: 103–107.

133. Oh S, Tanaka K, Warabi E, et al. Exercise reduces inflammation and oxidative stress in obesity-related liver diseases. *Med Sci Sports Exerc* 2013; 45(12): 2214–2222.

134. Kawanishi N, Yano H, Mizokami T, et al. Exercise training attenuates hepatic inflammation, fibrosis and macrophage infiltration during diet induced-obesity in mice. *Brain Behav Immun* 2012; 26: 931–941.

135. Campillo B, Fouet P, Bonnet JC, et al. Submaximal oxygen consumption in liver cirrhosis. Evidence of severe functional aerobic impairment. *J Hepatol 1990*; 10: 163–267.

136. Campillo B, Chapelain C, Bonnet JC, et al. Hormonal and metabolic changes during exercise in cirrhotic patients. *Metabolism* 1990; 39: 18–24.

137. DeLissio M, Goodyear LJ, Fuller S, et al. Effects of treadmill exercise on fuel metabolism in hepatic cirrhosis. *J Appl Physiol* 1991; 70: 210–216.

138. Dharancy S, Lemyze M, Boleslawski E, et al. Impact of impaired aerobic capacity on liver transplant candidates. *Transplantation* 2008; 86: 1077–1083.

139. Epstein SK, Ciubotaru RL, Zilberberg MD, et al. Analysis of impaired exercise capacity in patients with cirrhosis. *Dig Dis Sci* 1998; 43: 1701–1707.

140. Epstein SK, Freeman RB, Khayat A, et al. Aerobic capacity is associated with 100-day outcome after hepatic transplantation. *Liver Transpl* 2004; 10: 418–424.

141. Pieber K, Crevenna R, Nuhr MJ, et al. Aerobic capacity, muscle strength and health-related quality of life before and after orthotopic liver transplantation: preliminary data of an Austrian transplantation centre. *J Rehab Med* 2006; 38: 322–328.

142. Terziyski K, Andonov V, Marinov B, et al. Exercise performance and ventilatory efficiency in patients with mild and moderate liver cirrhosis. *Clin Exp Pharmacol Physiol* 2008; 35: 135–140.

143. Wiesinger GF, Quittan M, Zimmermann K, et al. Physical performance and health-related quality of life in men on a liver transplantation waiting list. *J Rehabil Med* 2001; 33: 260–265.

144. Wong F, Girgrah N, Graba J, et al. The cardiac response to exercise in cirrhosis. *Gut* 2001; 49: 268–275.

145. Andersen H, Borre M, Jakobsen J, et al. Decreased muscle strength in patients with alcoholic liver cirrhosis in relation to nutritional status, alcohol abstinence, liver function, and neuropathy. *Hepatology* 1998; 27: 1200–1206.

146. Tarter RE, Panzak G, Switala J, et al. Isokinetic muscle strength and its association with neuropsychological capacity in cirrhotic alcoholics. *Alcohol Clin Exp Res* 1997; 21: 191–196.

147. Jones JC, Coombes JS, Macdonald GA. Exercise capacity and muscle strength in patients with cirrhosis. *Liver Transplant* 2012; 18: 146–151.

148. Lemyze M, Dharancy S, Wallaert B. Response to exercise in patients with liver cirrhosis: implications for liver transplantation. *Dig Liver Dis* 2013; 45(5): 362–366.

149. Garcia-Pagan JC, Santos C, Barbera JA, et al. Physical exercise increases portal pressure in patients with cirrhosis and portal hypertension. *Gastroenterology* 1996; 111: 1300–1306.

150. Morrison W, Bouchier IA, Gibson JN, et al. Skeletal muscle and whole-body protein turnover in cirrhosis. *Clin Sci* 1990; 78: 613–619.
151. Stanca CM, Bach N, Krause C, et al. Evaluation of fatigue in US patients with primary biliary cirrhosis. *Am J Gastroenterol* 2005; 100: 1104–1109.
152. Wu L-J, Wu M-S, Lien G-S, et al. Fatigue and physical activity levels in patients with liver cirrhosis. *J Clin Nurs* 2012; 21: 129–138.
153. Zucker DM. An exercise intervention to prevent hepatitis related fatigue. *Hepatology* 2004; 40: 511A.
154. Bay Nielsen H, Secher NH, Clemmesen O, et al. Maintained cerebral and skeletal muscle oxygenation during maximal exercise in patients with liver cirrhosis. *J Hepatol* 2005; 43: 266–271.
155. Behrens G, Matthews CE, Moore SC, et al. The association between frequency of vigorous physical activity and hepatobiliary cancers in the NIH-AARP Diet and Health Study. *Eur J Epidemiol* 2013; 28: 55–66.
156. Piguet A-C, Saran U, Simillion C, et al. Regular exercise decreases liver tumor development in hepatocyte-specific PTEN-deficient mice independently of steatosis. *J Hepatol* 2015; 62(6): 1296–1303.
157. Crevenna R, Schmidinger M, Keilani M, et al. Aerobic exercise as additive palliative treatment for a patient with advanced hepatocellular cancer. *Wien Med Wochenschr* 2003; 153 (9–10): 237–240.
158. Rongies E, Speniewska S, Lewandrowska M, et al. Physical activity long-term after liver transplantation yields better quality of life. *Ann Transplant* 2011; 16(3): 126–131.
159. Bergasa NV, Mehlman J, Bir K. Aerobic exercise: a potential therapeutic intervention for patients with liver disease. *Med Hypoth* 2004; 62: 935–941.
160. Frith J, Day CP, Robinson L, et al. Potential strategies to improve uptake of exercise interventions in non-alcoholic fatty liver disease. *J Hepatol* 2010; 52: 112–116.
161. Kawaguchi T, Shiba N, Maeda T, et al. Hybrid training of voluntary and electrical muscle contractions reduces steatosis, insulin resistance, and IL-6 levels in patients with NAFLD: a pilot study. *J Gastroenterol* 2011; 46: 746–757.

3 Effects of physical activity on the gallbladder and biliary tract in health and disease

Introduction

This chapter looks at the impact of acute and chronic physical activity upon biliary function in both health and disease. Although physical activity modifies the secretions and emptying of the healthy gall bladder, the responses to exercise have greater significance for the prevention of disease than for the enhancement of human performance. After considering the prevalence, economic impact and factors contributing to gall bladder disease, and taking a brief look at the resting function of the gall bladder, the text examines the impact of exercise-induced changes in gallbladder emptying upon the risks of cholecystitis, gallstones and biliary tract tumours. In particular, it attempts to distinguish the direct effects of physical activity from changes due to reductions in body fat and blood cholesterol levels.

Prevalence and economic impact of biliary tract disorders

In Classical Greece, black and yellow bile were regarded as two of the body's four basic "humours", and an imbalance in their secretion was considered a cause of ill-health.[1]

Today, a major segment of people in the developed world still suffers from disorders of the biliary tract. Gallstones affect perhaps 25 million Americans, at estimated annual direct and indirect costs of over US$6 billion, and as many as 500,000 Americans undergo surgical removal of the gallbladder each year. Moreover, gallstones are equally prevalent in many other developed countries.[2–8] If untreated, the stones can provoke a gallbladder infection in up to 35% of affected individuals,[9] and if combined with stasis of the bile, such infection predisposes to gall bladder cancer. There are 2.5 cases of gallbladder cancer per 100,000 of the US population each year, and gallstones are found in 80% of those with gallbladder malignancies.[10]

Factors contributing to gallbladder disease

Important factors contributing to the development of gallbladder pathologies include an excessive secretion of mucus, supersaturation of the bile with cholesterol and other chemicals that can crystallize out, an aggregation of the cholesterol crystals provoked by mucin and a reduction of gallbladder motility.[3, 6, 22] As a young medical student, I was taught to suspect the presence of gallstones in a woman who was "fair, fat and forty". Consistent clinical concomitants of gall bladder disease include a low level of habitual physical activity, obesity, non-insulin dependent (maturity onset) diabetes mellitus and hyperlipidaemia (the last sometimes due to attempts at rapid weight loss), as well as the female sex and the number of children that a woman has borne.[23, 24] The potential benefits of physical activity as a means of augmenting emptying of the gallbladder, reducing stasis and protecting against biliary disease have as yet received surprisingly little attention. Nevertheless, a survey of the published literature found 11 reviews (Table 3.1) that concluded with varying enthusiasm that regular physical activity was helpful in preventing gallbladder disease. Commonly, this opinion was based upon two or three cross-sectional comparisons between active and inactive groups of individuals. Utter and Goss[21] concluded that regular aerobic activity had a beneficial effect upon gallbladder function, although the exact mechanism underlying the benefit was unclear.

Resting gallbladder function

Bile is a greenish-brown fluid produced in the liver. It serves as a surfactant and emulsifying agent, and is important to the intestinal digestion of fat. In its absence, fat remains largely unabsorbed and is excreted in the faeces. However, the gallbladder in itself is not essential to digestion, since the entire organ can be removed without obvious adverse effects upon the patient other than some dilatation of the bile ducts.

When a person is fasting, bile accumulates and is concentrated in the gall-bladder. Here, the concentration of its constituents is 3–11 times higher than in the fluid first secreted by the liver.[25, 26] Bile is released into the gut after a meal, through a combination of gallbladder contraction and relaxation of the sphincter of Oddi, located where the bile duct empties into the duodenum. Contraction of the gallbladder is probably initiated by the combined action of intrinsic nerve plexuses in its walls, a weak response to vagal[27] and alpha-adrenergic nerve fibres,[28] and the liberation of hormones (particularly cholecystokinin) from the intestinal wall.[29–32] Cholecystokinin induces gallbladder contraction via the para-sympathetic nerves, serving as a neurotransmitter for this component of the autonomic nervous system.[30] Its action can be countered by the drug loxiglumide, which blocks parasympathetic nerve receptors in the gallbladder wall.[33, 34]

Methods of visualizing gallbladder function include watching the emptying of a contrast medium in serial radiographs, following the excretion of radioisotopes, and the use of ultrasound.[35, 36] The last approach has the advantage that the subject is not exposed to radiation. Depending on age, sex and body size, the human gallbladder has a capacity of some 50 mL, but it typically contains less than 30 mL of bile.[35, 37] Even when fasting, the gallbladder shows both rhythmic contractions (with a frequency of 2–6/sec) and sustained contractions that persist for 5–30 minutes. When resting, some 10–30% of the gallbladder contents are emptied every one to two hours.[38] As much as 65% of the gallbladder contents can be expelled during the first 30–40 minutes following the ingestion of a fatty meal.[39]

Table 3.1 Published reviews suggesting a possible role for regular physical activity in protecting a person against chronic gallbladder disease

Authors	*Conclusions of reviewers*
Deibert et al.[11]	Brief discussion of the gall bladder in the context of sport, suggesting that the risk of cholelithiasis could be reduced by physical training
de Oliveira & Burini[12]	General review of exercise and the gastro-intestinal tract, commenting that mild to moderate intensity exercise protected against cholelithiasis
Hofmann[4]	Exercise was seen as allowing frequent meals without an excessive energy intake relative to energy expenditures, thus enhancing gallbladder emptying
Jeong et al.[13]	Emphasized the potential contribution of obesity to the development of gallbladder disorders
Khazaeina et al.[14]	Main focus was upon the impact of exercise upon the elimination of drugs, but noted that physical activity increased the rate of biliary excretion
Lammert and Matern[15]	Suggested that measures for the prevention of biliary disorders included physical activity, slow weight reduction, regular vitamin C supplementation and moderate coffee consumption
Moga[16]	Regular aerobic exercise was seen as an appropriate alternative to cholecystectomy
Peters & de Vries[17]	General review of physical activity and the gastrointestinal tract. Concluded that physical activity had beneficial effect upon cholelithiasis beyond its effect in reducing body mass
Rissanen and Fogelholm[18]	Concluded that some (but not all) studies of gallstones have shown a protective effect of regular physical activity
Shaffer[19]	Physical activity is mentioned as the final item among a list of potential measures to prevent gallstones
Simrén[20]	General review of physical activity and gastrointestinal tract. Concluded that physical activity seems to protect against cholelithiasis
Utter and Goss[21]	Concluded that aerobic exercise seemed beneficial in preventing gallstones, but the precise mechanism remained unclear

Most of the cholesterol found in the bile has been secreted by the liver. It remains unclear whether cholesterol is also excreted by the healthy gallbladder mucosa. However, cholesterol can accumulate in the gallbladder wall under pathological conditions. Inflammation reduces the ability of the gallbladder to concentrate bile, but it also increases its viscosity through a greatly increased secretion of mucinous material.[40]

Acute effects of physical activity on the gallbladder

An acute bout of vigorous physical activity could potentially stimulate emptying of the gallbladder by increasing the activity of vagal and sympathetic nerves, or by changing blood hormone concentrations. During prolonged endurance activity, effects might also arise from a progressive reduction in visceral blood flow. Empirical studies of acute responses are limited to one study of cholecys-tokinin levels and two studies of gallbladder function, one carried out on dogs and the other in healthy women (Table 3.2).

The study of dogs concluded that vigorous physical activity (4–5 h of treadmill running at an unspecified speed and slope) did not increase the quantity of bile secreted by previously sedentary animals. However, the pigment content was augmented, possibly because running increased the breakdown of red cells.[40] Philipp et al.[41] examined plasma levels of cholecystokinin in 11 male and 8 female marathon runners. Relative to control values collected a few weeks later, plasma cholecystokinin concentrations were elevated immediately before competition, apparently in anticipation of the run, and levels of this hormone showed a further modest increase immediately following completion of the event. Gallbladder function was not measured directly, but from the known effects of cholecystokinin one might anticipate an increase in emptying of the gallbladder in response to the run. Utter et al.[38] have made the only direct human obser-vations on gallbladder function in relation to exercise. They examined 12 healthy

Table 3.2 Acute effects of physical activity upon cholecystinin secretion and gallbladder function

Author	Subjects	Type of exercise	Findings
McMaster et al.[40]	Dogs	4–5 h of treadmill running in previously sedentary animals; speed and slope not specified	No increase in volume of bile secretion, but increase of pigment content (? due to red cell haemolysis)
Philipp et al.[41]	11 male, 8 female marathon runners	Competitive marathon run	Cholecystokinin increased in anticipation of event, further boosted after run
Utter et al.[38]	12 healthy females	30 min of recumbent cycle ergometer exercise to 65% of individual's maximal aerobic power	No significant effect on scintigraphic estimates of gallbladder emptying, either fasting or post-prandial

females, injecting a technetium-99m marker and recording images at five-minute intervals. The fractional emptying of the gall bladder, the latent period to the onset of emptying and the duration of ejection following 30 minutes of recumbent cycle ergometer exercise at 65% of peak aerobic power did not differ significantly from what had been observed at rest.

Blood concentrations of other hormones known to modify gallbladder motility are affected by physical activity (for instance, there are increases in gastrin, motilin, secretin and somatostatin, and decreases in pancreatic polypeptide and vasoactive intestinal peptide), but the possible impact upon gallbladder function of such widespread changes in the hormonal milieu has yet to be examined.

Chronic effects of physical activity on the gallbladder

The chronic effects of physical activity upon gallbladder function have been examined in two cross-sectional comparisons of obese versus more active individuals and two longitudinal exercise interventions, all involving relatively small groups of subjects (Table 3.3).

Table 3.3 Effects of chronic physical activity upon gallbladder function, as seen in both cross-sectional studies and longitudinal interventions

Authors	Subjects	Activity assessment	Findings
Cross-sectional studies			
Mathus-Vliegen et al.[43]	60 obese patients entering weight-loss programme	Subjects questioned about their physical activity	No effect of physical activity on gallbladder function
Vezina et al.[42]	18 morbidly obese individuals, 9 tall and 9 muscular people of similar body mass	No specific observations on physical activity	Gallbladder volumes and emptying rates similar in the 3 groups
Longitudinal interventions			
Sari et al.[45]	23 middle-aged obese women (no control group)	4 weeks of a walking intervention (45 min sessions at 60–80% of maximal heart rate) 5 days/week	Intervention led to small increase in late-phase post-prandial gallbladder motility, and decrease in late-phase post-prandial gallbladder volume, independent of changes in body mass
Utter et al.[44]	27 obese women (16 assigned to training programme)	12 weeks of aerobic training that increased peak oxygen intake by 9%	Non-significant trend to increase of gallbladder ejection fraction

Vezina et al.[42] used both ultrasound and the radio-isotope [99]-technetium diisopropyliminodiacetic acid to make inter-individual comparisons of gallbladder volumes and emptying rates. No significant differences were found between a group of 18 individuals who were morbidly obese and 9 tall and 9 muscular subjects who had a comparable body mass, but who presumably engaged in greater levels of physical activity. Mathus-Vliegen et al.[43] used ultrasonography to study inter-individual differences in the fasting and post-prandial gallbladder volumes of obese individuals who had entered a weight-loss programme. They concluded that body mass, fat-free mass, a central (abdominal) pattern of fat distribution and insulin levels were the main determinants of such functional characteristics of the gallbladder as fasting volume, ejection volume and ejection fraction. Subjects were also questioned about their habitual physical activity, but responses showed no significant association with any measures of gallbladder function.

Utter et al.[44] had 16 obese women engage in 12 weeks of aerobic training (30 min/day of recumbent cycle ergometer exercise at 65% of their individual peak aerobic power). This regimen increased their maximal oxygen intake by 9%. The ejection fraction of the gallbladder as measured by the radio-isotope Technetium-99m showed a tendency to increase by 15% after training, but this trend was not statistically significant relative to control subjects (who also showed a 5% increase in ejection fraction). In contrast to this equivocal result, Sari et al.[45] looked at the effects on gallbladder volume and motility of four weeks of walking (5 days/week for 45 minutes at 60–80% of the individual's maximal heart rate) in 23 middle-aged obese women. This uncontrolled study showed small but significant decreases in post-prandial volumes of the gallbladder following training, accompanied by 12–25% increases in the post-prandial ejection fraction; the main changes in response were seen 90–150 minutes after ingesting the test meal. The gain in peak aerobic power following the intervention was not specified; there was a 2.2 kg decrease of body mass, although weight changes were said to be unrelated to the changes in gallbladder function.

There is plainly some discrepancy between the significant changes of gallbladder motility observed in the uncontrolled trial of Sari et al.[45] and the statistically insignificant trends of similar magnitude described by Utter et al.[44] after a longer period of apparently comparable training. This issue needs to be resolved by further experimentation.

Physical activity and chronic gallbladder disease

Gallstone formation, cholecystitis and cholecystectomy are closely intertwined problems, and many reports have examined the influence of regular physical activity upon all three conditions. After discussing factors predisposing to gallstone formation, findings are thus analysed jointly for all three diagnoses, although a distinction is drawn between conclusions based upon cross-sectional, prospective and case-control studies and what is normally regarded as the optimal epidemiological approach of randomized controlled trials.

Factors predisposing to gallstone formation

Gallstones contain varying proportions of cholesterol, calcium and bilirubin. Factors predisposing to gallstone formation include not only biliary stasis, but also local infection, metabolic abnormalities and a failure of acidification of the bile.

A reduced motility of the gallbladder and resulting biliary stasis allows more time for crystal formation. As discussed above, there is some evidence that a reduction of biliary motility is associated with both obesity and the adoption of a sedentary lifestyle.

Under normal conditions, the gallbladder probably secretes some cholesterol. This process is stimulated by infection, and there is also an increased secretion and/or a reduced breakdown of a mucinous, protein-containing exudate,[46, 47] possibly with a reduction of bile salt concentrations. All of these changes predispose to gallstone formation.

Metabolic abnormalities of interest in the context of gallbladder disease include an increased uptake of cholesterol from the circulation, an increased hepatic synthesis of cholesterol, a reduced breakdown of cholesterol to bile salts and an increased intestinal reabsorption of cholesterol.[48] These several factors predispose to a bile that is super-charged with cholesterol and readily undergoes crystallization.[49, 50] Crystallization is associated with a decreased ratio of bile salts to cholesterol. The normal range is from 1:20 to 1:30, but stone formation occurs if the ratio drops below 1:13.[51, 52]

Failure of the diseased gallbladder epithelium to acidify an alkaline bile is a further adverse factor, leading to the precipitation of calcium carbonate,[53] an important component of gallstones.

Cross-sectional studies

Many cross-sectional studies have examined associations between habitual physical activity and some measure of gallbladder disease (often an ultrasonographic diagnosis of gallstones, but sometimes only a physician's report of gallbladder disease or a hospital record of a cholecystectomy) (Table 3.4). Some studies have found benefit from physical activity, but conclusions in other reports have been negative or equivocal. Among problems of interpretation, subject numbers have sometimes been small, the categorization of physical activity has often been quite crude and statistical analyses have not always made adequate adjustment for other important co-variates such as obesity.

Sarin et al.[54] commented on a relationship between the level of habitual physical activity and the type of gallstone that is formed. In 200 consecutive patients where an arbitrary three-level classification of habitual physical activity had been made, they noted that cholesterol stones (94% of the total) were typical of sedentary individuals, whereas pigmented stones were more frequent in active individuals, probably reflecting a contribution of exercise induced haemolysis to stone formation.

Table 3.4 Effects of habitual physical activity upon various manifestations of gallbladder disease as seen in cross-sectional studies

Authors	Subjects	Method of physical activity measurement	Indicator of disease	Covariates	Conclusions
Basso et al.[62]	512 pregnant women	Crude 3-level classification of physical activity	Ultrasono-graphic diagnosis of gallstones	No covariate adjustments	Gallstones found in 4.5% of sample; little relationship to habitual physical activity
Chuang et al.[63]	53 obese women	Questionnaire on sport, occupational activity and leisure activity	Ultrasono-graphic diagnosis of gallstones	BMI, HDL cholesterol	Sport participation, but neither occupational nor leisure activity associated with reduced risk of gallstones
Friedman [59]	5209 adults	Interview	Combination of hospital records and self reports of gallbladder disease	No data provided, but population activity said to be low	Habitual physical activity not related to gallbladder disease
GREPCO [64]	2325 Roman civil servants	4-item questionnaire on physical activity at leisure and work, active commuting and other walking	Ultrasono-graphic diagnosis of gallstones or history of cholecystec-tomy	Age, BMI, lipids, parity	Habitual physical activity showed no significant effect, even in univariate analyses
Jorgensen [60]	3608 Danish adults 30–60 years of age	4-level classification of occupational and leisure activity	Ultrasono-graphic diagnosis of gallstones and/or cholecystec-tomy	Cigarette smoking, coffee, BMI, weight change	No significant relationship between gallbladder disease and habitual physical activity
Kriska et al.[65]	2130 Puma Indians	Interviewer-conducted physical activity questionnaire	Ultrasono-graphic diagnosis of gallstones	BMI and other confounders	Gall stones significantly related to inactivity in cross-sectional analysis
Pagliarulo et al.[66]	1337 cases of diabetic mellitus	3-level estimate of habitual physical activity	Ultrasono-graphic diagnosis of gallstones	Age, obesity, family history	No significant relationship between gallstones and habitual physical activity

Table 3.4 continued

Authors	Subjects	Method of physical activity measurement	Indicator of disease	Covariates	Conclusions
Sakuta & Suzuki[67]	974 male members of Japanese defence forces	2-way classification of physical activity, based on reports of "sweat-producing activity"	Ultrasonographic diagnosis of gallstones	Cigarette smoking, vegetable intake	Gallstones related to total homocysteine levels, but not to habitual physical activity
Sarin et al.[54]	200 consecutive patients with gallstone disease	Arbitrary 3-level classification of habitual physical activity	Gallstones obtained at cholecystectomy		Cholesterol stones typical of sedentary individuals, pigmented stones found in more active individuals
Storti et al.[56]	8010 post-menopausal women	Modified Harvard alumni questionnaire	Self-report of cholecystectomy or gallbladder disease	Body mass and other risk factors	Lower 3 physical activity quartiles vs. top quartile, odds ratio of 1.57 for gallbladder disease
Utter et al.[68]	2088 Puma Indians	Interviewer administered questionnaire	Clinically diagnosed gallstones	Diabetes mellitus	Gradient of risk 14.2–4.7% from least to most active tertile of diabetic men. Unable to test in non-diabetic men or women
Walcher et al.[57]	2129 adults aged 18–65 years	Interviewer supervised physical activity questionnaire	Ultrasonographic diagnosis of gallstones	Age, BMI, cholesterol, Vitamin C ingestion	Odds ratio of physical activity >2h/week vs. <2h/week 0.65 (0.52–0.79)
Williams [55]	29,110 male, 11,953 female runners	Habitual physical activity and 10 km running speed	Self-reported, clinician-diagnosed gallbladder disease	BMI and running distance	Relative to least fit individuals, 75% reduction of risk in males running >4.75 m/s, 85% in females running >4 m/s

Table 3.4 continued

Authors	Subjects	Method of physical activity measurement	Indicator of disease	Covariates	Conclusions
Williams and Johnston [58]	97 rural Canadian women	Energy intake, 3 level classification of habitual physical activity	Ultrasono-graphic diagnosis of gallstones and/or cholecystec-tomy	Age, skinfold thicknesses	Low physical activity and low range of energy intake increased risk of gallbladder disease

Notes: BMI = body mass index; METs = metabolic equivalents

Positive findings

The study of Paul Williams[55] is the largest to report positive findings. He examined the independent effects of physical fitness (as inferred from 10 km race speed), habitual physical activity (the reported km/day of running) and body mass index on the risks of self-reported but clinician-diagnosed gallbladder disease in 29,110 male and 11,953 female runners. In this study, women with a body mass index >22. 5 kg/m² had a greater age-adjusted risk of gallbladder disease than that seen in the leanest women, and the risk accelerated sharply in those with a BMI above 27.5 kg/m². In terms of fitness, in men a running speed faster than 4.75 m/s reduced the risk by 83% (75% after adjusting for BMI and physical activity), and in women a speed >4 m/s reduced the risk by 93% (85% after adjusting for daily running distance and BMI) relative to individuals who were slower runners. The relationship of risk to habitual running distance (men: $p = 0.01$; females: $p = 0.008$) reflected largely the greater thinness of those who were running longer distances.

A second large study (Storti et al.[56]) carried out a logistic regression analysis on 8,010 post-menopausal women of average age 71 years, categorizing participants as either healthy or diseased (the latter group developing self-reported gallstones or requiring cholecystectomy). Modified Harvard questionnaire reports of habitual physical activity were divided into quartiles. Comparing the lowest two with the topmost physical activity quartile, the less active women had an odds-ratio of 1.57 (95% confidence interval 1.11–2.23) of developing gallbladder disease, after allowing statistically for the effects of body mass index and other known risk factors.

Walcher et al.[57] examined 2,129 adults. The overall prevalence of gallstones was 7.8%, and a multivariate analysis showed that the odds ratios for evidence of gallstones were 0.34 (95% CI 0.14–0.81) for those taking vitamin C supplements, 0.62 (CI 0.42–0.94) for those engaging in physical activity >2 h/week vs. <2 h/week, and 0.65 (CI 0.52–0.79) for those showing a high total cholesterol.

Finally, Williams and Johnston[58] looked at the prevalence of gallbladder disease in 97 rural Canadian women. The total daily energy intake was estimated from a four-day dietary record, and a three-level classification of habitual physical activity was made. After controlling for age, significant factors increasing the risk of gallbladder disease were skinfold thicknesses, reports of taking little physical activity and a limited range of energy intakes.

Negative findings

In contrast to the above reports, several quite large studies have failed to find significant associations between habitual physical activity and gallbladder disease. Friedman et al.[59] examined data from 5209 Framingham residents aged 30–62 years. Gallbladder disease was diagnosed from a combination of subjective reports and hospital records, and a simple classification of habitual physical activity was ascertained by interview. This investigation found no association between gallbladder disease and reported physical activity, but the authors admitted that analysis was made more difficult because there was little range of physical activity among their subjects.

Jorgensen[60, 61] made a four-level rating of both occupational and leisure activity in 3608 Danes aged 30–60 years. Body mass index (women), smoking (men only) and slimming treatment (men only) all showed significant associations with the risk of gallstones, but risk was unrelated to the simple index of habitual physical activity used in this investigation.

The Roman group for epidemiology and prevention of cholelithiasis (GREPCO)[64] undertook ultrasonographic examinations of 2325 Italian civil servants. A five-item questionnaire assessed habitual physical activity, but in a multivariate analysis, scores for this index showed no significant relationship to the risk of gallstones.

Pagliarulo et al.[66] studied risk factors for ultrasonographic evidence of gallstones in 1337 patients with diabetes mellitus. In this study, risk was linked to age, obesity and family history, but not to a three-level estimate of habitual physical activity.

Among other, smaller studies, Basso et al.[62] examined 512 pregnant women. A crude three-level classification of physical activity ("a lot", "a little" or "none") showed little relationship to the presence of gallstones as seen on ultrasound. Sakuta and Suzuki[67] examined risk factors for ultrasonographic evidence of gallstones in 974 male members of the Japanese defence forces. Gallstones were found in only 39 members; stones were associated with total homocysteine concentrations (but not with total cholesterol concentrations) after adjusting the data for lifestyle factors that included cigarette smoking, vegetable intake and habitual physical activity (a two-way classification, based on reports of undertaking sweat-producing activity). However, no comment was made about any association of risk with habitual physical activity.

Equivocal reports

Chuang et al.[63] studied 53 obese women who were undergoing gastric by-pass surgery. After allowing for the effects of BMI and HDL cholesterol levels, sport participation but not occupational or leisure activity reduced the odds of discovering gallstones during surgery.

Utter et al.[68] studied relationships among physical activity (as determined by an interviewer-administered questionnaire), diabetes mellitus and gallbladder disease in Puma Indians, a population with a high prevalence of clinically diagnosed gallstones. Among the men with diabetes, there was a clear decrease in incidence of gallstones from the least to the most active tertiles (14.1%, 6.1% and 4.7%). However, there were few gallstones among the non-diabetic men and an insufficient range of physical activity among the women to examine risks for the other categories of subject.

Longitudinal studies

Longitudinal studies have the advantage of greatly increasing the number of person-years of experience, and both habitual physical activity and the onset of gallbladder disease can often be determined more precisely. Three of four major trials have shown a substantial inverse association between physical activity and the risk of gallbladder disease (Table 3.5), and in two of the three trials, the level of physical activity was well known, since it was reassessed every two years. Banim et al.[69] carried out a 14-year prospective trial on 25,639 volunteers aged 40–74 years. The risk of developing gallstones was evaluated against an initial four-level categorization of occupational and leisure physical activity. Comparing the most active quartile against the three less active quartiles, the hazard ratio for the development of gallstones was a statistically significant 0.3 at 5 years, and a non-significant 0.70 (95% CI 0.49–1.01) at 14 years. The authors speculated that after ten years, their initial classification of physical activity was probably no longer valid for many subjects, thus explaining the weakening of the association.

Leitzmann et al.[70] completed an eight-year prospective study on 45,813 medical professionals, initially aged 40–75 years; 828 members of the group developed gallstones or underwent cholecystectomy over the course of the investigation. Comparing extremes of physical activity as determined by a detailed questionnaire, and allowing for multiple confounding variables that included diabetes mellitus, body mass index and the use of cholesterol-lowering drugs, the relative risk of gallbladder disease in the most active quintile (an estimated energy expenditure of 32.6 metabolic equivalents (MET)-h/week) was 0.65 in those aged <65 years and 0.75 in those aged >65 years. Risk was also independently associated with sedentary behaviour. Comparing those who watched >40 h of television per week with those who watched less than 6 h/wk, the risks of gallbladder disease for the sedentary individuals in 1.58 for younger men and 3.32 in older men.

Table 3.5 Longitudinal studies relating the onset of gallbladder disease to initial assessments of habitual physical activity

Authors	Subjects	Activity measurement	Diagnostic criterion	Covariates	Findings
Banim et al.[69]	25,639 volunteers	4-level categorization of occupational and leisure activity at entry to study	Medical diagnosis of biliary disease and/or ultra-sonography	BMI and other risk factors	Most active quartile vs. remaining quartiles; risk of gallstones in active quartile 0.3 at 5 years and 0.7 at 10 years
Kriska et al.[65]	2130 Puma Indians	Interviewer-conducted physical activity questionnaire at entry to study	Ultra-sonographic diagnosis of gallstones over 3–4 years	BMI and other confounding variables	Gallstones significantly related to inactivity, but relationship only statistically significant in those free of diabetes mellitus
Leitzmann et al.[70]	45,813 medical profes-sionals	Detailed physical activity questionnaire, reassessed every 2 years	History of gallstones or cholecystec-tomy	Diabetes, body mass index, use of cholesterol-lowering drugs	Relative risk (most active quintile, 32.6 MET-h/wk) vs. least active quintile) 0.65 if aged <65 yr, 0.75 if aged >65 yr. Adverse effects of TV watching (>40 vs <6h/wk) 1.58 (younger), 3.32 (older men)
Leitzmann et al.[71]	60,290 nurses initially aged 40–65 yr	Recreational physical activity and sedentary behaviour reassessed every 2 years for 10 years	Cholecystec-tomy	BMI and weight change	Relative risk of cholecystectomy, highest vs. lowest physical activity quintile, 0.69. Sitting time (>60 h vs. <6h) relative risk 2.32
Sahi et al.[72]	16,785 male Harvard alumni	Harvard physical activity questionnaire	Self-reported physician-diagnosis of gallbladder disease	BMI, cigarette smoking	No significant relationship between gallbladder disease in 1972 or 1977 and habitual physical activity as assessed in 1962–1966

Leitzmann et al.[71] collected reports of physical activity every two years for ten years in a study of 60,290 nurses who were initially aged 40–65 years. Using a multivariate analysis, they showed that the relative risk of cholecystectomy was 0.69 in the most active quintile relative to those in the least active quintile. The relative risk of cholecystectomy in those sitting >60 h/week vs. those sitting <6 h/week was also 2.32. Further, the risks associated with low physical activity and sedentary behaviour persisted after statistical adjustments for the effects of body mass index and changes of body mass.

Sahi et al.[72] made a prospective study of 16,785 male Harvard alumni, initially aged 15–24 years. Within this sample, body mass index and cigarette smoking but not physical activity as assessed for the period 1962–1966 were significant risk factors for self-reported, physician-diagnosed gallbladder disease as recorded in 1972 and 1977. As in the study of Banim et al.,[69] it is possible that relationships with physical activity were obscured by a change of lifestyle between 1962–1966 and 1977.

Kriska et al.[65] carried out a three to four year prospective trial on 2130 American Indians who were initially free of gallstones. Ultrasonography was undertaken at follow-up, and 650 of the sample were found to have developed gallbladder disease over the course of the trial. After adjusting for confounding variables including body mass index, gallbladder disease was inversely related to habitual physical activity as determined by an interviewer-conducted question-naire. However, this relationship was only statistically significant in those individuals who were free of diabetes (about a half of the total sample).

Case-control studies

With the exception of the investigation of Hou et al.[73], case-control studies have involved relatively small samples of subjects, with a corresponding limitation in their power to detect statistically significant benefits from a physically active lifestyle (Table 3.6).

Positive findings

Hou and associates[73] compared 8485 women with a self-reported physician diagnosis of gallstones versus 16,970 controls, matched by year of birth and age at diagnosis. Positive odds of developing gallbladder disease were associated with the highest vs. the lowest body mass index, with large waist and hip circum-ferences (3.82, 95% CI 2.47–5.23) and with the time spent sitting at work (p = 0.01). Negative odds were associated with questionnaire estimates of occupational (p = 0.03) and domestic (p = 0.02) physical activity, regardless of the individual's level of adiposity.

Two other studies presented positive findings. Ortega et al.[74] compared 54 patients with gallstones against 46 matched controls. Physical activity habits were assessed from a simple questionnaire based on the time spent in activities such as vigorous walking and sleeping. The controls were substantially more active than those with gallstones, but the two groups did not differ in body mass index. Ostrowska et al.[75] compared 169 patients with cholelithiasis and 203 controls. Preventive value was found in a moderate intensity of physical activity, both at work and in leisure time.

Table 3.6 Case-control trials of physical activity and gallbladder disease

Authors	Subjects	Physical activity or fitness indicator	Indicator of disease	Covariates	Findings
Hou et al.[73]	8485 cases, 16,970 controls	Questionnaire of occupational, commuting and domestic activity	Self-reported physician diagnosis of gallbladder disease	BMI, waist-hip circum-ferences	Gallstones positively related to sitting time and negatively associated with occupational and domestic activity
Ko et al.[76]	205 pregnant women with gallstones vs. 443 controls	Questionnaire and interviews	Ultra-sonographic diagnosis of gallbladder disease	BMI, HDL cholesterol, insulin resistance	Data was co-varied for physical activity, but any influence not stated
Linos et al.[79] Misciagna[80]	100 cases, 290 controls	10-item physical activity questionnaire	Ultra-sonographic diagnosis of gallbladder disease	Various constituents of diet	Energy expenditure of cases 7.05 MJ/d vs. 7.76 MJ/d in controls (p = 0.06)
Ortega et al.[74]	54 cases, 46 controls	Questions on walking time and sleeping time	Ultra-sonographic diagnosis of gallbladder disease	BMI	Controls substantially more physically active than cases
Ostrowska et al.[75]	54 patients, 46 controls	Simple questionnaire on walking and sleeping habits	Ultra-sonographic diagnosis of gallbladder disease	BMI	Controls show substantially more physical activity than those with gallstones
Sarles et al.[77]	101 female patients, 101 controls	Two simple questions on habitual physical activity	Radiology and/or surgery		No difference in body mass or response to physical activity questions
Wheeler et al.[78]	396 cases of chole-lithiasis, 397 controls	Physical activity inferred from total energy intake	"Proven gallstones"		Trend to lower physical activity in men developing gallstones; no difference in women

Negative findings

Ko and colleagues[76] compared 205 women who showed evidence of new gallbladder sludge or stones during pregnancy against 443 controls. A logistic
analysis showed that the effect of body mass index was attenuated after adjusting
for insulin resistance. Insulin resistance was a predictor of cholelithiasis, even
after adjusting for body mass index, HDL cholesterol and habitual physical
activity. Although physical activity was assessed in this study, there was no
discussion of its impact upon the risk of gallbladder disease; however, habitual
physical activity would likely have modified both body mass index and insulin
resistance.

Sarles et al.[77] compared 101 female patients where cholelithiasis was found at
operation or on radiography with 101 controls. The patients with gallstones had a
greater energy intake than the controls, but neither physical activity (as assessed
by questions such as "how active is your life?" and "do you like walking?") nor
body mass differed significantly between cases and controls.

Equivocal findings

Wheeler et al.[78] compared 396 patients with clinically-proven cholelithiasis
against 397 controls. The main focus of their study was upon diet, but physical
activity levels were inferred from total energy intakes; there was an insignificant
trend to a lower energy intake (and thus presumably a lower level of physical
activity) in the men who had developed gallstones, but no differences of energy
intake were found between female cases and controls.

Linos and associates[79] compared 100 small-town Italians with gallstones
against 290 matched control subjects. A multiple regression analysis that also
included dietary characteristics showed a nearly significant trend to an
association between gallstones and a lack of physical activity (as assessed by a
ten-item physical activity questionnaire). Other significant risk factors were a diet
rich in animal fats and refined sugars but poor in vegetables. The estimated
energy expenditures for cases and controls were 7.05 and 7.76 MJ/d, respectively
($p = 0.06$). Misciagna et al.[80] reported further details on what appear to have been
the same 100 cases and 290 controls, reaching essentially the same conclusions.

Randomized controlled trials

There have as yet been only three small-scale randomized controlled trials of
physical activity as a means of reducing the risk of developing gallstones in
individuals who were initially free of gallbladder disease (Table 3.7). In each
study, subjects in the intervention group were encouraged to increase their weekly
volume of physical activity, but the change in behaviour relative to control
subjects was quite modest. Moreover, given the sample sizes, even with a ten-
year follow-up, the number of patients developing gallstones was too small to
anticipate strong statistical evidence of health benefit.

Table 3.7 Randomized controlled trials relating physical activity to the risk of developing gallbladder disease

Authors	Subjects	Experimental approach	Diagnostic criterion	Covariates	Findings
Randomized controlled trials (humans)					
Ko et al.[82]	Pregnant women (591 intervention, 605 controls)	Physical activity of intervention group increased by motivational materials and small group instruction	Ultra-sonographic diagnosis of gallstones		No difference of sludge or stones at 18 or 36 weeks (but increases of physical activity quite modest)
Rexroad et al.[81]	171 post-menopausal women, half assigned to a walking programme	Walking group energy expenditures 4.9 vs. 2.8 MJ/week for control group	Not stated	Age, body mass	10-year incidence of gallbladder disease 4.8% vs. 9.1% (n.s.)
Storti et al.[56]	182 elderly women aged 74 years	7-year walking intervention, objective activity monitor	Self-report of gallbladder surgery or physician-diagnosed gallstones	BMI, hormone use, smoking and other risk factors	Odds ratio 1.13 lowest vs. highest tertile of walking activity
Randomized controlled trial (mice)					
Wilund et al.[83]	50 gallstone-sensitive (C57/L/J) mice	Experimental group ran for 12 weeks, 45 min/d at 15 m/min	Collective weight of gallstones at euthanasia		Sedentary vs. exercised animals 143 vs. 57 g of gallstones

Note: n.s. = non-significant.

Rexroad et al.[81] carried out a ten-year follow up of 171 post-menopausal women who were initially free of gallbladder disease. Subjects were randomly assigned to a walking programme or a control group. At the end of the trial, the respective reported walking energy expenditures were 4.9 and 2.8 MJ/week. There was a statistically non-significant tendency ($p = 0.27$) to a difference in the number of diagnoses of gallbladder disease over the ten years (4.8% vs. 9.1%, 4 vs. 8 cases), and this difference became larger and statistically significant ($p < 0.05$) when a post-hoc comparison was drawn between highly active members of the intervention group vs. low active members of the control group (2.1% vs. 13.9%, 1 vs. 5 cases). Adjustment for age and body mass did not diminish these effects.

Storti et al.[56] carried out a randomized controlled trial of a walking intervention on 182 elderly women (average age 74 years). They followed their subjects for seven years. Women in the lowest tertile of habitual physical activity as determined by an objective electronic monitor had a higher risk of self-reported physician diagnosed gallstone disease than those in the top tertile (odds ratio 1.13, 95% confidence interval 1.01–1.28; 6 vs. 0 cases).

Ko et al.[82] randomized pregnant women between what was intended as a moderate exercise intervention (n = 591) and a control group (n = 605). The intervention (motivational materials and participation in small group educational sessions) produced only modest increases in reported physical activity, and the incidence of gallbladder sludge and/or stones in the experimental subjects was unchanged relative to that in the control group at either the 18th or the 36th week of pregnancy (25 vs. 20 cases).

Animal experiments

Animal experiments have the advantage that the daily dose of physical activity can be closely controlled. However, it is not easy to transfer the conclusions to humans. The enforced exercise is often stressful for the animal, there are substantial differences of anatomy and physiology between laboratory animals and humans, and it is difficult to evaluate effects from differences of body size and life span.

Wilund and associates[83] carried out a small controlled trial on a sample of 50 gallstone-sensitive (C57-L/J) mice. Animals in the experimental group ran on a treadmill for 12 weeks, 45 min/day at a speed of 15 m/min, and they were then euthanized. The pooled weight of gallstones was 2.5 times greater in the animals that had remained sedentary than in the experimental group (a total weight of 153 vs. 57 mg). However, by the end of the experiment, the sedentary animals were also more obese than those in the experimental group, and the accumulation of fat could have contributed to the greater gallstone formation in control animals.

Overall conclusions

The overall findings are by no means unanimous. In cross-sectional comparisons, some have seen a reduced frequency of gallbladder disease in individuals who were physically more active,[55–58] but others have reported equivocal findings[63, 65, 68] or have observed no such association.[59–62, 64, 66, 67] Nevertheless, studies finding a significant effect were mostly those with the largest sample size.[55–57] Possibly, the absence of a significant effect in other cross-sectional studies could reflect an inadequate sample size and/or a weak assessment of habitual physical activity. Longitudinal studies generally support the cross-sectional work, with three of four major investigations showing substantial benefit to the physically active group. Leitzmann et al.[70] concluded that the risk of gallstone disease could be reduced 34% by taking as little as 30 minutes of aerobic exercise five times/week.

Case-control studies provide further tentative support for the health benefits of regular physical activity; three reports (including by far the largest of seven studies[73]) showed positive effects, and in two other papers there were non-significant trends towards benefit. One small study with a weak measure of physical activity showed no benefit, and in the final study there was no comment on any possible effect of physical activity.

Randomized controlled trials have not to date resolved these controversies. The increases of habitual physical activity achieved by experimental interventions have been quite small, and with the sample sizes used, the number of cases developing gallstones have been too few to demonstrate a statistically significant effect. There are many differences between laboratory animals and human subjects, but a single trial in mice supports the view that regular exercise reduces the risk of gallstones.

Neverthelss, the weight of evidence seems to point towards a reduced risk of gallbladder disease in those who are active, and this seems one more reason for clinicians to urge adoption at least the minimum recommended levels of daily physical activity.

Possible mechanisms of altered risk

If indeed the risk of gallbladder disease is diminished by engaging in regular physical activity, what are the likely mechanisms of benefit? One tempting explanation is a reduction of biliary stasis, brought about by an increase of gallbladder motility[44, 84, 85] that is mediated through increased neural stimulation, cholecystokinin secretion[86, 87] and/or an increase of gastro-intestinal transit rates.[84] However, the empirical data supporting any decrease in biliary stasis are by no means conclusive. Regular exercise could also address other major risk factors, including obesity, a high serum cholesterol level and type 2 diabetes mellitus. Moreover, a focus upon individuals who adopt an active lifestyle could identify health-conscious people who have favourable dietary practices and avoid cigarette smoking. However, some published trials have controlled for such co-variates, and these studies suggest that regular physical activity reduces the risk of cholelithiasis beyond any effects attributable to the control of body mass, diet and other risk factors.[69-71] Regular physical activity speeds gastro-intestinal transit[84] and this could decrease the resorption of cholesterol from the large intestine,[84, 88] thus reducing the risk of a supersaturation of the bile.[49, 63, 87] Finally, regular physical activity could act upon the liver, modifying the synthesis of cholesterol phospholipids and bile acids and/or altering their excretion into the bile.[83]

Studies in mice bred for their susceptibility to gallbladder disease have shown that training also increases the hepatic expression of two genes (*LDLr* and *SRB1*) that are known to be involved in the clearance of cholesterol. Exercised mice demonstrate an up-regulation of the protein Cyp27 that is associated with the hepatic production of bile acids.[83] The net effect of exercise upon the intestinal reabsorption of cholesterol remains less clear. Trained animals show a reduced expression of NPC1L1 (which would reduce cholesterol reabsorption), but at the same time there is a reduction in the expression of ABCG5 and G8 (which would have the effect of increasing cholesterol reabsorption).[83]

Physical activity and gallbladder cancer

Gallbladder cancer accounts for 80–95% of malignant lesions of the biliary tract. The incidence in North America is quite low (about 1.5/100,000 people). Three papers have examined associations between habitual physical activity and the risk of developing such neoplasms (Table 3.8). In order to accumulate an adequate number of cases, investigators have needed to follow very large populations for long periods, and the measures of habitual physical activity have been correspondingly weak.

Behrens et al.[89] examined data on 507,981 participants in the National Institutes of Health-Association of Aging and Retired Persons (NIH-AARP) Diet and Health Study. They looked at the association between the frequency per week of physical activity (lasting >20 min and of sufficient intensity to work up a sweat) and the risk of hepato-biliary cancer. Over a ten-year follow-up, there were 317 cases of incident biliary cancer. A multivariate analysis compared the most active (vigorously active >5/week) with the least active individuals (never or rarely engaging in vigorous activity). When data were simply adjusted for age

Table 3.8 Prospective studies showing a possible association between habitual physical activity or fitness level and the risk of gallbladder or biliary tract cancer

Author	Subjects	Measure of activity or fitness	Covariates	Conclusions
Behrens et al.[89]	507,981 individuals initially aged 50–71 years	Frequency of activity bouts lasting >20 min and of sufficient intensity to develop a sweat	Multiple variables, including BMI	317 cases of biliary cancer in 10 year follow-up; most active quartile vs. 3 least active quartiles, relative risk 0.63 (0.33–1.21)
Peel et al.[91]	38,801 men attending Cooper Aerobics Center	Treadmill endurance time	Age, smoking, alcohol consumption, diabetes, family history of cancer, BMI	7 cases of gallbladder cancer over up to 28 years. Non-significant trend favouring fit over unfit individuals (RR 0.83, 0.09–7.74)
Yun et al.[90]	444,693 men aged >40 years	2-level classification of habitual physical activity	Dietary preferences	Almost significant reduction of risk of gallbladder cancer for those with moderate or vigorous physical activity (RR 0.81, 0.65–1.02)

and sex, there was a suggestion of benefit (odds ratio 0.47 for the active individuals), but with a fuller multivariate analysis that included other known risk factors, somewhat favourable trends were no longer statistically significant for tumours in the extra-hepatic bile duct (0.86, 95% CI 0.45–1.65), the ampulla of Vater (0.66, 95% CI 0.29–1.48) or the gallbladder itself (0.63, 95% CI 0.33–1.21).

Yun et al.[90] made a six-year follow up of 444,693 Korean men aged >40 years, including their reported dietary preferences as co-variates in the analysis. A two-level classification of habitual physical activity yielded an almost significant reduction in the risk of gallbladder cancer among those who habitually engaged in moderate or vigorous physical activity (risk ratio 0.81, 95% CI 0.65–1.02).

Peel et al.[91] used treadmill endurance times as a measure of attained aerobic fitness and a presumed surrogate of habitual physical activity in a study of 38,801 men attending the Cooper Aerobics Center in Dallas, Texas. Over a 28-year follow-up there were only seven cases of gallbladder cancer, but these cases showed a weak non-significant trend favouring the fit over unfit individuals (relative risk 0.83, 95% CI 0.09–7.74).

Thus, all three prospective studies of habitual physical activity and biliary tract cancer showed a non-significant trend to a reduced risk of gallbladder cancer in the more active individuals. Further investigation with even larger samples and/or a meta-analytic combination of data from several studies may in the future provide a statistically more convincing proof that regular physical activity has significant value in preventing cancer of the biliary tract. If indeed the reduced risk is confirmed by further study, possible mechanisms of benefit could include not only a lesser frequency of cholecystitis, but also a reduction of body mass, an increase of insulin sensitivity, a reduction of oxidant stress and a lesser likelihood of cigarette consumption among regular exercisers.[89]

Areas for further research

There is scope for further study of cholecystokinin concentrations, coupling this data with measures of gallbladder emptying.[41] Moreover, further investigations are needed to clarify conflicting evidence concerning the effects of physical activity and gallbladder function.[44, 45]

In terms of gallbladder disease, objective pedometer/accelerometer monitoring could be used to provide more accurate information on the volume of physical activity undertaken in cross-sectional, prospective and case-control trials. Such monitors are now sufficiently inexpensive that it is possible to collect data on large population samples, particularly older individuals whose main form of daily activity is walking. There is also scope for more randomized controlled trials, both in humans and in animals. In human trials, the incidence of gallbladder disease could possibly be increased by focusing on recruiting high-risk groups, as in the animal experiments of Wilund et al.[83] A meta-analysis of closely similar trials might also serve to accumulate sufficient data to demonstrate statistically significant effects. Meta-analysis certainly seems the only approach that is likely to yield an adequate number of cases to test the effects if physical activity upon gallbladder cancer.

Practical implications and conclusions

Gallstones form if supersaturated biliary fluid remains in the gallbladder for too long. Gallstones predispose to chronic infection and cancerous change in the biliary tract. Current evidence suggests that an acute bout of physical activity may increase the motility and emptying of the gallbladder, thus reducing the risk of gallstone formation and limiting exposure of the gallbladder to carcinogenic chemicals. Although many investigations have now examined the influence of acute and chronic physical activity upon gallbladder function and susceptibility to disease, the findings remain suggestive rather than conclusive. In terms of gall-bladder motility and biliary stasis, one uncontrolled report suggested a modest benefit from four weeks of aerobic exercise, and a second study found a similar change following 12 weeks of roughly equivalent physical activity, but any change was not significant relative to control subjects. Many cross-sectional, prospective and case-control studies have pointed towards some reduction in the risk of gallbladder disease among physically more active individuals, but randomized controlled trials have lacked the statistical power to confirm these observations. Nevertheless, observations on gallstone-sensitive mice support the overall inference from human studies that there is indeed some benefit from regular physical activity.

The potential clinical value of exercise programmes in preventing gallstone formation could be substantial. One prospective five-year study of 25,639 adults suggested that after adjusting for other risk factors, individuals with the highest level of physical activity had a 70% lower risk of symptomatic gallstones than those who were sedentary.[69] This particular report left unclear whether physical activity had actually reduced the risk of gallstone formation, or whether it had merely made the onset of symptoms less likely. However, other studies with ultrasonographic monitoring of gallstone formation[12] have provided good evidence that not only are symptoms reduced, but the prevalence of gallstones is lower among individuals who engage in regular physical activity.

The practicality of encouraging greater physical activity in those who are at risk is less clearly established. The person who develops gallstones is typically an obese middle-aged woman, and it is not easy to bring about and sustain a substantial increase of physical activity in such a population. The prospective study of Banim et al.[69] estimated that 161 patients would have to be treated in order to avert a single case of symptomatic gallstones. Possibly, programmes should be justified in part on the basis of the remaining 160 people who make substantial increases in their habitual physical activity and who thus gain important health advantages unrelated to changes in gallbladder function.

Chronic gallbladder infection also predisposes to cancer of the biliary tract, and a limited number of prospective studies suggest that regular physical activity may reduce this risk.

References

1. Shephard RJ. An *illustrated history of health and fitness, from pre-history to our post-modern world*. Cham, Switzerland: Springer 2015.
2. Attili AF, Carulli N, Roda E, et al. Epidemiology of gallstone disease in Italy; prevalence data of the Multicenter Italian study on cholelithiasis. *Am J Epidemiol* 1995; 141: 158–165.
3. Bowen JC, Brenner HI, Ferrante WA, et al. Gallstone disease. *Med Clin N Am* 1992; 76(5): 1143–1157.
4. Hofmann AF. Primary and secondary prevention of gallstone disease. Implications for patient management and research priorities. *Am J Surg* 1993; 165: 541–548.
5. Kratzer W, Mason RA, Kachele V. Prevalence of gallstones in sonographic surveys worldwide. *J Clin Ultrasound* 1999; 27: 1–7.
6. Patanakar R, Ozmen MM, Bailey IS, et al. Gall bladder motility, gallstones and the surgeon. *Dig Dis Sci* 1995; 40(11): 2323–2335.
7. Sandler RS, Everhart JE, Donowitz M, et al. The burden of selected digestive diseases in the United States. *Gastroenterology* 2002; 122: 1500–1511.
8. Stinton LM, Shaffer AA. Epidemiology of gallbladder disease: cholelithiasis and cancer. *Gut Liver* 2012; 6(2): 172–187.
9. Schirmer BD, Winters KL, Edlich RF. Cholelithiasis and cholecystitis. *J Long Term Eff Med Implants* 2005; 15(3): 329–338.
10. Trivedi V, Gumaste VV, Liu S, et al. Gallbladder cancer. *Gastroenterol Hepatol* 2008; 4(10): 735–737.
11. Deibert P, König D, Allgaier H-P, et al. Sport und Verdauungssystem (sport and the digestive system). *Dtsch Med Wochenschr* 2007; 132(4): 155–160.
12. de Oliveira EP, Burini RC. The impact of physical exercise on the gastrointestinal tract. *Curr Opin Clin Nutr Metabol Care* 2009; 12: 533–538.
13. Jeong SU, Lee SK. [Obesity and gallbladder diseases]. [Review] [Korean]. *Kor J Gastroenterol* 2012; 59(1): 27–34.
14. Khazaeinia T, Ramsey AA, Tam YK. The effect of exercise on the pharmacokinetics of drugs. J *Pharm Pharmaceut Sci* 2000; 3(3): 292–302.
15. Lammert F, Matern S. Evidenzbasierte Prävention der Cholezystolithiasis (evidence-based prevention of cholecystoliathis). *Dtsch Med Wochenschr* 129(28): 1548–50.
16. Moga MM. Alternative treatment of gallbladder disease. *Med Hypoth* 2003; 60(1): 143–147.
17. Peters HPF, deVries WR. Potential benefits and hazards of physical activity and exercise on the gastrointestinal tract. *Gut* 2001; 48: 435–439.
18. Rissanen A, Fogelholm M. Physical activity in the prevention and treatment of other morbid conditions and impairments associated with obesity: current evidence and research issues. *Med Sci Sports Exerc* 1999; 31(11 Suppl): S635–S645.
19. Shaffer E. Gallstone disease: epidemiology of gallbladder stone disease. *Best Pract Res Clin Gastroenterol* 2006; 20(6): 981–986.
20. Simrén M. Physical activity and the gastrointestinal tract. *Eur Rev Gastroenterol Hepatol* 2002; 14: 1053–1056.
21. Utter AC, Goss F. Exercise and gall bladder function. *Sports Med* 1997; 23(4): 218–227.
22. Portincasa P, Stolk MF, Van Erpecum KJ, et al. Cholesterol gallstone formation in man and potential treatments of the gallbladder motility defect. *Scand J Gastro-emterol* 1995; 30 Suppl. 212: 63–78.

23. Cuevas A, Miquel JF, Reyes MS, et al. Diet as a risk factor for cholesterol gallstone disease. *J Am Coll Nutr* 2004; 23: 187–196.

24. Everhart JD, Khare M, Hill M, et al. Prevalence and ethnic differences in gallbladder disease in the United States. *Gastroenterology* 1999; 117: 632–639.

25. Hammarsten O, Mandel JA. *Textbook of physiological chemistry*. New York, NY, J. Wiley, 1906.

26. McMaster PD. Studies on the total bile. VI. The influence of diet upon the output of cholesterol in the bile. *J Exp Med* 1924; 40(1): 25–42.

27. Fisher RS, Rock E, Malmud S. Choilinergic effects on gall bladder emptying in humans. *Gastroenterology* 1985; 89: 716–722.

28. Amer MS. Studies with cholecystokinin in vitro. III: mechanism of the effect on the isolated gall bladder strips. *J Pharmacol Exp Ther* 1972; 183(3): 527–534.

29. Ivy AC, Oldberg E. A hormone mechanism for gallbladder contraction and evacuation. *Am J Physiol* 1928; 86: 599–613.

30. Strah KM, Melendez RL, Pappas TN, et al. Interactions of vasoactive intestinal polypeptide and cholecystokinin octapeptide on the control of gall bladder contraction. *Surgery* 1986; 99(4): 469–473.

31. O'Donnell LJ, Fairclough PD. Gall stones and gall bladder motility. *Gut* 1993; 34(4): 440–443.

32. Malagelada JR, Holtermuller KH, Sizemore GW, et al. The influence of hypercalcemia on basal and CCK stimulated pancreatic, gall bladder and gastric function in man. *Gastroenterology* 1976; 71: 405–408.

33. Meyer BM, Werth BA, Berlinger C, et al. Role of cholecystokinin in regulation of gastrointestinal motor function. *Lancet* 1989; 2(8653): 12–15.

34. Tierney S, Pitt HA, Lillemoe KD. Physiology and pathophysiology of gall bladder motility. *Surg Clin North Am* 1993; 37(6): 1267–1291.

35. Kapicioglu S, Gürbüz S, Danalioglu A, et al. Measurement of gallbladder volume with ultrasonography in pregnant women. *Can J Gastroenterol* 2000; 14(5): 403–405.

36. Palframan A, Meire HB. Real-time ultrasound. A new method for studying gallbladder kinetics. *Br J Radiol* 1979; 52: 801–803.

37. Akintomade AO, Eduwem DU. Ultrasonograpohic assessment of the fasting gallbladder volume in healthy adults in Calabar; correlatiion with body weight. *IOSR J Dent Med Sci* 2013; 4(6): 64–68.

38. Utter AC, Goss FL, Whitcomb DC, et al. The effects of acute exercise on gall bladder function in an adult female population. *Med Sci Sports Exerc* 1996; 28(3): 280–284.

39. Donald JJ, Fache JS, Buckley AR, et al. Gallbladder contractility: variation in normal subjects. *Am J Roentgenol* 1991; 157(4): 753–756.

40. McMaster PD, Broun GO, Rous P. Studies on the total bile: 1. The effects of operation, exercise, hot weather, relief of obstruction, intercurrent disease, and other normal and pathological influences. *J Exp Med* 1923; 37(3): 395–420.

41. Philipp E, Wilckens T, Friess E, et al. Cholecystokinin, gastrin and stress hormone responses in marathon runners. *Peptides* 1992; 13(1): 125–128.

42. Vezina WC, Paradis RL, Grace DM, et al. Increased volume and decreased emptying of the gallbladder in large (morbidly obese, tall normal, and muscular normal) people. *Gastroenterology* 1990; 98: 1000–1007.

43. Mathus-Vliegen EMH, Van Ierland-Van Leeuwen ML, Terpstra A. Determinants of gallbladder kinetics in obesity. *Dig Dis Sci* 2004; 49(1): 9–16.

44. Utter AC, Whitcomb DC, Butterworth DE, et al. Effects of exercise training on gallbladder function in an obese female population. *Med Sci Sports Exerc* 2000; 32(1): 41–45.

45. Sari R, Balci N, Balci MK. Effects of exercise on gallbladder volume and motility in obese women. *J Clin Ultrasound* 2005; 33(5): 218–222.

46. Choi J, Klinkspoor JH, Yoshida T, et al. Lipopolysaccharide from Escherichia coli stimulates mucin secretion by cultured dog gallbladder epithelial cells. *Hepatology* 1999; 29(5): 1352–1357.

47. Marschall HU, Einarsson C. Gallstone disease. *J Intern Med* 2007; 261(6): 529–542.

48. Wang DQ, Zhang I, Wang HH. High cholesterol absorption efficiency and rapid biliary secretion of chylomicron remnant cholesterol enhance cholelithogenesis in gallstone susceptible mice. *Biochem Biophys Acta* 2005; 1733(1): 90–99.

49. Portincasa P, Van Erpecum KJ, Vaberge-Hengouwen GP. Cholesterol crystallization in bile. *Gut* 1997; 41: 138–141.

50. Portincasa P, Moschetta A, Palasciano G. Cholesterol gallstone disease. *Lancet* 2006; 368: 230–239.

51. Vennemann NG, Van Erpecum KJ. Pathogenesis of gallstones. *Gastroenterol Clin N Am* 2010; 39: 171–183.

52. Carey MC, Lamont JT. Cholesterol gallstone formation. 1. Physical chemistry of bile and biliary lipid secretion. *Prog Liver Dis* 1992; 10: 139–163.

53. Plevris JN, Bouchier IAD. Defective acid base regulation by the gallbladder epithelium and its significance for gallstone formation. *Gut* 1995; 37: 127–131.

54. Sarin SK, Kapur BML, Tandon RK. Cholesterol and pigment stones in Northern India: A prospective analysis. *Dig Dis Sci* 1986; 31(10): 1041–1045.

55. Williams PT. Independent effects of cardiorespiratory fitness, vigorous physical activity, and body mass index on clinical gallbladder disease risk. *Am J Gastroenterol* 2008; 103(9): 2239–2247.

56. Storti KL, Brauch JS, Fitzgerald SJ, et al. Physical activity and decreased risk of clinical gallstone disease among post-menopausal women. *Prev Med* 2005; 41(3–4): 772–777.

57. Walcher T, Haenle MM, Kron M, et al. Vitamin C supplement use may protect against gallstones: an observational study on a randomly selected population. *BMC Gastroenterol* 2009; 9: 74.

58. Williams CN, Johnston JL. Prevalence of gallstones and risk factors in Caucasian women in a rural Canadian community. *Can Med Assoc J* 1980; 120: 664–668.

59. Friedman GD, Kannel WB, Dawber TR. The epidemiology of gall bladder disease: observations in the Framingham study. *J Chron Dis* 1966; 19: 273–292.

60. Jørgensen T. Gall stones in a Danish population. Relation to weight, physical activity, smoking, coffee consumption,and diabetes mellitus. *Gut* 1989; 30: 528–534.

61. Jørgensen T, Jørgensen L. Gallstones and diet in a Danish population. *Scand J Gastroenterol* 1989; 24: 821–826.

62. Basso L, McCollum PT, Darling MRN, et al. A descriptive study of pregnant women with gallstones, relation to dietary and social habits, education, physical activity, height and weight. *Eur J Epidemiol* 1992; 8(5): 629–633.

63. Chuang CZ, Martin LF, LeGardeur BY, et al. Physical activity, biliary lipids, and gallstones in obese subjects. *Am J Gastroenterol* 2001; 96: 1860–1865.

64. GREPCO. The epidemiology of gallstone disease in Rome, Part II: factors associated with the disease. *Hepatology* 1988; 8(4): 907–13.

65. Kriska AM, Brach JS, Jarvis BJ, et al. Physical activity and gallbladder disease determined by ultrasonography. *Med Sci Sports Exerc* 2007; 39(11): 1927–1932.
66. Pagliarulo M, Fornari F, Fraquelli M, et al. Gallstone disease and related risk factors in a large cohort of diabetic patients. *Dig Liv Dis* 2004; 36(2): 130–134.
67. Sakuta H, Suzuki T. Plasma total homocysteine and gallstone in middle-aged Japanese men. *J Gastroenterol* 2005; 40(11): 1061–1064.
68. Utter AC, Kriska AM, Fernandes RJ, et al. The association between physical activity and gallbladder disease among Pima Indians. *Med Sci Sports Exerc* 1995; 32(5 Suppl.): S57.
69. Banim PJR, Luben RN, Wareham NJ, et al. Physical activity reduces the risk of symptomatic gallstones: a prospective cohort study. *Eur J Gastroenterol Hepatol* 2010; 22(8): 983–988.
70. Leitzmann MF, Giovannucci EL, Rimm EB, et al. The relation of physical activity to risk for symptomatic gallstone disease in men. *Ann Int Med* 1998; 128(6): 417–425.
71. Leitzmann MF, Rimm EB, Willett WC, et al. Recreational physical activity and the risk of cholecystectomy in women. *N Engl J Med* 1999; 341: 777–784.
72. Sahi T, Paffenbarger RS, Gsieh CC, et al. Body mass index, cigarette smoking, and other characteristics as predictors of self-reported, physician-diagnosed gallbladder disease in male college alumni. *Am J Epidemiol* 1998; 147(7): 644–651.
73. Hou L, Shu X-O, Gao Y-T, et al. Anthropometric measurements, physical activity, and the risk of symptomatic gallstone disease in Chinese women. *Ann Epidemiol* 2009; 19(5): 344–350.
74. Ortega RM, Fernandez-Azuela M, Encinas-Sortillos A, et al. Differences in diet and food habits between patients with gallstones and controls. *J Am Coll Nutr* 1999; 16: 88–95.
75. Ostrowska L, Karczewski J, Serwin AB. Wpływ społeczno-zawodowa w trakcie kamicy żółciowej [Occupational-social influence in the course of cholelithiasis]. *Med Pr* 1996; 47(5): 461–465.
76. Ko CW, Beresford SAA, Schilte SJ, et al. Insulin resistance and incident gallbladder disease in pregnancy. *Clin Gastroenterol Hepatol* 2008; 6(1): 76–81.
77. Sarles H, Chabert C, Pommeau Y, et al. Diet and cholesterol gallstones: A study of 101 patients with cholelithiasis compared to 101 matched controls. *Am J Dig Dis* 1969; 14(8): 531–537.
78. Wheeler M, Hills LL, Laby B. Cholelithiasis: a clinical and dietary survey. *Gut* 1970; 11: 430–437.
79. Linos AS, Daras V, Linos DA, et al. Dietary and other risk factors in aetiology of cholelithiasis: A case control study. *HPB Surgery* 1989; 1: 221–227.
80. Misciagna G, Centonze S, Leoci C, et al. Diet, physical activity, and gallstones – a population-based, case-control study in southern Italy. *Am J Clin Nutr* 1999; 69(1): 120–126.
81. Rexroad AR, Fitzgerad AS, Pereira MA, et al. Effect of walking intervention on ten-year cumulative incidence of gallbladder disease. *Med Sci Sports Exerc* 1998; 30(5 Suppl): S134.
82. Ko CW, Napolitano PG, Lee SP, et al. Physical activity, maternal metabolic measures, and the incidence of gallbladder sludge or stones during pregnancy: a randomized trial. *Am J Perinatol* 2014; 31(1): 39–48.
83. Wilund KR, Feeney LA, Tomayko EJ, et al. Endurance exercise training reduces gallstone development in mice. *J Appl Physiol* 2008; 104: 761–765.

84. Oettle GJ. Effect of moderate exercise on bowel habit. *Gut* 1991; 32: 941–949.

85. Veysey MJ, Thomas LA, Mallet AI, et al. Prolonged large bowel transit time increases serum deoxycholic acid: a risk factor for octreide induced gallstones. *Gut* 1999; 44: 675–681.

86. Sullivan SN, Champion MC, Christofides ND, et al. Gastrointestinal regulatory peptide responses in long distance runners. *Phys Sports Med* 1984; 12(7): 77–82.

87. Reshetnyak VI. Concept of the pathogenesis and treatment of cholelithiasis. *World J Hepatol* 2012; 4(2): 18–34.

88. Meissner M, Havinga R, Boverhof R, et. al. Exercise enhances whole-body cholesterol turnover in mice. *Med Sci Sports Exerc* 2010; 42(8): 1460–1468.

89. Behrens G, Matthews CE, Moore SC, et al. The association between frequency of vigorous physical activity and hepatobiliary cancers in the NIH-AARP Diet and Health Study. *Eur J Epidemiol* 2013; 28(1): 55–66.

90. Yun YH, Lim MK, Won YJ, et al. Dietary preference, physical activity, and cancer risk in men: national health insurance corporation study. *BMC Cancer* 2008; 8: 366.

91. Peel JB, Sui X, Matthews CE, et al. Cardiorespiratory fitness and digestive cancer mortality: findings from the aerobics center longitudinal study. *Cancer Epidemiol Biomarkers Prev* 2009; 18(4): 1111–1117.

4 Physical activity and kidney function in health and disease

Introduction

This chapter examines the impact of physical activity upon the normal functioning of the kidneys, and explores such manifestations of temporary dysfunction as exercise-induced microproteinuria and microhaematuria. It also considers the potential of developing acute renal failure during a prolonged bout of exhausting exercise and the possibility of chronic renal damage in athletes with an excessive intake of creatine supplements or non-steroidal anti-inflammatory drugs (NSAIDs). Turning to issues of renal disease, it then examines the place of exercise programmes in the rehabilitation of patients who are undergoing dialysis or who have received renal transplants, and it considers the possibility that regular physical activity may reduce the risk of renal cancer. Finally, it looks at the impact of physical activity upon the endocrine function of the kidneys and the development of kidney stones. The following chapter discusses the tricky clinical issue of advice that should be given to the competitive athlete who has only a single kidney.

Physiological background

The kidneys play an important role in the maintenance of fluid and electrolyte homeostasis at rest, and this function becomes even more critical when equilibrium is challenged by the demands of athlete who engages in vigorous physical activity. An interplay between renal artery perfusion pressure and sodium excretion influences the renin-angiotensin-aldosterone system, thus making an important contribution to the regulation of systemic blood pressure. However, the impact of acute and chronic physical activity upon function of the healthy kidney has received relatively little attention in physiological texts, and even less is known about interactions between habitual physical activity and long-term renal health.

When writing *The Physiology of Muscular Exercise* in 1919, Francis Bainbridge[1] did not discuss renal issues. Other books on exercise physiology written from the 1930s to the 1970s[2–5] also gave scant recognition to the impact of physical activity upon the renal system, although there were some exceptions.

Sir Charles Lovatt Evans[6] commented in a general physiology text "a small trace of albumin will often be found in the urine which is passed shortly after taking muscular exercise, but it has no pathognomic significance". Laurence Wesson[7] also contributed a brief chapter on kidney function to a text on exercise and sports medicine, emphasizing the adjustments of renal plasma flow and glomerular filtration rates that were seen during a bout of vigorous exercise, and David Lamb[8] devoted an 11-page chapter to the kidneys in his exercise physiology text.

Others have focused on such overt responses to vigorous physical activity as proteinuria, haemoglobinuria and myoglobinuria.[9-11] In 1878, von Leube[12] noted proteinuria in 14 of 119 soldiers after they had completed a strenuous 1–3 day march, and in 1910 J.H. Barach[13] commented on microscopic haematuria in 18 of 19 marathon runners shortly after they had completed their event. Barach pointed out that runners with the highest blood pressures at the end of the race excreted the most protein. In contrast, Hellebrandt attributed albuminuria to the drop in blood pressure that commonly followed a bout of strenuous exercise.[14] Edwards et al.[15] observed that 13 of 13 football players had albuminuria after 45–60 minutes of play. Jundell and Fries emphasized that at any given intensity of effort, the extent of proteinuria was reduced after subjects had undergone aerobic training.[16]

The diversion of renal plasma flow from the kidneys to the working muscles was first inferred by Edwards and colleagues[17] on the basis of an exercise-related reduction of urea clearance, a phenomenon noticed earlier by Addis and Drury[18] and by MacKay.[19] The magnitude of such changes was first estimated by Barclay et al.[20], using a diodrast clearance technique. A full-speed 400 m run caused a 45% decrease in glomerular filtration and a 39% decrease in renal blood flow. White and Rolf confirmed these observations, noting that while light jogging induced little change, heavy exercise could reduce renal perfusion by up to 80%, with a five-fold increase of renal vascular resistance.[21] Observations by Chapman et al.[22] and Grimby[23] demonstrated the impact of both absolute and relative exercise intensity on the reduction of plasma flow, with persistence of the flow deficit for as long as 40 minutes following exercise. Robinson and colleagues further demonstrated that that these adverse changes were exacerbated if an athlete was dehydrated or exercising in a hot environment.[24, 25]

In 1921, Campbell and Webster introduced the idea of measuring glomerular filtration in terms of creatinine excretion.[26, 27] Their attempts to determine how filtration was affected by physical activity led to inconclusive results, but subsequent authors have used both creatinine[28] and inulin[20, 29] clearance techniques to demonstrate that there is a substantial decrease of glomerular filtration in response to vigorous physical activity.

Physical activity and renal blood flow

In humans, renal blood flow has commonly been estimated by the clearance of diodrast or para-amino hippurate. Other options have included thermodilution (using a thermistohr to measure intravascular temperature following injection of a warm solution), positron emission tomography (collecting the gamma rays as a marker perfuses the kidney), radionuclide angiography (detecting the emissions from a ^{99m}Technetium infusion) and Doppler ultrasound. Animal experiments have commonly been based on the passage of radio-labelled microspheres through the kidneys. Other techniques used in animal research have included a thermo-stromuhr (a small intravascular electrical heater positioned between two thermocouples), an electromagnetic flow transducer, Doppler ultrasound and Technetium clearance (Table 4.1).

Under resting conditions, the kidneys receive about a quarter of the total cardiac output, a perfusion rate of some 4 ml/min per gram of renal tissue. Flow is directed mainly to the renal cortex, where a high flow rate persists over a wide range of systemic blood pressures. The efferent blood vessels leading from the renal glomeruli are smaller than the afferents. Thus, the hydrostatic pressure within the glomeruli is high, and this tends to force small molecules (water, glucose, amino acids, sodium chloride and urea) across the glomerular membrane from the renal capillaries into the nephrons. This process of molecular transfer is termed glomerular filtration and it is commonly evaluated in terms of creatinine clearance (the rate of creatinine excretion, divided by the plasma creatinine concentration). Some 15% of renal plasma flow is filtered into the glomeruli under resting conditions.[30] However, filtration tends to fall during physical activity, as a means of enhancing muscle blood flow.[31] Much of the material excreted into the glomeruli is normally reabsorbed in the renal tubules, but in very vigorous exercise, the process of reabsorption may either become over-loaded because of increased leakage of protein into the glomeruli, or it may be impaired by a local oxygen lack associated with the physical activity itself.

In humans, indirect measurements of renal plasma flow using diodrast and para-amino hippurate clearance techniques suggest that exhausting endurance exercise quickly initiates a general visceral vasoconstriction. Renal vascular resistance can increase as much as fivefold.[21] Renal blood flow is reduced by 70% or more[32–34] (Table 4.1), depending on the intensity of exercise,[22, 35] with the extent of vasoconstriction exacerbated by heat exposure or dehydration.[25] Changes seem related to the release of epinephrine and dopamine,[36] and they can persist for a substantial time following a sustained bout of exercise.[20, 22] One comparison of young and elderly men found little difference in flow reduction with age, but in this study the two groups had surprisingly similar levels of maximal oxygen intake,[37] suggesting that the older individuals were unusually fit. The flow reduction is abolished by the vasodilator dihydralazine.[38]

Most studies have involved dynamic forms of physical activity, although vigorous static muscular contractions also decrease renal blood flow.[40, 41] The renal vasoconstriction of endurance exercise seems a manifestation of sympathetic nerve activity. Likewise, the vascular constriction associated with static handgrip exercise is largely absent in humans who have received kidney transplantation and thus lack a renal autonomic nerve supply.[41]

Table 4.1 Changes of renal plasma flow associated with physical activity

Author	Subjects	Methodology	Findings	Comments
Human studies				
Barclay et al.[20]	9 male, 1 female student	Diodrast technique	402 m run reduced renal plasma flow 39%, from 736 mL/min to 447 mL/min	Flow remained reduced after exercise
Bucht et al.[39]	8 medical students or nurses	Para-amino hippurate	Supine cycle ergometry to oxygen consumption of 0.5, 1.0 L/min; heavier work reduced renal blood flow 20%	
Castenfors & Piscator[35]	11 males	Para-amino hippurate	Supine cycle ergometry, 67–200 W, decreased PAH clearance 32% with light and 53% with heavy exercise	Renal plasma flow reduction proportional to exercise intensity
Castenfors et al.[38]	10 males	Para-amino hippurate	Supine cycle ergometry for 45 min at 76% PWC170 reduced renal blood flow 50%	Effect abolished by vasodilator dihydralazine
Chapman et al.[22]	9 young males	Continued diodrast and para-amino hippuric acid injection	4.8 km/h 0% slope to 5.6 km/h 10% slope treadmill exercise reduced renal blood flow by 30% from resting 610 mL/min	Effect intensity dependent, blood flow recovered over 40 min post-exercise
Grimby[23]	15 males	Inulin and para-amino hippuric acid clearance	Supine cycle ergometry, 45 min at 25–150 W; renal blood flow dropped from 17% to 2.5–5% of cardiac output	Filtration fraction increased during exercise
Kenny & Ho[37]	6 young, 6 old men	para-amino hippurate	Cycle ergometer exercise at 60% of peak oxygen intake gives similar reduction of renal flow in young and old (25, 21%)	Both groups had similar peak oxygen intakes

Table 4.1 continued

Author	Subjects	Methodology	Findings	Comments
Middlekauf et al.[40]	20 males, 9 females	Positron emission tomography	Graded handgrip exercise gives 17% decrease of renal blood flow	Possibly a reaction to increased systemic blood pressure
Momem et al.[41]	7 transplant patients (2–27 months post-op.), 11 matched controls	Doppler ultrasound	Fatiguing handgrip (40% of voluntary maximum) led to 4-fold greater increase of vascular resistance in controls than in transplants	
Radigan & Robinson[24]	5 males	Para-amino hippurate	Treadmill, 4.2 km/h, 5% grade; renal blood flow decreased 39–42% when exercising in cool, fell 39% at rest in heat, and further 31% fall when exercising in heat	Glomerular filtration fraction increased when exercising
Rowell[33]	17 males	Dye injection	Overall splanchnic blood flow reduced up to 75% in vigorous exercise	
Smith et al.[25]	4 males (2 un-acclimatized subjects excluded)	Para-amino hippurate	Treadmill, 4.2 km/h, 5% slope reduced renal plasma flow 22% in cool, 31% at 50°C, 56% with heat + dehydration	
Suzuki et al.[34]	6 males	Radionuclide angiography (^{99m}Tech-netium)	Cycle ergometry to exhaustion gave 53% decrease of renal blood flow	Flow remained reduced 17.5% 30 min after exercise
Tidgren et al.[36]	8 males	Thermo-dilutioin technique	Supine exercise to 90% of capacity caused progressive 47% decrease of renal blood flow	Increase of renal vascular resistance related to epinephrine and dopamine release
White & Rolf[21]	4 healthy males	Inulin and para-amino hippuric acid	Running 9.1–11.2 km/h for 11–19 min; renal vascular resistance increased 5-fold in heaviest exercise	

Table 4.1 continued

Author	Subjects	Methodology	Findings	Comments
Animal studies				
Armstrong & Laughlin[42]	80 trained and untrained Sprague-Dawley rats	Radio-labelled microspheres	Trained rats maintained higher renal blood flows during 15 min treadmill exercise (−14% vs. −52%)	
Blake[43]	3 trained female dogs	Para-amino hippuric acid	Treadmill exercise, 4–8 km/h	Exercise had no effect upon renal function
Gleadhill et al.[31]	5 thorough-bred horses	99mTechnetium clearance	Trotting reduced glomerular perfusion 40–50%	Changes began as soon as horses walked
Hales & Ludbrook[44]	5 rabbits	Radioactive microspheres	60 sec treadmill exercise at 13 m/min caused 20% reduction of renal flow	Flow reduction not seen if baro-denervated
Herrick et al.[45]	5 dogs 12–22 kg	Thermo-stromuhr	Decrease of renal flow in 4 of 26 experiments, but increase in 11/26 with treadmill running (15% slope)	Treadmill speed not specified
Hohimer & Smith[46]	12 baboons	Electro-magnetic flow transducer	4 min of dynamic leg exercise induced 19% decrease of renal blood flow	Rapid recovery of normal flow post-exercise
Kregel[47]	16 mature and 16 elderly rats	Pulsed Doppler flowmeter	Treadmill running, 10–30 m/min, 0% grade; flow reduction in heavy exercise greater in older than in younger rats	
Millard et al.[48]	13 male mongrel dogs	Doppler ultrasound	Maximal sustainable exercise did not change renal flow after transient drop at onset of activity	Decrease of flow seen in dogs with experimentally induced congestive heart failure
Musch et al.[49]	25 trained female rats and 25 controls	Radio-labelled microspheres	6 weeks of sprint training did not change 63% renal flow reduction with exercise	

Table 4.1 continued

Author	Subjects	Methodology	Findings	Comments
Parks & Manohar[50]	11 adult ponies	Radio-labelled microspheres	Heavy treadmill exercise reduced renal blood flow 81%	
Rushmer et al.[51]	7 20–30 kg dogs	Pulsed ultrasonic flowmeter	Treadmill 4.2–7.2 km/h, 12% slope produced initial drop, then return to normal renal blood flow	Slight decreases of renal blood flow during spontaneous activity
Sanders et al.[52]	14 miniature swine aged 6–9 months	Radio-labelled microspheres	Exercise at 4.8–7.2 km/h, 0–10% grade; 34% flow reduction with moderate, 70% reduction with severe exercise	
Stebbins & Symons[53]	12 miniature swine	Radio-labelled microspheres	20 min exercise at 80% of heart rate reserve reduced renal blood flow 36% (31% if treated with Losartan)	Losartan is an angiotensin II antagonist
Van Citters & Franklin[54]	18 sled dogs	Doppler ultrasound/ telemetry	Sledge hauling did not change renal blood flow	
Vatner et al.[55, 56]	9 adult baboons	Doppler ultrasound	Blood flow to kidneys showed minor reductions during spontaneous exercise in outdoor enclosure	

Miniature swine trained to run on a treadmill show a 70% reduction of renal blood flow during vigorous physical activity.[52, 53] Horses and ponies also show a 50% reduction of renal blood flow as soon as they begin to walk.[31, 50] However, the response of dogs and baboons[43, 45, 46, 48, 51, 54–56] apparently differs from that of humans; conscious animals of these species sometimes show an immediate decrease of renal blood flow, but resting values return as the exercise continues, even if the animal is engaged in such heavy exercise as pulling a sled or running 2.4 km at a speed of about 32 km/hr. Millard and colleagues[48] suggested that in dogs, any vasoconstriction occurred in the face of blockade of the autonomic nerves, and thus was a form of auto-regulation. However, in rabbits the early reduction of renal blood flow was not seen after denervation of the baro-receptors,[44] suggesting that the immediate stimulus to renal vasoconstriction was an exercise-induced rise of systemic blood pressure.

Training reduced the renal vasoconstriction of exercise in one study of rats,[42] but another report found no difference in response after six weeks of sprint training.[49] The impact of exercise was greater in elderly than in young adult animals.[47]

Physical activity and glomerular filtration

Glomerular filtration is the process whereby fluid and solutes are filtered from the renal capillaries into the renal glomeruli and nephrons. It is usually measured in terms of the clearance of a marker such as inulin that is freely filtered by the kidneys, and does not undergo subsequent metabolism, secretion or reabsorption in the renal tubules. In humans, vigorous physical activity leads to a progressive drop in the glomerular filtration rate (GFR) as renal perfusion decreases.[57] Changes in both renal blood flow and glomerular filtration are apparently proportional to the intensity of effort,[23, 58, 59] and are greater in young than in older subjects.[60] GFR decreased by 18% following a half-marathon event[61] and a 230 km Alpine cycle event,[62] by 25% after a 525 km Alpine ultra-marathon ride[63] and by 30% after an 81 km Nordic ski race.[20, 64] A bout of circuit training also reduced the estimated GFR by 8–10%.[65] Values may fall to 60% of resting figures during maximal exercise, with substantial associated decreases in creatinine and urea clearance. In one of the studies cited above, the GFR had largely normalized within six hours of ceasing exercise,[61] but decreases of GFR have persisted for 24 hours following both a 21 km run[66] and two endurance cycle races.[62, 63]

The decrease in GFR is usually somewhat smaller than that for renal blood flow. Thus, the GFR per unit of blood flow (i.e. the filtration fraction) increases progressively from a resting figure of 15% to 25% or more during a severe bout of exercise.[20, 38, 67]

Physical activity and other aspects of renal physiology

Physical activity usually has a marked anti-diuretic effect, as the pituitary gland attempts to maintain plasma volume in the face of fluid losses in sweat by increasing plasma concentrations of anti-diuretic hormone. However, this compensatory mechanism is not always sustained during prolonged heavy exercise.[20, 30] There is also an increased secretion of the hormone aldosterone; this facilitates the reabsorption of sodium ions in the glomerular tubules, counteracting increases in the secretion of atrial natriuretic peptides that would otherwise have increased glomerular flow rate and sodium excretion.[58, 68] Other factors limiting the action of atrial natriuretic peptides during heavy exercise likely include greater renal sympathetic nerve activity, and increased blood levels of angiotensin II and catecholamines.[57] Urodilatin is a hormone similar to the atrial natriuretic peptides and it causes diuresis by augmenting renal blood flow. The kidneys increase the output of this substance during physical activity.[69] Further research is needed to clarify the respective contributions of urodilatin and atrial natriuretic peptides to the exercise response.

Despite large increases in plasma lactate concentrations during exhausting activity, renal mechanisms of lactate excretion quickly become saturated and urinary excretion is a minor consideration in the metabolism of lactate during exercise.[70, 71] Only minor quantities of lactate have been found in the urine after such activities as mountain climbing[72] or five hours of hard work.[27] Some of the lactate entering the renal glomeruli is actively reabsorbed in the proximal renal tubules.[73] A part is reconverted to glucose,[74] although the gluconeogenic capacity of the renal cortex is only about a fifth of that of liver tissue. There is some evidence that the acidosis associated with vigorous exercise stimulates a doubling of the activity of the kidney enzymes involved in this process.[75]

If the exercise has been very severe, there may be a rise of serum creatinine. Creatinine concentrations >0.3 mg/dl or >50% over baseline usually indicate acute renal dysfunction,[76–78] although in athletes with well-developed muscles and a large muscle mass, care must be taken to interpret absolute concentrations relative to the individual's body mass index.[79]

Given extensive losses of sodium ions in sweat, it is important to reduce the renal excretion of sodium during vigorous physical activity. During a marathon run, the renal excretion of sodium ions decreases by 30–50%.[57] Commonly, the change is larger than can be explained by a decrease in glomerular filtration; altered secretions of the hormones renin-angiotensin and aldosterone are probably involved, as well as a direct action of the renal sympathetic nerves.[80]

Other changes in renal function during physical activity can include an oliguria (defined clinically as a urinary secretion in the range 80–400 mL/day) and a rise of serum potassium levels. Unless an athlete drinks large volumes of fluid during a prolonged event, urine output decreases by 50% or more. There is generally an associated increase in urinary acidity and electrolyte concentrations, although very heavy physical activity may impair a person's ability to concentrate the urine.[81, 82] If the antidiuretic effect of exercise is combined with an over-enthusiastic drinking of water or hypotonic fluids and exposure to a cool environment, this can potentially induce the dangerous condition of hyponatraemia;[83] the normal lower limit of plasma sodium is 135 mE/L and symptoms are likely if the sodium ion concentration falls below 130 mE/L.

Exercise-induced proteinuria

Proteinuria may reflect either an increased glomerular filtration of protein molecules or a slowing in their tubular resorption.[84, 85] The rate of protein filtration depends upon the health of the kidneys and the balance of hydrostatic and osmotic pressures across the glomerular membrane.[86] Thus, an exercise-induced increase of systemic blood pressure can increase protein filtration. An accumulation of acids (including lactic acid) in the renal tissue may also increase protein loss,[14, 87] and the abolition of proteinuria following administration of indomethacin suggests that prostaglandins may be involved in the process.[88]

At rest, urinary protein excretion averaged over a 24-hour period is less than 80 mg/L, and values >100 mg/L are suggestive of a renal pathology.[89] Alternative definitions of abnormality are a total urinary protein loss >150 mg/day[90] or >100 mg/day[91] and/or an albumin loss >30 mg/day.[91] It is important to draw a clinical distinction between microalbuminuria and macroalbuminuria. Microalbuminuria is a normal phenomenon in those who engage in prolonged and vigorous physical activity. It is characterized by a protein loss in the range 30–300 mg/day, with a urinary albumin/creatinine ratio of >3.5mg/mmol in women and >2.5mg/mmol in men. Hohwü-Christensen and Högberg[92] found a post-exercise proteinuria in almost all top Swedish cross-country skiers (Table 4.2), and Gardner[84] found protein in 45% of urine specimens collected from 47 football players. Others have described proteinuria following participation in various sports with the magnitude of protein loss being proportional to the intensity of effort.[59, 94, 98–101] Gardner[84] coined the term "athletic pseudonephritis" for his findings, since the red cell and broad granular casts he observed in the urinary sediment had previously been considered (erroneously) as a sign of renal disease; these findings disappeared quickly after completion of the athletic season[84] and he thus reasoned they had little clinical significance.

For most investigators, macroalbuminuria implies a protein loss >300 mg/day and values[59, 93–97] in excess of this threshold are harbingers of underlying renal disease.[87] Cubeddu et al.[102] noted that a protein excretion substantially smaller than 300 mg/day was sometimes still associated with various cardiac risk factors and could be corrected by reductions in obesity, hypertension and insulin resistance. They thus suggested that clinicians should set the limit of normality much lower than 300 mg/day; in their view, urinary protein losses of 10–29 mg/day were associated with an adverse prognosis.

Most urinary protein is in the form of relatively small molecules (molecular weights <200,000 Daltons). Some 20 mg consists of pre-albumin and albumin, and the residue includes transferrin (an iron carrying glycoprotein), the k and g light chains of immunoglobulin, Tamm Horsfall mucoproteins (secreted by the renal tubules) and a and g immunoglobulins (probably derived from the renal tubules).[107] Although well-standardized laboratory assays of urinary protein are now available,[107, 108] assessments are commonly based on the colour changes seen during a simple urine dipstick test (Albustix). This detects albuminuria reasonably well, but is less effective in measuring the loss offlow molecular weight proteins, gamma globulins and haemoglobin. Estimates of protein loss can also be compromised if urine is retained in the bladder following exercise, and rather than expressing protein loss per unit volume of urine, it is preferable to relate it to the excretion of creatinine.[109, 110]

Techniques involving paper electrophoresis[106] and the use of immune antisera[111] have allowed identification of the various proteins and thus to infer glomerular and tubular contributions to the observed protein loss.[112] Glomerular proteinuria yields a urine with a high proportion of plasma constituents and is commonly assessed in terms of albumin loss. A normal albumin excretion but an increased excretion of alpha-1-microglobulin suggests that the disorder is of

Table 4.2 Reports of proteinuria following vigorous physical activity

Author	Subjects	Findings	Comments
Alyea & Parish[103]	Participants in various sports	70–100% showed albuminuria in track, lacrosse, crew, football and distance swimming	Red cells and casts also seen in 60–80% of athletes
Bailey et al.[94]	369 athletes	Proteinuria frequent, incidence increased with intensity of exertion	42 of 369 athletes had positive occult blood test
Barach et al.[104]	19 Marathon runners	18/19 developed proteinuria immediately following their event	
Coye & Rosandich[95]	10 football players	Protein content of urine increased 2–15-fold in 24 hours following a game	Larger increase in albumin than in globulin
Edwards et al.[15]	42 Harvard football players (male)	Incidence of proteinuria rises from 4/9 (first period) to 13/13 (final period)	Proteinuria estimated from turbidity in nitric acid test; average degree of turbidity rises as match continues
Gardner[84]	47 football players, 424 urine specimens	45% of samples showed proteinuria	Unusual formed elements in 27 of 424 samples, gross haematuria in 1 sample
Hellebrandt et al.[14]	Cycle ergometry, load ~120 Watts	Exhausting exercise gives immediate proteinuria; prolonged exercise gives proteinuria during post-exercise hypotension	Sulpho-salicyclic acid turbidity method
Hohwü-Christensen and Högberg[92]	204 top cross-country skiers	Almost all (92%) showed proteinuria immediately after skiing	Also haematuria in 28% of skiers
Javitt & Miller[105]	5 healthy university students	Proteinuria peaked 5 minutes after 3–22 min vigorous treadmill runs	Protein loss correlated with both decreased glomerular filtration and renal acidity
Kachadorian et al.[97]	51 20 km runners	Proteinuria in 41/51	Proteinuria associated with cast formation
Nedbal & Seliger[106]	41 normal young men	All showed proteinuria after 5 min treadmill run	Protein fractions show similar distribution to that in blood
Perlman et al.[98]	499 males, progressive treadmill test to exhaustion	Incidence of proteinuria (average 10.6%) increased with age to 4th decade	Albustix method
Poortmans & Labilloy[99]	15 men, 100m, 400m and 3000m runs	5-, 25- and 18-fold increase of protein excretion	Protein loss influenced by intensity and thus lactate accumulation

Table 4.2 continued

Author	Subjects	Findings	Comments
Todorović et al.[101]	11 male physical education students	Cycle ergometer exercise to heart rate of 170–180 beats/min; proteinuria in 10/11 constant effort and 11/11 variable intensity	Proteinuria related to lactate accumulation, greater with variable intensity effort
von Leube[12]	119 soldiers	14/19 showed proteinuria after 1–3 day march	

tubular origin.[91] Tubular proteinuria usually reflects a saturation of reabsorption mechanisms by a high rate of glomerular protein leakage, with the urine containing a large fraction of normally reabsorbed low molecular weight proteins such as lysozymes and the beta-2 microglobulins.[113] Defects of tubular reabsorption can be demonstrated by examining the changes in proteinuria following lysine perfusion; lysine blocks the normal tubular reabsorption of protein.[114, 115]

Protein reabsorbed in the renal tubules may be metabolized locally, or it may be returned to the circulation as intact protein molecules, polypeptides and amino acids.[116]

Clinical significance of resting microglobinuria

Under resting conditions, even a low-level microglobinuria can be the harbinger of an adverse prognosis.[102] In children, the extent of daily protein loss is, paradoxically, inversely related to the individual's obesity. Possibly, this is because thin children have a much higher level of daily physical activity and are therefore more likely to boost their average protein excretion by periods of exercise-related proteinuria.[117] In adults, resting microglobinuria merits a careful examination of the patient, since it is associated with an increased risk of many chronic conditions, including the metabolic syndrome,[118, 119] atherosclerotic heart disease,[120–132] hypertension,[133–137] ischaemic stroke,[138–140] left ventricular hypertrophy,[141] cardiomyopathy,[142] cardiovascular death,[143, 144] all-cause mortality,[145] diabetic nephropathy,[146] chronic obstructive pulmonary disease,[147, 148] cancer (particularly bladder and lung cancer[149]) and systemic inflammation as indicated by high blood levels of c-reactive protein.[150, 151]

The pathological bases for associations between resting urinary protein loss and chronic disease remain unclear.[125] When predicting prognosis in chronic renal disease, the estimated GFR is a stronger predictor of mortality than the extent of proteinuria. Cardiorespiratory fitness also remains a significant predictor of mortality, irrespective of the individual's GFR.[152] The detection of exercise proteinuria has some value in indicating the likelihood of developing persistent microproteinuria in diabetes,[153] but microalbuminuria is not usually associated with impaired insulin sensitivity[125] or with exercise proteinuria.[154]

Physical activity and microhaematuria

Microhaematuria is defined as the presence in the urine of >3 red cells per high-power microscopic field,[155, 156] or more than 50 red cells per mL of fluid.[157] Estimates of the prevalence of microhaematuria in the general population range from 0.19% to 16.1%.[158] Exercise-related microhaematuria is most commonly seen in distance runners. Haematuria was found in 9 of the 50 marathoners immediately following their event, although all initially had a normal urine; the blood disappeared in all 9 individuals within 48 hours.[159] Others have set the prevalence of microhaematuria in those running distances of 21–90 km at 20–25%.[160, 161] Red cells are usually seen in the first specimen of urine collected after a run, and findings are apparently independent of the intensity of effort. Potential explanations include repeated impacts of the posterior wall of the bladder against its base (particularly during running on hard surfaces) and glomerular bleeding due to local hypertension, vascular spasm and hypoxic damage.[160, 162, 163] One report suggested that haematuria could be avoided if the bladder was not completely emptied prior to a run; it was hypothesized that the residual urine provided a hydrostatic cushion, reducing impacts of the posterior bladder wall with the base.[163]

The presence of haemoglobin or myoglobin can also cause the secretion of a red-coloured urine, as in acute renal failure (below). In acute rhabdomyolysis, myoglobin may be found in the absence of haemoglobin.[157]

Although microhaematuria can be precipitated by vigorous physical activity, a careful history, physical examination and a laboratory evaluation that include an estimate of glomerular filtration rate are required to rule out both menstruation and potentially dangerous causes of haematuria such as infection, renal disease, viral illnesses, trauma and recent urological procedures.[164] Particular concern should be shown if the haematuria does not resolve within 72 hours of ceasing exercise. The red cells should be inspected critically for abnormal cells and casts that may indicate renal disease. In individuals over the age of 35 years, cystoscopy is also advisable to check for a possible tumour in the bladder or urinary tract.

Physical activity and acute and chronic renal failure

Severe exercise, particularly if it is performed under hot conditions with an inadequate supply of fluids can occasionally lead to an acute renal failure. An excessive intake of creatine can cause chronic renal failure, but as discussed below, chronic problems more commonly arise from damage to the renal blood vessels due to diabetes mellitus or chronic high blood pressure.

Acute exercise-induced renal failure

The patho-physiology of acute, exercise-induced renal failure may involve either an exertional breakdown of muscle tissue (rhabdomyolysis), with myoglobinuria and a blockage of the renal tubules, or an excessive reduction of renal blood flow with ischaemic damage to the kidney tissue, sometimes exacerbated by the direct toxic effects of myoglobin.[165] There may also be an increase in serum creatinine.[166] An acute renal failure of this type is quite rare. In the very demanding 90 km Comrades ultra-marathon race in South Africa, there have been only ten cases of acute renal failure among more than 20,000 competitors.[167] One option in further reducing this risk would seem to focus on countering mechanisms that cause excessive renal vascular constriction. However, additional research is needed to determine whether the emphasis should be on reducing renal sympathetic nerve activity, increasing nitric oxide availability or countering prostaglandin release[168, 169] as a means of decreasing vasoconstriction.

Adverse effects of creatine supplements and anti-inflammatory drugs

In 1998, concerns were raised that the prolonged ingestion of large doses of creatine supplements by athletes could cause chronic renal damage.[170] In theory, the conversion of excess creatine to sarcosine could lead to the formation of methylamine, with toxic end-products of formaldehyde and hydrogen peroxide.[171] A watch should certainly be kept for this danger, although as yet studies have not confirmed the fear that long-term creatine supplements produce toxic levels of methylamine, formaldehyde and hydrogen peroxide.[172]

A large intake of anti-inflammatory drugs can also have adverse effects on the kidney, particularly in individuals whose bodies normally rely on an increased prostaglandin secretion to counter a reduced renal blood flow. Occasionally, an excessive reliance on NSAIDS may cause an acute deterioration of renal function, but provided that is detected, this can be reversed by stopping the use of such medication.[173]

Physical activity and end-stage renal disease

A Canadian survey set the prevalence of chronic renal disease at 12.5% of adults.[174] The affected patient initially compensates for the diseased kidney tissue by increasing glomerular filtration in those glomeruli that are still functional. However, as the condition progresses, a growing proportion of glomeruli show a thickening of their basement membranes, and later they collapse, to be replaced by hyaline material. Cells in the renal tubules also undergo a fatty degeneration, and the loss of excretory power leads to a progressive increase in blood urea, with weakness, fatigue, loss of appetite, a high blood pressure, anaemia and impaired cardiac function.[175]

End-stage renal disease is unfortunately progressive, and eventually the decrease in glomerular filtration and the rise of blood urea are such that the patient requires treatment by either regular dialysis sessions or a renal transplant. The threshold for initiating dialysis is commonly a glomerular filtration rate of less than 15 mL/min.[176] At this stage, the individual's physical condition is usually poor, and the quality of life can be improved by participation in a regular exercise programme, conveniently arranged concurrently with dialysis sessions.

Chronic exercise enhances overall body function and it may also improve renal function by its action upon other systems, inducing changes in visceral perfusion, sympathetic nerve activity and hormonal secretions at any given intensity of exercise.

Patients requiring thrice weekly dialysis typically enter treatment with a peak oxygen intake and a peak working capacity as low as 55–75% of normal (Table 4.3). Some authors have attributed the impairment of oxygen transport to a low haemoglobin level[180, 185, 189, 190] and others to cardiac dysfunction.[177, 183, 186, 187] Probably, both factors are involved. Another potential limiting factor is a generalized muscle weakness.[191] Exercise is unwise immediately before dialysis because serum potassium levels are then high, and immediately following dialysis the patient often feels too fatigued to engage enthusiastically in an exercise programme. However, patients can usefully undertake moderate cycle ergometer training to occupy their time while dialysis is proceeding.

Well-designed aerobic training can increase the working capacity of a dialysis patient by 25%[192] (Table 4.4). Exercise is thus an important component of treatment at all stages of care. Even prior to enrolment in dialysis, it can increase a patient's maximal walking distance.[193] As treatment continues, specific efforts are needed to increase strength and endurance and to encourage incorporation of the patient into an on-going community rehabilitation programme. The effects of such conditioning can be reinforced by the administration of erythropoietin to counter the low haemoglobin level.[192] Long-term studies are still needed to demonstrate that such interventions increase longevity, but existing data show a substantial impact upon the individual's immediate quality of life.[192]

Physical activity and renal transplantion

Exercise-induced changes in glomerular filtration rate in the transplanted kidney are very similar to those seen in a normal individual, but those with a renal transplant show a less marked exercise-induced excretion of albumin, possibly because a lack of innervation abolishes the normal increase in plasma renin activity.[194] Patients sometimes have a near normal maximal aerobic power and functional capacity following recovery from a successful renal transplantation[187, 195–197] but often a continuing lack of interest in physical activity keeps their maximal oxygen intake below the anticipated level for their age.[198, 199] Further, evaluation is not easy because weakness and a low oxidative capacity in the muscles often limit attainment of a plateau of oxygen consumption during exercise testing.[200] One study of patients over the age of 60 years found little gain of muscle strength in the year following renal transplantation.[201] In contrast, a vigorous 24-week training programme increased the maximal oxygen intake of 16 renal transplant patients from 29 to 38 ml/[kg.min], and it also yielded 25–56% gains in their isokinetic strength.[200]

Table 4.3 Physical working capacity in patients with chronic renal disease

Author	Subjects	Measure	Effects of chronic renal disease	Comments
Barnea et al.[177]	22 patients undergoing dialysis	Peak cycle ergometer test	Peak working capacity was 52% of normal	Poor performance attributed to lactate accumulation and early muscle fatigue
Clyne et al.[178, 179]	20 pre-dialysis patients	Maximal cycle ergometer test	Maximal working capacity 74% of normal	Loss or work capacity correlated with low haemoglobin (67% normal)
Clyne et al.[180]	38 men, 20 women with GFR of 3–32 mL/min	Maximal cycle ergometer test	Maximal working capacity 40–143% of expected norm	Working capacity correlated with total haemoglobin after allowing for sex, age and GFR
Clyne & Jogestrand[181]	5 M, 3 F uremic patients, pre-dialysis	Maximal cycle ergometer test	Maximal working capacity 80% of normal	Working capacity increased to 92% normal with erythro-poietin treatment
Clyne et al.[182]	11 uraemic patients	Maximal cycle ergometer test	Maximal working capacity 67% normal	Working capacity increased to 78% of normal after transplantation
Lundin et al.[183]	9 men, 1 woman, dialysis >5 yr	Maximal oxygen intake (Bruce treadmill test)	8 of 10 patients said to be normal but max.oxygen intake averaged only 28.6 ml/[kg.min] at average age of 32.7 years	2/10 had cardiac enlargement, myocardial ischaemia in 1/10
Lundin et al.[184]	7 men, 3 women on haemo-dialysis	Maximal oxygen intake (Bruce treadmill test)	Maximal oxygen intake 15.1 ml/[kg.min] at average age of 44 yr	Max oxygen intake increased to 22.7 ml/[kg.min] with erythropoietin treatment
Mayer et al.[185]	13 patients on dialysis, haemoglobin 5.1–12.2 mg/100 mL	Maximal cycle ergometer test	Oxygen consumption at anaerobic threshold and maximal oxygen intake (53% of normal)	Decrease in both variables correlated with low haemoglobin level

Table 4.3 continued

Author	Subjects	Measure	Effects of chronic renal disease	Comments
Metra et al.[186]	10 patients receiving chronic dialysis treatment	Peak cycle ergometer test	Peak oxygen intake 55% of predicted value	Max oxygen intake boosted from 21.4 to 26.6 ml/[kg.min] with 3 months erythropoietin treatment
Painter et al.[187]	18 haemo-dialysis, 12 chronic ambulatory peritoneal dialysis patients	Maximal treadmill stress tests	Maximal oxygen intake 64, 62% of normal	
Sagiv et al.[188]	10 end-stage renal disease patients	Graded treadmill test to exhaustion	Maximal oxygen intake averaged 22.6 ml/[kg.min] at age 30 years	Oxygen transport not limited by pulmonary capacity or lactate accumulation

Note: GFR = glomerular filtration rate

Physical activity and the risk of renal cancer

The incidence of renal cancer varies substantially from one country to another. In British Colombia, tumours of the renal parenchyma are found in 6.5/100,000 in men and 3.2/100,000 in women, with corresponding figures of 0.6 and 0.3/100,000 for the rarer type of lesions affecting the renal pelvis.[203] Available reports offer a tantalizing suggestion that regular physical activity may protect against renal parenchymal cancers[203] (Table 4.5), although there does not seem

Table 4.4 Responses to training in patients before or during dialysis

Author	Subjects	Treatment	Response	Comments
Clyne et al.[202]	7 men, 3 women, predialytic, uraemic	Exercise 3/wk for 3 months vs. 9 controls	9.4% increase in peak work capacity in exercised group	No change in controls
Painter[192]	Patients on dialysis	Aerobic training	25% gain of working capacity	No erythropoietin administered
Zabetakis et al.[190]	5 haemodialysis patients	10 wk aerobic treadmill training at anaerobic threshold	21% increase in peak oxygen intake	Also increase in anaerobic threshold of experimental group

Table 4.5 Habitual physical activity and the relative risk of renal parenchymal cancer

Author	Sample	Findings	Comments
Bergström et al.[204]	3.28 million men, 3.35 million women, 18-year follow-up	4-level classification of occupational activity, RR of sedentary job 1.25 in men, no effect in women	Few women had active jobs
Bergström et al.[205]	17,241 twin-pairs, 20 yr follow-up	102 cases of renal cell cancer, risk of tumours unrelated to occupational or leisure activity	
Brownson et al.[206]	17,174 male cancer patients (449 renal cases)	No reduction of risk of renal cancers in those with active occupations	
Choi et al.[207]	576,562 men followed for 6 years	92 deaths from renal cancer; hypertension gave mortality risk of 2.43; risk for exercisers 0.9 (CI 0.6–1.4)	Prime focus of experiment on hypertension rather than exercise
Chiu et al.[208]	406 cases, 2434 controls	In women, OR of cancer with exercise <1/month vs. >1/day 2.5; no significant effect of physical activity in men	Substantial effect from BMI, but little interaction between physical activity and BMI
Chow et al.[209]	363,392 men long-term follow up, 759 renal cell and 136 renal pelvic cancers	Top third of BMI distribution doubled cancer risk	Prime focus on obesity, not exercise
Goodman et al.[210]	189 M, 79 F cases of renal cell carcinoma vs. matched controls	3-level leisure activity categorization and occupational activity unrelated to risk of cancer	BMI is associated with cancer in both sexes
Lindblad et al.[211]	Structured interviews, 379 cases of renal cell cancer, 353 controls	Physical activity at work reduced risk in men but not in women; men showed dose-response effect, greatest if related to physical activity at age 40 years	Body mass and BMI weak risk factors in men, but important in women
Mahabir et al.[212]	29,133 male smokers	210 cases of renal cell cancer seen over 12-year follow-up. Vigorous leisure activity gave relative risk of 0.46, no effect of occupational activity	Dose-related effect of leisure activity

Table 4.5 continued

Author	Sample	Findings	Comments
Mellemgaard et al.[213]	368 cases, 396 matched controls	Questionnaire on activity at work and leisure. No effect of physical activity on cancer risk	Relative weight was an important risk factor
Menezes et al.[214]	Cases (173 M, 133 F) and matched controls	Women (highest vs. least physical activity) RR 0.41, report of strenuous recreation RR 0.40; in men, RR 0.49	Moderate physical activity of little benefit in women. In men, greatest effect from activity as an adolescent.
Moore et al.[215]	482,386 adults	1,238 cases of renal cancer in 8.2 yr follow-up; multivariate risk ratios (highest vs. lowest activity) 0.77 (current activity), 0.82 (as adolescent)	
Nicodemus et al.[216]	34,637 women followed for 15 years	124 cases of renal cancer; benefit of physical activity seen with age-adjusted data but not in multivariate model	Central adiposity a major risk factor
Pan et al.[217]	810 cases, 3106 controls	Recreational physical activity 2 years earlier had no effect on risk of cancer	Large risk associated with high BMI
Paffenbarger et al.[218]	51,977 men, 4706 women	Risk of renal cancer unrelated to former participation in university sports teams	Only 29 cases of cancer
Pukkala et al.[219]	Comparison of 1449 physical education and 8619 language teachers	RR of renal cancer 0.29 in physical education teachers	Only 15 cases of cancer
Setiawan et al.[220]	161,126 adults, 8.3 year follow-up	Relative risk of renal cell cancer in obesity: 1.76 (M), 2.27 (F), with hypertension 1.42 (M), 1.58 (F), current smokers 2.3 (M), 1.7 (F)	Significant dose-related trend to reduction of risk with physical activity (METS/day) in women only
Tavani et al.[221]	767 cases, 1534 controls	Occupational activity reduces risk at all ages from 15–60 years (OR 0.65–0.70). No effect of leisure activity	Controlled for BMI, smoking and alcohol consumption

Table 4.5 continued

Author	Sample	Findings	Comments
Van Dijk et al.[222]	Case-cohort study, 120,852 adults. 9.3 year follow-up	275 histologically confirmed cases of renal cell cancer. Energy intake unrelated to risk, but in men RR 0.52 if leisure activity 30–60 min/day	High BMI a risk in both sexes. Leisure activity does not show dose-related gradient

Notes: BMI = body mass index; CI = confidence interval; RR = relative risk.

any information concerning the possible effects of exercise on the risk of pelvic lesions. Unfortunately, many studies have been based on relatively few cases of renal cancer, limiting the possibility of demonstrating a statistically significant benefit. Moreover, measurements of physical activity have often been weak, some samples have included few individuals who were vigorously active, either at work or in their leisure hours, and the period when activity was examined may not have coincided with the time when the carcinogenic change is likely to have occurred.

Prospective and cohort studies

There have been eight large-scale prospective trials. Six of the eight have found some relationship between renal parenchymal cancer and leisure or occupational activity, although the relationship has not always been demonstrated in both sexes. Setiawan et al.[220] completed a prospective study of 161,126 adults over a period averaging 8.3 years. In a multivariate analysis, there were substantial relative risks of renal cell cancer associated with current smoking (2.3 [M], 1.7 [F]), obesity (1.76 [M], 2.27 [F]) and hypertension (1.42 [M], 1.58 [F]). Question-naire estimates of physical activity (MET/day) were also significantly related to cancer risk in women (with an inverse dose-related association between habitual physical activity and renal cancer), but a physically active lifestyle conferred no benefit in men. It was suggested that the sex difference in response might reflect residual confounding of the data by effects of exercise upon obesity. Bergström et al.[204] conducted an 18-year prospective study of Swedes (3.28 million men and 3.35 million women), noting diagnoses of renal cell cancer in relationship to a four-level categorization of occupational activity. A significant dose-response relationship was observed in men, disadvantaging those in the more sedentary jobs (a relative risk averaging 1.25 after adjusting for socio-economic status, area of residence and year of follow-up). However, perhaps because of lesser job demands or confounding from substantial domestic physical demands, a heavy occupation provided no protection to the women.

A 12-year follow-up of 29,133 male smokers found 210 cases of renal cell cancer.[212] In a multivariate analysis, the risk was unrelated to occupational activity, but was strongly related to reported leisure activity, with a dose-related risk ratio of 0.46 favouring the most active individuals.

Nicodemus et al.[216] followed 34,637 women for 15 years. Most women reported little physical activity, but nevertheless in an age-adjusted model 124 cases of renal cancer showed an inverse relationship to participation in vigorous leisure activity (RR 0.37). Relative weight was also a major risk factor, and after including this and other co-variates in the analysis, leisure activity no longer had a statistically significant effect.

Moore et al.[215] questioned 482,386 adults about their current leisure activity and their physical activity as an adolescent. During an 8.2-year follow-up there were 1238 cases of renal cancer. Risk was reduced both with current leisure activity (RR 0.77) and with reported physical activity as an adolescent (0.82).

The case-cohort study of van Dijk et al.[222] followed 120,852 adults for 9.3 years. There were 275 histologically confirmed cases of renal cell cancer over this period. Risk was unrelated to energy intake, but in the men there was a substantial inverse relationship to leisure activity; those taking 30–60 minutes of such activity per day had a relative risk of 0.52 relative to those who were inactive (although with no evidence of a dose-response gradient).

Bergström et al.[205] followed 17,241 twin pairs for 20 years. There were 102 cases of renal cell cancer in their sample, but risk was not associated with either occupational or leisure activity. Brownson et al.[206] made a general survey of occupational classifications in 17,174 male cancer cases, including 449 individuals with renal tumours. They also found no relationship between occupational classification and the renal lesions.

Case-control studies

Of nine case-control studies, five have shown a reduced risk of renal cancer in the more active individuals. Lindblad et al.[211] conducted a case-control study that compared 379 cases of renal cell cancer with 353 controls. A structured interview found a strong inverse dose-related relationship between relative risk and a four-level classification of job activity in men, the greatest benefit being associated with vigorous activity at the age of 40 years (a risk of 0.37 relative to the least active workers); however, occupational activity had no significant impact upon the relative risk of renal cancer in women. Menezes et al.[214] compared 173 male and 133 female cases of renal cancer with matched controls. After adjustment for age, BMI and smoking habits comparisons of the most active vs. the least active women yielded a relative risk of 0.41, and reports of strenuous leisure activity were also associated with a relative risk of 0.40; however, little reduction of risk was seen among those reporting only moderate physical activity. In the men, both total recreational activity and moderate physical activity yielded risk ratios of 0.49, with the greatest effects being seen from physical activity undertaken as an adolescent. The study of Chiu et al.[208]

included 406 cases of renal cancer and 2434 controls. In the women, the odds of developing renal cancer for those reporting exercise <1 time/month versus those who were exercising at least once per day was 2.5; there was also a substantial risk associated with a high body mass index, but apparently little interaction between the two variables. However, in the men, no significant benefit was associated with reports of frequent physical activity.

Tavani et al.[221] studied 767 individuals with renal tumours and 1534 controls. After controlling for BMI, smoking and alcohol consumption, there was a beneficial effect from occupational activity, irrespective of the age when it was undertaken (odds ratio 0.65–0.7), but no effect of leisure activity was observed. Pukkala et al.[219] compared 1449 physical education teachers with that of 8619 (presumably physically less active) language teachers. The relative risk of renal cancer in the physical education teachers was 0.29 relative to the language teachers, although the entire study included only 19 individuals with renal cancer.

Other case-control studies reached negative conclusions. Paffenbarger et al.[218] examined relationships between renal cancer and prior membership of university sports teams. There were only 29 cases of renal cancer in this series and these incidents bore no relationship to the rather tenuous measure of habitual physical activity provided by affiliation to an athletic team as a young adult. Goodman et al.[210] made a three-level categorization of leisure activity and a categorization of occupational activity in a small sample. The risk of renal cell cancer was strongly related to body mass index, but was unrelated to either leisure or occupational physical activity. Likewise, Mellemgaard et al.[213] compared 368 histologically verified cases of renal cancer with 396 controls, finding an association between tumours and relative weight, but no relationship of cancers to physical activity either at work or in leisure time. Finally, in a comparison between 810 cases of renal cancer and 3106 controls, Pan et al.[217] found no effect from recreational activity that had been undertaken two years prior to the diagnosis of malignancy.

Conclusions

Despite the difficulties associated with this type of investigation, six of eight prospective trials and five of nine case-control studies have suggested that habitual physical activity is associated with a reduced risk of renal cancer. Possible mechanisms include a reduction in body mass and body fat, a lowering of blood pressure and reductions of chronic inflammation and oxidative stress.[223, 224]

Physical activity and prevention of renal calculi

The lifetime risk of renal stones is about 19% in men and 9% in women. To the extent that a prolonged and vigorous physical activity causes dehydration and increases urinary calcium concentrations, it can increase the immediate risk of developing renal calculi. In contrast, an eight-year follow-up of 84,225 initially healthy post-menopausal women suggested that regular moderate physical activity decreased the overall risk of kidney stones. The threshold of protection was three hours of moderate walking per week, and the reduction of risk rose to 31% among those who engaged in >10 MET-h/wk of leisure activity.[225] Suggested mechanisms of overall risk reduction include an activity-stimulated increase of fluid intake, a decreased sodium excretion and a decreased sympathetic nerve activity. Weight-bearing activity might also encourage the deposition of calcium in the bones, rather than its excretion in the urine. In contrast, a high body mass index is associated with an increased risk of renal stones.

Physical activity and endocrine functions of the kidney

An exercise training programme can have a positive effect upon health in many other parts of the body by modulating the endocrine functions of the kidney,[226] increasing the secretion of erythropoietin, calcitrol (which modulates the uptake of calcium from the gut and thus bone health) and renin-angiotensin (important in hypertension and congestive heart failure).

Areas for further research

Human studies consistently show a large reduction of renal blood flow during vigorous physical activity. In contrast, exercise may induce an initial vasoconstriction in dogs, but renal blood flow returns to its resting value as effort continues. It would be interesting to explore reasons for this species difference. Is it an expression of the greater contribution of the spleen to the maintenance of blood volume in the dog, or is it simply an artifact, due to differences in the methods used to measure regional blood flow in humans and in dogs?

A variety of mechanisms regulate renal blood flow during physical activity and there is scope to explore these control processes in greater detail. How far is the vascoconstriction related to altered levels of hormones such as urodilatin, atrial natriuretic peptides, renin-angotensin and aldosterone, and how far does control operate more directly via the renal sympathetic nerves? This is a question that could be examined after local denervation in animals or by the study of humans with a kidney transplant. A greater understanding of control systems could help in the prevention of the acute exercise-induced renal failure associated with excessive vasoconstriction. Should the focus of preventive efforts be on reducing renal sympathetic nerve activity, on increasing nitric oxide availability or even on countering prostaglandin release?

Exercise rehabilitation certainly enhances renal functional capacity and the immediate quality of life in patients who are undergoing dialysis, but long-term studies are still needed to demonstrate whether such interventions increase longevity and/or the quality adjusted life expectancy.

Other areas meriting further investigation include the possible role of habitual physical activity in reducing the risks of urinary calculi and renal parenchymal cancer.

Practical implications and conclusions

A drastic reduction of renal blood flow may be anticipated during prolonged endurance exercise. Although this normally causes no more than a slight and rapidly reversed urinary loss of protein and red cells, in a hot environment it is important to monitor water intake and to avoid the dehydration that could precipitate acute renal failure. Further, the risk of renal failure seems to be exacerbated by the frequent administration of NSAIDs, and athletes should be advised against excessive self-medication with such drugs. In those with chronic renal failure, functional capacity is generally low; an early assessment of physical capacity is advisable in such individuals, and thereafter, they should be enrolled in a progressive rehabilitation programme. Finally, the likely relationship between sedentary living and renal parenchymal cancer is one more good reason to encourage everyone to adopt an active lifestyle.

References

1.   Bainbridge FA. *The physiology of muscular exercise*. London, UK: Longmans Green, 1919.
2.   Dawson PM. *The physiology of physical education for physical educators and their pupils*. Baltimore, MD: Williams & Wilkins, 1935.
3.   Redman SR. *The physiology of work and play*. Oak Brook, IL: Dryden Press, 1950.
4.   Schneider EC. *Physiology of muscular exercise* (3rd ed). Philadelphia, PA: Saunders, 1933.
5.   Simonson E. *Physiology of work capacity and fatigue*. Springfield, IL: C.C. Thomas, 1971.
6.   Starling EH, Evans CAL, Hartridge H. *Starling's principles of human physiology*. London, UK: J & A Churchill, 1941.
7.   Wesson LG. Kidney function in exercise. In: Johnson WR, (ed.) *Science and medicine of exercise and sports*. New York, NY: Harper, 1960, pp. 270–284.
8.   Lamb D. *Physiology of exercise: responses and adaptations* (1st ed). New York, NY: Macmillan, 1978.
9.   Gardner K. Exercise and the kidney. In: Appenzeller O, (ed.) *Sports medicine*. Baltimore, MD: Urban & Schwarzenberg, 1988, pp. 189–195.
10. Goldszer R, Siegel A. Renal abnormalities during exercise. In: Strauss R (ed.) *Sports medicine*. Philadelphia, PA: Saunders, 1984, pp. 130–139.
11. Rasch P, Dodd Wilson I. Other body systems and exercise. In: Falls H (ed.) *Exercise physiology*. New York, NY: Academic Press, 1978, pp. 129–151.
12. von Leube W. Uber ausscheidung von Eiweiss in urin des gesunden Menschen. [On the excretion of albumin in the urine of healthy men]. *Virchow's Arch Pathol Anat Physiol* 1878; 72: 145–147.
13. Barach JH. Physiological and pathological effects of severe exertion on the circulatory and renal systems. *Arch Int Med* 1910; 5: 382–405.
14. Hellebrandt FA. Studies on albuminuria following exercise. 1. Its incidence in women and its relationship to the negative phase in pulse pressure. *Am J Physiol* 1932; 101: 357–364.
15. Edwards HT, Richards TK, Dill DB. Blood sugar, urine sugar and urine protein in exercise. *Am J Physiol* 1931; 98: 352–356.

16. Jundell I, Fries KAE. Die Anstrenungsalbuminurie. [Intensity of work and albumniuria]. *Nord Med Ark* 1911; 44(Suppl. 2): 1–154.

17. Edwards HT, Cohen M, Dill DB. Renal function in exercise. *Arbeitsphysiol* 1937 9: 610–618.

18. Addis T, Drury DR. The rate of urea excretion. VII. The effect of various other factors than blood urea concentration on the rate of urea excretion. *J Biol Chem* 1923; 55: 629–638.

19. Mackay EM. Studies of urea excretion in normal individuals and patients with Bright's diseasse. The diurnal variation of urea excretion in normal individuals and patients with Bright's disease. *J Clin Invest* 1928; 8(3): 505–516.

20. Barclay JA, Cooke WT, Kenney RA, et al. The effects of water diuresis and exercise on the volume and composition of the urine. *Am J Physiol* 1947; 148: 327–337.

21. White HL, Rolf D. Effects of exercise and of some other influences on renal circulation in man. *Am J Physiol* 1948; 152: 505–516.

22. Chapman C, Henschel A, Minckler J, et al. The effect of exercise on renal plasma flow in normal male subjects. *J Clin Invest* 1948; 27: 639–644.

23. Grimby G. Renal clearances during prolonged supine exercise at different loads. *J Appl Physiol* 1965; 20: 1294–1298.

24. Radigan L, Robinson S. Effects of environmental heat stress and exercise on renal blood flow and filtration rate. *J Appl Physiol* 1949; 2: 185–191.

25. Smith J, Robinson S, Percy M. Renal responses to exercise, heat and dehydration. *J Appl Physiol* 1952; 4: 659–665.

26. Campbell J, Webster T. Day and night urine during complete rest, laboratory routine, light muscular work and oxygen administration. *Biochem J* 1921; 15: 660–664.

27. Campbell J, Webster T. Effects of severe muscular work on the composition of the urine. *Biochem J* 1922; 16: 106–110.

28. Covian F, Rehberg P. Uber die Nierenfunktion während schwerer Muskelarbeit. [On renal function during heavy muscular work]. *Skand Arch Physiol* 1936; 75: 21–37.

29. Merrill A, Cargill W. The effect of exercise on the renal plasma flow and filtration rate of normal and cardiac subjects. *J Clin Invest* 1948; 27: 272–277.

30. Castenfors J. Renal function during prolonged exercise. *Ann N Y Acad Sci* 1977; 301: 151–159.

31. Gleadhill A, Marlin D, Harris PA, et al. Reduction of renal function in exercising horses. *Equine Vet J* 2000; 32(8): 509–514.

32. Johnson JM. Endurance exercise and the regulation of visceral and cutaneous blood flow. In: Shephard RJ, Åstrand P-O (eds) *Endurance in sport* (2nd ed). Oxford, UK: Blackwell 2000, pp. 103–117.

33. Rowell LB. Cardiovascular adjustments to thermal stress. Suppl. 8. *Handbook of physiology; the cardiovascular system, peripheral circulation and organ blood flow.* Hoboken, NJ: Wiley, 2011.

34. Suzuki M, Sudoh M, Matsuhara S, et al. Changes in renal blood flow measured by radionuclide angiography following exhausting exercise in humans. *Eur J Appl Physiol* 1996; 74: 1–7.

35. Castenfors J, Piscator M. Renal haemodynamics, urine flow and urinary protein excretion during exercise in supine position at different loads. *Acta Med Scand* 1967; 171 (Suppl. 472): 231–244.

36. Tidgren B, Hjemdahl P, Theodorsson E, et al. Renal neurohormonal and vascular responses to dynamic exercise in humans. *J Appl Physiol* 1991; 70(5): 2279–2286.

136   *Kidney function in health and disease*

37. Kenney WL, Ho C-W. Age alters regional distribution of blood flow during moderate-intensity exercise. *J Appl Physiol* 1995; 79: 1112–1119.
38. Castenfors J. Renal function during exercise. Acta Physiol Scand 1967; 70(Suppl. 293): 1–43.
39. Bucht H, Ek J, Eliasch H, et al. The effect of exercise in the recumbent position on the renal circulation and sodium excretion in normal individuals. *Acta Physiol Scand* 1953; 28: 95–100.
40. Middlekauf HR, Nitzsche EU, Nguyen AH, et al. Modulation of renal cortical blood flow during static exercise in humans. *Circ Res* 1997; 80: 62–68.
41. Momen A, Bower D, Leuenberger UA, et al. Renal vascular response to static handgrip exercise: sympathetic vs. autoregulatory control. *Am J Physiol* 2005; 289(4): H1770–H1776.
42. Armstrong RB, Laughlin MH. Exercise blood flow patterns within and among rat muscles after training. *Am J Physiol* 1984; 246: H59–H68.
43. Blake W. Effect of exercise and emotional stress on renal hemodynamics, water and sodium excretion in the dog. *Am J Physiol* 1951; 165: 149–157.
44. Hales JRS, Ludbrook J. Baroreflex participation in redistribution of cardiac output at onset of exercise. *J Appl Physiol* 1988; 64(2): 627–634.
45. Herrick JF, Grindlay JH, Baldes EJ, et al. Effect of exercise on the blood flow in the superior mesenteric, renal and common iliac arteries. *Am J Physiol* 1939; 128: 338–344.
46. Hohimer AR, Smith OA. Decreased renal blood flow in the baboon during mild dynamic exercise. *Am J Physiol* 1979; 236(1): H141–H150.
47. Kregel KC. Augmented mesenteric and renal vasoconstriction during exercise in senescent Fischer 344 rats. *J Appl Physiol* 1995; 79(3): 706–712.
48. Millard RW, Higgins CB, Franklin D, et al. Regulation of the renal circulation during severe exercise in normal dogs and dogs with experimental heart failure. *Circ Res* 1972; 31: 881–888.
49. Musch TL, Terrell JA, Hilty MR. Effects of high-intensity sprint training on skeletal muscle blood flow in rats. *J Appl Physiol* 1991; 71: 1387–1395.
50. Parks CM, Manohar M. Distribution of blood flow during moderate and strenuous exercise in ponies (*Equus caballus*). *Am J Vet Res* 1983; 44(10): 1861–1866.
51. Rushmer RF, Franklin DL, Van Citters EL, et al. Changes in peripheral blood flow distribution in healthy dogs. *Circ Res* 1961; 9: 675–687.
52. Sanders M, Rasmussen S, Cooper D, et al. Renal and intrarenal blood flow distribution in swine during severe exercise. *J Appl Physiol* 1976; 40: 932–935.
53. Stebbins LC, Symons JD. Role of angiotensin II in hemodynamic response to dynamic exercise in miniswine. *J Appl Physiol* 1995; 78(1): 185–190.
54. Van Citters RL, Franklin DL. Cardiovascular performance of Alaska sled dogs during exercise. *Circ Res* 1969; 24: 33–42.
55. Vatner S, Pagani M. Cardiovascular adjustments to exercise: Hemodynamics and mechanisms. *Progr Cardiovasc Dis* 1976; 19: 91–108.
56. Vatner S. Effects of exercise and excitement on mesenteric and renal dynamics in conscious, unrestrained baboons. *Am J Physiol* 1978; 234: H210–H214.
57. Zambraski EJ. Renal regulation of fluid homeostasis during exercise. In: Gisolfi CV, Lamb DR, (eds) *Perspectives in exercise science and sports medicine*, vol 3; fluid homeostasis during exercise. Carmel, IN: Benchmark 1990, pp. 247–276.
58. Freund B, Shizuru E, Hashiro G, et al. Hormonal, electrolyte and renal responses to exercise are intensity dependent. *J Appl Physiol* 1991; 70: 900–906.

59. Kachadorian WA, Johnson RE. Athletic pseudonephritis in relation to rate of exercise. *Lancet* 1970; 1(7644): 472.

60. Poortmans JR, Ouchinsky M. Glomerular filtration rate and albumin excretion after maximal exercise in aging sedentary and active men. *J Gerontol* (Med Sci) 2006; 61A(1): 1181–1185.

61. Lippi G, Schena F, Salvagno GL, et al. Acute variation of estimated glomerular filtration rate following a half-marathon run. *Int J Sports Med* 2008; 29: 948–951.

62. Neumayr G, Pfister R, Hoertrtnagl H, et al. The effect of marathon cycling on renal function. *Int J Sports Med* 2003; 24: 131–137.

63. Neumayr G, Pfister R, Hoertrtnagl H, et al. Renal function and plasma volume following ultramarathon cycling. *Int J Sports Med* 2005; 26: 2–8.

64. Castenfors J, Mossfeldt F, Piscator M. Effect of prolonged exercise on renal function and urinary protein excretion. *Acta Physiol Scand* 1967; 70: 194–206.

65. Amorim MZ, Machado M, Hackney AC, et al. Sex differences in serum CK activity but not in glomerular filtration rate after resistance exercise: is there a sex dependent renal adaptative response? *J Physiol Sci* 2014; 64(1): 31–36.

66. Tian Y, Tong TK, Lippi G, et al. Renal function parameters during early and late recovery periods following an all-out 21-km run in trained adolescent runners. *Clin Chem Lab Med* 2011; 49(6): 993–997.

67. Poortmans JR, Vanderstraeten J. Kidney function during exercise in healthy and diseased humans: an update. *Sports Med* 1994; 18(6): 419–437.

68. Cappellin E, De Palo EF, Gatti R, et al. Effect of prolonged physical exercise on urinary proANP1-30 and proANP31-67. *Clin Chem Lab Med* 2004; 42(9): 1058–1062.

69. Schmidt W, Bub A, Meyer M, et al. Is urodilatin the missing link in exercise-dependent renal sodium retention? *J Appl Physiol* 1998; 84: 123–128.

70. Johnson RE, Edwards HT. Lactate and pyruvate in blood and urine after exercise. *J Biol Chem* 1937; 118: 427–432.

71. McKelvie RS, Lindinger MI, Heigenhauser GFl, et al. Renal responses to exerise-induced lactic acidosis. *Am J Physiol* 1989; 257: R102–R108.

72. Jerusalem E. Ueber ein neuer Verfahren zur quantitativen Bestimmung der Milchensäure in Organen und tierischen Flüssigkeiten .[About a new method for the quantitative determination of lactic acid in organs and animal fluids]. *Biochem Ztschr Berlin* 1908; 12: 361–389.

73. Dies F, Ramos G, Avelar E, et al. Renal excretion of lactic acid in the dog. *Am J Physiol* 1969; 216: 106–111.

74. Krebs HA, Yoshida T. Muscular exercise and gluconeogenesis. *Biochem Z* 1963; 338: 241–244.

75. Sanchez-Medina F, Sanchez-Urrutia L, Medina JM, et al. Effect of short-term exercise on gluconeogenesis by the rat kidney cortex. *FEBS Letters* 1972; 26: 25–26.

76. Hou DH, Bushinsky DA, Wish JB, et al. Hospital-acquired renal insufficiency. *Am J Med* 1983; 74: 243–248.

77. Molitoris BA, Levin A, Warnock DG, et al. Improving outcomes of acute kidney injury: report of an initiative. *Nat Clin Pract Nephrol* 2007; 3: 439–442.

78. Waikar DS, Bonventre JV. Creatinine kinetics and the definition of acute kidney injury. *J Am Soc Nephrol* 2009; 20(3): 672–679.

79. Banfi G, Colombini A, Lombardi G, et al. Metabolic markers in sports medicine. *Adv Clin Chem* 2012; 56: 1–54.

80. Dibona GF, Kopp UC. Neural control of renal function. *Physiol Rev* 1997; 77: 75–197.

81. Refsum HE, Strømme SB. Renal osmol clearance during prolonged heavy exercise. *Scand J Clin Lab Invest* 1977; 38(1): 19–22.
82. Wade CE, Claybaugh J. Plasma renin activity, vasopressin concentration, urinary excretory responses to exercise in men. *J Appl Physiol* 1980; 49: 930–936.
83. Noakes TD, Goodwin N, Rayer BL, et al. Water intoxication: A possible complication during endurance exercise. *Med Sci Sports Exerc* 1985; 17: 370–375.
84. Gardner KD. Athletic pseudonephritis; alterations of urine sediment by athletic competition. *JAMA* 1956; 161: 1613–1617.
85. Javitt NB, Miller AT. Mechanism of exercise proteinuria. *J Appl Physiol* 1952; 4: 834–839.
86. Shephard RJ. *Physiology and biohemistry of exercise*. New York, NY: Praeger Publications, 1982.
87. Viarnaud G. Contribution à l'étude de l'albuminurie d'effort. [Contribution to the study of exercise albuminuria.] Ph.D. thesis, Université de Lyon, 1944.
88. Mittelmann KD, Zambrasky RJ. Exercise-induced proteinuria is attenuated by indomethacin. *Med Sci Sports Exerc* 1992; 24: 1069–1074.
89. Bellinghieri G, Savica V, Santoro D. Renal alterations during exercise. *J Ren Nutr* 2008; 18(1): 158–164.
90. Bergstein JM. A practical approach to proteinuria. *Pediatr Nephrol* 1999; 13: 697–700.
91. Bergón E, Granados R, Fernández-Segoviano P, et al. Classification of renal proteinuria: a simple algorithm. *Clin Chem Lab Med* 2002; 40(11): 143–150.
92. Hohwü-Christensen E, Högberg P. Physiology of skiing. *Arbeitsphysiol* 1950; 14: 292–303.
93. Alyea EP, Boone AW. Urinary findings resulting from non-traumatic exercise. *Southern Med J* 1957; 50: 905–910.
94. Bailey RR, Dann E, Gillies AH, et al. What the urine contains following athletic compettion. *NZ Med J* 1976; 83: 309–313.
95. Coye RD, Rosandich RR. Proteinuria during the 24 hour period following exercise. *J Appl Physiol* 1960; 15: 592–594.
96. Kachadorian WA, Johnson RE. Renal response to various rates of exercise. *J Appl Physiol* 1970; 28(6): 748–752.
97. Kachadorian WA, Johnson RE, Buffington E, et al. The regularity of athletic pseudonephrits after heavy exercise. *Med Sci Sports* 1970; 2(3): 142–145.
98. Perlman LV, Cunningham D, Montoye H, et al. Exercise proteinuria. *Med Sci Sports* 1970; 2: 20–23.
99. Poortmans JR, Labilloy D. The influence of work intensity on postexercise proteinuria. *Eur J Appl Physiol* 1988; 57: 260–263.
100. Taylor A. Some characteristics of exercise proteinuria. *Clin Sci* 1960; 19: 209–217.
101. Todovorić B, Nikolić B, Brdarić R, et al. Proteinuria following submaximal work and vascular responses to dynamic exercise in humans. *Int Z angew Physiol* 1972; 30: 151–160.
102. Cubeddu LX, Alfieri AB, Hoffmann IS. Lowering the threshold for defining microalbuminuria: effects of a lifestyle-metformin intervention in obese "normoalbuminuric" non-diabetic subjects. *Am J Hypertens* 2008; 21(1): 105–110.
103. Alyea EP, Parish HH. Response to exercise-urinary findings. *JAMA* 1958; 167(7): 807–813.
104. Barach JH. Physiological and pathological effects of severe exertion on the circulatory and renal systems. *Arch Int Med* 1910; 5: 382–405.

105. Javitt NB, Miller AT. Mechanism of exercise proteinuria. *J Appl Physiol* 1952; 4: 833–839.
106. Nedbal J, Seliger V. Electrophoretic analysis of exercise proteinuria. *J Appl Physiol* 1958; 13(2): 244–246.
107. Naderi AS, Reilly RF. Primary care approach to proteinuria. *J Am Board Fam Med* 2008; 21: 569–574.
108. Leung AKC, Robson WL. Evaluating the child with proteinuria. *J Roy Soc Prom Health* 2000; 120(1): 16–22.
109. Carroll MF, Temte JL. Proteinuria in adults: a diagnostic approach. *Am Fam Phys* 2000; 62(6): 1333–1340.
110. Cirillo M. Evaluation of glomerular filtration rate and of albuminuria/proteinuria. *J Nephrol* 2010; 23(2): 125–132.
111. Rowe DS, Soothill JF. The proteins of postural and exercise proteinuria. *Clin Sci* 1961; 21: 87–91.
112. Poortmans JR, Vancalck B. Renal glomerular and tubular impairment during strenuous exercise in young women. *Eur J Clin Invest* 1978; 8: 175–178.
113. Miyai T, Ogata M. Changes in the concentrations of urinary proteins after physical exercise. *Acta Med Okayama* 1990; 44: 263–266.
114. Mogensen CE, Solling K. Studies on renal tubular absorption: partial and near complete inhibition by certain amino acids. *Scand J Clin Lab Invest* 1977; 37: 477–486.
115. Poortmans JR, Brauman H, Staroukine M, et al. Indirect evidence of glomerular/tubular postexercise proteinuria in healthy humans. *Am J Physiol* 1990; 254: F277–F283.
116. Maack T. Renal handling of low molecular weight proteins. *Am J Med* 1975; 58: 57–64.
117. Hirschler V, Molinari C, Maccallini G, et al. Is albuminuria associated with obesity in school children? *Pediatr Diabetes* 2010; 11(5): 322–330.
118. Ford ES, Li C, Zhao G. Prevalence and correlates of metabolic syndrome based on a harmonious definition among adults in the US. *J Diabetes* 2010; 2(3): 180–193.
119. Hoebel S, de Ridder JH, Malan L. The association between anthropometric parameters, the metabolic syndrome and microalbuminuria in black Africans: the SABPA study. *Cardiovasc J Afr* 2010; 21(3): 148–152.
120. Bianchi S, Bigazzi R, Amoroso A, et al. Silent ischemia is more prevalent among hypertensive patients with microalbuminuria and salt sensitivity. *J Hum Hypertens* 2003; 17(1): 13–20.
121. Böhm M, Thoenes M, Danchin N, et al. Association of cardiovascular risk factors with microalbuminuria in hypertensive individuals: the i-SEARCH global study. *J Hypertens* 2007; 25(11): 2317–2324.
122. Chang A, Kramer H. Should GFR and albuminuria be added to the Framingham risk score? Chronic kidney disease and cardiovascular disease risk prediction. *Nephron Clin Pract* 2011; 19(2): 171–177.
123. Choi SW, Yun WJ, Kim HY, et al. Association between albuminuria, carotid atherosclerosis, arterial stiffness, and peripheral arterial disease in Korean type 2 diabetic patients. *Kidney Blood Press Res* 2010; 33(2): 111–118.
124. Diercks GF, van Boven AJ, Hillege JL, et al. The importance of microalbuminuria as a cardiovascular risk indicator: a review. *Can J Cardiol* 2002; 18(5): 525–535.
125. Jensen JS, Borch-Johnsen K, Jensen G, et al. Insulin sensitivity in clinically healthy individuals with microalbuminuria. *Atherosclerosis* 1996; 119(1): 69–76.

126. Foster MC, Hwang SJ, Larson MG, et al. Cross-classification of microalbuminuria and reduced glomerular filtration rate: associations between cardiovascular disease risk factors and clinical outcomes. *Arch Intern Med* 2007; 167(13): 1386–1392.
127. Jensen JS, Feldt-Rasmussen B, Strandgaard S, et al. Arterial hypertension, microalbuminuria, and risk of ischemic heart disease. *Hypertension* 2000; 35: 898–903.
128. Liu CS, Pi-Sunyer FX, Li CI, et al. Albuminuria is strongly associated with arterial stiffness, especially in diabetic or hypertensive subjects: a population-based study (Taichung Community Health Study, TCHS). *Atherosclerosis* 2010; 211(1): 315–321.
129. McKenna K, Thompson C. Microalbuminuria: a marker to increased renal and cardiovascular risk in diabetes mellitus. *Scott Med J* 1997; 42(4): 99–104.
130. Rutter MK, McComb JM, Brady S, et al. Silent myocardial ischemia and microalbuminuria in asymptomatic subjects with non-insulin-dependent diabetes mellitus. *Am J Cardiol* 1999; 83(1): 27–31.
131. Yildirimtürk O, Kiliçgedik M, Tuğcu A, et al. Tip 2 diyabetli asemptomatik hastalarda sol ventrikül fonksiyonları ve sessiz miyokart iskemisi mikroalbüminüri ilişkisi [The relationship of microalbuminuria with left ventricular functions and silent myocardial ischemia in asymptomatic patients with type 2 diabetes]. *Turk Kardiyol Dern Ars* 2009; 37(2): 91–97.
132. Waldron JS, Baoku Y, Hartland AJ, et al. Urine microalbumin excretion in relation to exercise-induced electrocardiographic myocardial ischaemia. *Med Sci Monit* 2002; 8(11): CR725–727.
133. Cerasola G, Cottone S, Mulé G, et al. Microalbuminuria, renal dysfunction and cardiovascular complication in essential hypertension. *J Hypertens* 1996; 14(7): 915–920.
134. Forman JP, Fisher ND, Schopick EL, et al. Higher levels of albuminuria within the normal range predict incident hypertension. *J Am Soc Nephrol* 2008; 19(10): 1983–1988.
135. Habbal R, Sekhri AR, Volpe M, et al. Prevalence of microalbuminuria in hypertensive patients and its associated cardiovascular risk in clinical cardiology: Moroccan results of the global i-SEARCH survey – a sub-analysis of a survey with 21,050 patients in 26 countries worldwide. *Cardiovasc J Afr* 2010; 21(4): 200–205.
136. Hornych A, Asmar R. Microalbuminurie et l'hypertension artérielle. [Microalbuminuria and arterial hypertension]. *Presse Med* 1999; 28(11): 597–604.
137. Tsiachris D, Tsioufis C, Syrseloudis D, et al. Impaired exercise tolerance is associated with increased urine albumin excretion in the early stages of essential hypertension. *Eur J Prev Cardiol* 2012; 19(3): 452–459.
138. Beamer NB, Coull BM, Clark WM, et al. Microalbuminuria in ischemic stroke. *Arch Neurol* 1999; 56(6): 699–702.
139. Madison JR, Spies C, Schatz IJ, et al. Proteinuria and risk for stroke and coronary heart disease during 27 years of follow-up: the Honolulu Heart Program. *Arch Intern Med* 2006; 166(8): 884–809.
140. Sander D, Weimar C, Bramlage P, et al. Microalbuminuria indicates long-term vascular risk in patients after acute stroke undergoing in-patient rehabilitation. *BMC Neurol* 2012; 12:102. doi: 10.1186/1471-2377-12-102.
141. Salmasi AM, Jepson E, Grenfell A, et al. The degree of albuminuria is related to left ventricular hypertrophy in hypertensive diabetics and is associated with abnormal left ventricular filling: a pilot study. *Angiology* 2003; 54(6): 671–678.

142. Mbanya JC, Sobngwi E, Mbanya DS, et al. Left ventricular mass and systolic function in African diabetic patients: association with microalbuminuria. *Diabetes Metab* 2001; 27(3): 378–382.

143. Nerpin E, Ingelsson E, Risérus U, et al. The combined contribution of albuminuria and glomerular filtration rate to the prediction of cardiovascular mortality in elderly men. *Nephrol Dial Transplant* 2011; 26(9): 2820–2827.

144. Valmadrid CT, Klein R, Moss SE, et al. The risk of cardiovascular disease mortality associated with microalbuminuria and gross proteinuria in persons with older-onset diabetes mellitus. *Arch Intern Med* 2000; 160(8): 1093–1100.

145. Romundstad S, Holmen J, Kvenild K, et al. Microalbuminuria and all-cause mortality in 2,089 apparently healthy individuals: a 4.4-year follow-up study. The Nord-Trøndelag Health Study (HUNT), Norway. *Am J Kidney Dis* 2003; 42(3): 466–473.

146. Agarwal RP, Thanvi I, Vachhani G, et al. Exercise-induced proteinuria as an early indicator of diabetic nephropathy. *J Assoc Physicians India* 1998; 46(9): 772–774.

147. Casanova C, de Torres JP, Navarro J, et al. Microalbuminuria and hypoxemia in patients with chronic obstructive pulmonary disease. *Am J Respir Crit Care Med* 2010; 182(8): 1004–1010.

148. Kömürcüoğlu A, Kalenci S, Kalenci D, et al. Microalbuminuria in chronic obstructive pulmonary disease. *Monaldi Arch Chest Dis* 2003; 59(4): 269–272.

149. Jørgensen L, Heuch I, Jenssen T, et al. Association of albuminuria and cancer incidence. *J Am Soc Nephrol* 2008; 19(5): 992–998.

150. Kuo HK, Al Snih S, Kuo YF, et al. Cross-sectional associations of albuminuria and C-reactive protein with functional disability in older adults with diabetes. *Diabetes Care* 2011; 34(3): 710–717.

151. Kuo HK, Al Snih S, Kuo YF, et al. Chronic inflammation, albuminuria, and functional disability in older adults with cardiovascular disease: the National Health and Nutrition Examination Survey, 1999–2008. *Atherosclerosis* 2012; 222(2): 502–508.

152. Gulati M, Black HR, Arnsdorf MF, et al. Kidney dysfunction, cardiorespiratory fitness, and the risk of death in women. *J Womens Health* (Larchmt) 2012; 21(9): 917–924.

153. O'Brien SF, Watts GF, Powrie JK, et al. Exercise testing as a long-term predictor of the development of microalbuminuria in normoalbuminuric IDDM patients. *Diabetes Care* 1995; 18(12): 1602–1605.

154. Bognetti E, Meschi F, Pattarini A, et al. Post-exercise albuminuria does not predict microalbuminuria in type 1 diabetic patients. *Diabet Med* 1994; 11(9): 850–855.

155. Froom P, Ribak J, Benbassat J. Significance of of microhaematuria in young adults. *BMJ* 1984; 288: 20–22.

156. Jones GR, Newhouse I. Sport-related hematuria: a review. *Clin J Sports Med* 1997; 7: 119–125.

157. Patel DR, Torres AD, Greydanus DE. Kidneys and sports. *Adolesc Med Clin* 2005; 16(1): 111–119.

158. Woolhandler S, Pels RJ, Bor DH, et al. Dipstick urinalysis screening of asymptomatic adults for urinary tract disorders. I. Hematuria and proteinuria. *JAMA* 1989; 262: 1214–1219.

159. Siegel AJ, Hennekens CH, Solomon HS, et al. Exercise-related hematuria. Findings in a group of marathon runners. *JAMA* 1979; 241(4): 391–392

160. Reid RJ, Hosking DH, Ramsey EW. Haematuria following a marathon run: source and significance. *Br J Urol* 1987; 59: 133–136.

161. Kallmeyer JC, Miller NM. Urinary changes in ultra long-distance marathon runners. *Nephron* 1993; 64: 119–121.

162. Abarbanel J, Benet AE, Lask D, et al. Sports hematuria. *J Urol* 1990; 143(5): 887–890.

163. Blacklock NJ. Bladder trauma in the long-distance runner: '10000 metres haematuria'. *Br J Urol* 1977; 49: 129–132.

164. Grossfeld GD, Wolf JS, Litwin MS, et al. Asymptomatic microscopic hematuria in adults: summary of the AUA best practice policy recommendations. *Am Fam Physician* 2001; 63(6): 1145–1155.

165. De Francesco Daher E, da Silva HB, Brunetta DM, et al. Rhabdomyolysis and acute renal failure after strenuous exercise and alcohol abuse: case report and literature review. *Sao Paulo Med J* 2005; 123(1): doi.org/10.1590/S1516-318020050001 00008.

166. Ohta T, Sakano T, Ogawa T, et al. Exercise-induced acute renal failure with renal hypouricemia: a case report and a review of the literature. *Clin Nephrol* 2002; 58(4): 313–316.

167. MacSearraigh ETM, Kallmeyer JC, Schiff HB. Acute renal failure in marathon runners. *Nephron* 1979; 24: 236–240.

168. Farquhar W, Morgan A, Zambraski E, et al. Effects of acetaminophen and ibuprofen on renal function in the stressed kidney. *J Appl Physiol* 1999; 86: 598–604.

169. Zambraski EJ. The kidney and body fluid balance during exercise. In: Buskirk E, Puhl S, (eds) *Body fluid balance during exercise and sport.* Boca Raton, FL: CRC Press, 1996, pp. 75–95.

170. Pritchard N, Kalra P. Renal dysfunction accompanying oral creatine supplemen-tations. *Lancet* 1998; 351: 1252–1253.

171. Sale C, Harris RC, Florence J, et al. Urinary creatine and methylamine excretion following 4 x 5 g.day^{-1} or 20 x 1 g.day^{-1} of creatine monohydrate for 5 days. *J Sports Sci* 2009; 27: 759–766.

172. European Food Safety Association. Creatine monohydrate for use in foods for particular nutritional uses. *EFSA J* 2004; 36: 1–4.

173. Whelton A, Hamilton CW. Nonsteroidal anti-inflammatory drugs: effects on kidney function. *J Clin Pharmacol* 1991; 31(7): 588–598.

174. Arora P, Vasa P, Brenner D, et al. Prevalence estimates of chronic kidney disease in Canada: results of a nationally representative survey. *Can Med Assoc J* 2013; 185(9): E417–E423.

175. Poortmans JR, Niset G, Godefroid C, et al. Responses to exercise and limiting factors in hemodialysis and renal transplant patients In: Rieu M (ed) *Physical work capacity in organ transplantation.* Basel, Switzerland, Karger, 1998, pp. 113–133.

176. Tatterstall J, Dekker F, Heimbürger O, et al. When to start dialysis: updated guidance following publication of the Initiating Dialysis Early and Late (IDEAL) study. *Nephrol Dial Transplant* 2011; 26(7): 2082–2086.

177. Barnea N, Drory Y, Iaina C, et al. Exercise tolerance in patients on chronic hemodialysis. *Isr J Med Sci* 1980; 16: 17–21.

178. Clyne N, Jogestrand T, Lins L-E, et al. Factors limiting physical working capacity in predialytic uraemic patients. *Acta Med Scand* 1987; 222: 183–190.

179. Clyne N, Jogestrand T, Lins LE, et al. Physical working capacity in uraemic patients. *Scand J Urol Nephrol* 1996; 30: 247–252.

180. Clyne N, Jogenstrand T, Lins LE, et al. Progressive decline in renal function induces a gradual decrease in total hemoglobin and exercise capacity. *Nephron* 1994; 67: 322–326.

181. Clyne N, Jogestrand T. Effect of erythropoietin treatment on physical exercise capacity and on renal function in predialytic uremic patients. *Nephron* 1992; 60: 390–396.

182. Clyne N, Jogestrand T, Lins LE, et al. Factors influencing physical working capacity in renal transplant. *Scand J Urol Nephrol* 1989; 23: 145–150.

183. Lundin AP, Stein RA, Frank F, et al. Cardiovascular status in long-term hemodialysis patients: An exercise and echocardiography study. *Nephron* 1981; 28: 234–238.

184. Lundin AP, Akerman MJH, Chesler RM, et al. Exercise in hemodialysis patients after treatment with recombinant erythropoietin. *Nephron* 1991; 58: 315–319.

185. Mayer G, Thum J, Graf H. Anaemia and reduced exercise capacity in patients on chronic haemodialysis. *Clin Sci* 1989; 76(3): 265–268.

186. Metra M, Cannella G, La Canna G, et al. Improvement in exercise capacity after correction of anemia in patients with end-stage renal disease. *Am J Cardiol* 1991; 68: 1060–1066.

187. Painter P, Messer-Rehak D, Hanson P, et al. Exercise capacity in haemodialysis, CAPD, and renal transplant patients. *Nephron* 1986; 42: 47–51.

188. Sagiv M, Rudoy J, Rotstein A, et al. Exercise tolerance of end-stage renal disease patients. *Nephron* 1991; 57: 424–427.

189. Clyne N, Jogestrand T, Lins L-E. Factors limiting working capacity in predialytic uraemic patients. *Acta Med Scand* 1987; 222(2): 183–90

190. Zabetakis PM, Gleim GW, Pasternack FL. Long-duration submaximal exercise conditioning in hemodialysis patients. *Clin Nephrol* 1982; 18: 17–22.

191. Diesel W, Noakes TD, Swanepoel C, et al. Isokinetic muscle strength predicts maximum exercise tolerance in renal patients on chronic hemodialysis. *Am J Kidney Dis* 1990; 16: 109–114.

192. Painter P. The importane of exercise training in rehabilitation of patients with end-stage renal disease. *Am J Kidney Dis* 1994; 24(Suppl. 1): S2–S9.

193. Fitts S, Guthrie MR, Blagg CR. Exercise coaching and rehabilitation counseling improve quality of life for predialysis and dialysis patients. *Nephron* 1999; 82: 115–121.

194. Poortmans JR, Hermans L, Vandervliet A, et al. Renal responses to exercise in heart and kidney transplant patients. *Transplant Int* 1997; 10: 323–327.

195. Evans R, Mammen D, Garrison L, et al. The quality of life of patients with end-stage renal disease. *N Engl J Med* 1985; 312: 553–559.

196. Feber J, Dupuis JM, Chapuis F, et al. Body composition and physical performance in children after renal transplantation. *Nephron* 1997; 75: 13–19.

197. Painter P, Hanson P, Messer-Rehak D, et al. Exercise tolerance changes following renal transplantation. *Am J Kidney Dis* 1987; 10: 452–456.

198. Hamiwaka L, Cantell M, Crawford S, et al. Physical activity and health-related quality of life in children following kidney transplantation. *Pediatr Transplant* 2009; 13: 861–867.

199. Matteucci C, Calzolari A, Pompei E, et al. Abnormal hypertensive response during exercise test in normotensive transplanted children and adolescents. *Nephron* 1996; 73: 201–206.

200. Kempeneers G, Noakes TD, van Zyl-Smit R, et al. Skeletal muscle limits the exercise tolerance of renal transplant recipients: Effects of an exercise training program. *Am J Kidney Dis* 1990; 16: 57–65.

201. Nyberg G, Hallste G, Norden G, et al. Physical performance does not improve in elderly patients following successful kidney transplantation. *Nephrol Dial Transplant* 1995; 10: 86–90.
202. Clyne N, Ekholm J, Jogestrand T, et al. Effect of exercise training in predialytic uremic patients. *Nephron* 1991; 59: 84–89.
203. Chow E-H, Dong LM, Devesa SS. Epidemiology and risk factors for kidney cancer. *Nat Rev Urol* 2010; 7(5): 245–257.
204. Bergström A, Moradi T, Lindblad P, et al. Occupational physical activity and renal cell cancer: a nation-wide cohort study in Sweden. *Int J Cancer* 1999; 83: 186–191.
205. Bergström A, Terry P, Lindblad P, et al. Physical activity and risk of renal cell cancer. *Int J Cancer* 2001; 92: 155–157.
206. Brownson RC, Chang JC, Davis JR, et al. Physical activity on the job and cancer in Missouri. *Am J Public Health* 1991; 81: 639–642.
207. Choi MY, Jee SH, Sull JW, et al. The effect of hypertension on the risk for kidney cancer in Korean men. *Kidney Internat* 2005; 67(2): 647–652.
208. Chiu B-H, Gapstur SM, Chow W-H, et al. Body mass index, physical activity, and risk of renal cell carcinoma. *Int J Obesity* 2006; 30: 940–947.
209. Chow W-H, Gridley G, Fraumeni JF, et al. Obesity, hypertension, and the risk of kidney cancer in men. *N Engl J Med* 2000; 343: 1305–1311.
210. Goodman MT, Morgernstern H, Wynder EL. A case-control study of factors affecting the development of renal cell cancer. *Am J Epidemiol* 1986; 124: 926–941.
211. Lindblad P, Wolk A, Bergström R, et al. The role of obesity and weight fluctuations in the etiology of renal cell cancer: a population-based case-control study. *Cancer Epidemiol Biomarkers Prev* 1994; 3: 631–639.
212. Mahabir D, Leitzman MF, Pietinen P, et al. Physical activity and renal cell cancer risk in a cohort of male smokers. *Cancer* 2004; 108: 600–605.
213. Mellemgaard A, Engholm G, McLaughlin JK, et al. Risk factors for renal-cell carcinoma in Denmark. III. Role of weight, physical activity and reproductive factors. *Int J Cancer* 1994; 2: 66–71.
214. Menezes RJ, Tomlinson G, Kreiger N. Physical activity and risk of renal cell carcinoma. *Int J Cancer* 2003; 107: 642–646.
215. Moore SC, Chow W-H, Schatzkin A, et al. Physical activity during adulthood and adolescence in relation to renal cell cancer. *Am J Epidemiol* 2008; 168: 149–157.
216. Nicodemus KK, Sweeney C, Folsom AR. Evaluation of dietary, medical and lifestyle risk factors for incident kidney cancer in postmenopausal women. *Int J Cancer* 2004; 108: 115–121.
217. Pan SY, DesMeules M, Morrison H, et al. Obesity, high energy intake, lack of physical activity, and the risk of kidney cancer. *Cancer Epidemiol Biomarkers Prev* 2006; 15: 2453–2460.
218. Paffenbarger RS, Lee I-M, Wing AL. The influence of physical activity on the incidence of site-specific cancers in college alumni. *Adv Exp Med Biol* 1992; 322: 7–15.
219. Pukkala E, Poskiparta M, Apter D, et al. Life-long physical activity and cancer risk among Finnish female teachers. *Eur J Cancer Prev* 1992; 2: 369–376.
220. Setiawan VW, Stram DO, Nomura AM, et al. Risk factors for renal cell cancer: the multiethnic cohort. *Am J Epidemiol* 2007; 166: 932–940.
221. Tavani A, Zucchetto A, Dal ML, et al. Lifetime physical activity and the risk of renal cell cancer. *Int J Cancer* 2007; 120: 1977–1980.

222. van Dijk BAC, Schouten LJ, Kiemeney LA, et al. Relation of height, body mass, energy intake, and physical activity to risk of renal cell carcinoma: results from the Netherlands Cohort Study. *Am J Epidemiol* 2004; 160: 1159–1167.
223. Pialoux V, Brown AD, Leigh R, et al. Effect of cardiorespiratory fitness on vascular regulation and oxidative stress in postmenopausal women. *Hypertension* 2009; 54: 1014–1020.
224. Solomon TPJ, Haus JM, Kelly KR, et al. Randomized trial on the effects of a 7-d low-glycemic diet and exercise intervention on insulin resistance in older obese humans. *Am J Clin Nutr* 2009; 90: 1222–1229.
225. Sorensen MD, Chi T, Shara NM, et al. Activity, energy intake, obesity, and the risk of incident kidney stones in postmenopausal women: a report from the Women's Health Initiative. *J Am Soc Nephrol* 2014; 25(2): 362–369.
226. Henderson J, Henderson IW. The endocrine functions of the kidney. *J Biol Educ* 1994; 28(4): 245–254.

5 Implications of a single kidney for the young athlete

Introduction

The kidneys play a vital role in maintaining the "milieu intérieur".[1, 2] In the view of Claude Bernard, the *"constancy of the internal environment (milieu intérieur) is the condition of free and independent life"*.[3] The previous chapter examined the reactions of the healthy kidneys to acute and chronic physical activity. In this chapter, we consider responses in the individual who has only a single kidney, looking at the advice that the clinician should offer to the young athlete with only one kidney.

Although the kidneys are normally paired organs, kidney donors typically live as long as their peers. Within two weeks of kidney removal, resting function based upon the remaining kidney is running at 70% of pre-operative levels, and eventually excretory capacity may reach 85% of that for the paired organs.[4] Other causes of a unilateral kidney include a birth defect (renal agenesis, affecting between 1 in 500 and 1 in 1800 infants),[5] and surgical removal of a kidney because of a neoplasm, injury or disease. Despite the generally favourable prognosis for those with a single kidney, it is important to maintain the health of the remaining organ; regular physical activity can contribute to renal health by reducing the risks of hypertension, diabetes mellitus and other kidney-damaging diseases.

The main objectives of this chapter are to weigh conflicting opinions on the risks of renal injury associated with an active lifestyle and to suggest principles that should guide the clinical management of children with a single kidney. Specific issues include (1) permissible types of physical activity for individuals who have only a single kidney, (2) the overall risk of renal injury during various types of physical activity, (3) factors modifying this risk, including the absence of one kidney, (4) a close examination of the purported dangers associated with "contact" sports, and (5) practical issues in the management of renal injuries and the communication of risk levels to anxious parents.

Current opinions on sport participation with a single kidney

There is currently a wide division of opinion among health professionals on the wisdom of sport participation by those with a solitary kidney. In Italy, an annual medical certification is required to participate in any type of organized sport, and such certification is denied to those with a solitary kidney.[17] In North America, also, many physicians are reluctant to recommend that such individuals participate in sport, particularly if body contact is anticipated, because of the perceived risk of trauma to the remaining kidney. It is argued that even minor cumulative damage from repeated trauma could shorten the useful lifespan of the remaining kidney, and if any one injury were severe enough to require a nephrectomy, the only option left for the patient would be to perform dialysis several times per week, with the hope that a suitable kidney donor might eventually be found. Even following renal transplantation, the patient would face on-going treatment with immune-suppressant drugs; this would cause a greatly reduced overall resistance to infectious diseases and a reduced overall quality of life.

Given these potentially serious adverse prospects, a survey of the American Society of Pediatric Nephrology found that 86% of respondents banned children with a single kidney from playing American football, although surprisingly only 5% were prohibited from cycling.[7] A similar survey of the Urology Section of the American Academy of Pediatrics found 68% of members prohibiting all types of contact sports for individuals with a single kidney.[16] Again, only 42% of members of the American Medical Society for Sports Medicine would allow one of their own children with a solitary kidney to practice unrestricted sports.[5, 18] Many review articles have appeared (Table 5.1), but unfortunately there is as yet no consensus on an appropriate policy.[12] Moreover, decisions to date have generally been based on expert clinical opinions rather than on hard epidemiological evidence.

The American Academy of Pediatrics[19] and the American and the Canadian Urological Associations[11] have recently looked critically at the available statistics, suggesting that the constraints commonly applied may be excessive, and run counter to the best interests of a child's overall health. The American Academy of Pediatrics[13–16, 19] has pointed out that the risk of renal injury in contact sports is in fact very low. It seems that many physicians continue to make cautious recommendations about sport participation more because of fears of litigation in the event of an injury than because of an objective assessment of the true costs and benefits. As Psooy has underlined,[9–11] the risk of a catastrophic injury to the head is far greater than the risk of injury to a solitary kidney. Psooy has thus argued that sport should be allowed for those with a solitary kidney, after a careful and documented explanation of risks to both the participant and the next of kin and the adoption of appropriate protective measures. Other authors who have made an objective analysis of injury statistics[7, 8, 17, 20, 21] have concluded that widely prevalent and draconian restrictions on sport participation for the child with a single kidney are unwarranted. Styn and Wan[21] further noted that there is no evidence of an over-representation of individuals with solitary kidneys among reported cases of renal injury, although this could reflect either low risk or a restriction of sport participation by the individuals concerned.

Table 5.1 Review articles making recommendations concerning sport participation for the patient with a single kidney

Authors	Information source	Recommendation
Favourable		
Bernard[6]	Literature review	Sports participation is generally safe, with very minimal risk to the remaining kidney
Grinsell et al.[7]	Search of medical and sports literature	Restricting participation of patients with a single, normal kidney from contact/collision sports is unwarranted
Johnson et al.[8]	National paediatric trauma registry	Prohibition of contact sports with a solitary kidney overly protective, needs to be re-evaluated
Psooy[9-11]	Nine recent articles	Risk of renal injury a fifth of that for head injury; most dangerous sports are bicycling, sledding, downhill skiing/snowboarding and horse-related activities
Rice[19]	Council on Sports Medicine & Fitness, American Academy of Pediatrics	Athlete needs individual assessment for contact, collision and limited-contact sports. Protective equipment may reduce the risk of injury to the remaining kidney sufficiently to allow participation in most sports, providing such equipment remains in place during activity
Styn & Wan[21]	Literature review	Risk of sport participation very low, but not zero. No evidence that risk of renal injury greater if solitary rather than bilateral kidneys
Neutral		
Patel et al.[12]	Review of major articles	No consensus on participation in contact or collision sports by adolescents with one kidney
Sacco et al.[20]	Literature review	Sports responsible for 13% of genitourinary trauma, but renal trauma usually Grade I–II, not requiring surgical treatment; significant injury rare if solitary kidney
Risser; Washington [13, 14]	Am. Acad. Pediatrics, consensus report	Athlete needs individual assessment for contact, collision and limited-contact sports
Unfavourable		
Dyment[15]	Consensus of American Academy of Pediatrics	No contact or collision sports should be allowed
Sharp et al.[16]	Survey of American Academy of Pediatrics, Urology Section	68% of respondents recommended no contact sport if solitary kidney, although recognizing that the risk was low (<1%)
Speafico et al.[17]	Study of survivors of renal tumours	Need to avoid lifestyles and behaviours potentially dangerous to remaining kidney; but current Italian blanket prohibition of competitive organized sports seems unjustified

Risks of renal injury during sport and physical activity

Renal injury is in itself a rare occurrence, accounting for about 3% of all trauma, and despite the fears of some physicians, sport accounts for only a small fraction of injuries involving the kidneys. In adults, a survey of 9119 individuals with blunt renal injuries found that 63% of these were caused directly by motor vehicle collisions, and a further 4% by cars hitting pedestrians; 14% were due to falls and only 11% were attributed to sport participation.[28] In the paediatric portion of the sample, motor vehicles caused 30% of cases directly and 13% were caused by a motor vehicle hitting the child; falls caused a further 27% of incidents and only 12% were due to sports participation. Other authors have found recreational sports responsible for 2–28% of renal injuries[21, 23] (Table 5.2).

Table 5.2 The incidence and severity of renal injury during sports participation

Authors	Sample	Findings
Berqvist et al.[22]	1354 cases of abdominal trauma in Skaraborg County (Sweden), 1950–1979	59 sport-related injuries to kidneys; approximate incidence 8 per million person-years, apparently rising. Nephrectomy needed in 2 cases, hemi-nephrectomy in 1 case over 30 years of experience
Gerstenbluth et al.[23]	68 children with blunt renal trauma (14 due to sport)	5 cycling and 1 sports injuries grade IV or V damage to kidneys
Grinsell et al.[7]	American Organ Procurement and Transplantation Network	96,000 patients awaiting a renal transplant. None due to sport participation
Grinsell et al.[24]	US National Athletic Trainers' Association High-School injury survey, 1995–1997; 4 million athletic exposures	18 renal injuries, but none resulted in nephrectomy or permanent renal injury. Renal injuries in basketball 2.3 (M), 2.6 (F) per million exposures; soccer 2.5 (M), 6.0 (F) per million exposures. Risk lower than head or spinal injury
Johnson et al.[8]	US national pediatric trauma registry, 49,561 cases	92 incidents due to cycling, 88 to sports participation (approximate incidence 8 and 7 per million children-years). Only 4 sports injuries required nephrectomy
McAleer et al.[25]	San Diego trauma registry 1984–2000, 14,763 patients	113 renal injuries due to various physical activities (7 per year); no single-kidney cases, no nephrectomies required
Wan et al.[26]	Trauma registry, 4921 injured children aged 5–18 yr, Western New York State, 1993–2000	Recreational kidney injury 6.9 per million children-years. Recreational injuries requiring nephrectomy 0.4 per million children-years
Wan et al.[27]	National pediatric trauma registry, 81,923 cases aged 5–18 yr, 1990–1999	42 renal injuries due to sport, mainly in older children, 4.2 per year. No injuries required nephrectomy

Not only is the risk of renal trauma during sport low, but many of the recorded injuries associated with sport are only a minor bruising of the kidneys, with full and rapid recovery of normal function. Only a small fraction of those who are injured require a nephrectomy. Wan et al.[26] studied 4921 children aged 5–18 years listed in the Western New York State Trauma Registry for 1993 to 2000. The total incidence of recreational kidney injuries was 6.9 per million children-years, and catastrophic injuries needing nephrectomy occurred only 0.4 times per million children-years. The same authors[27] examined data from the US national paediatric trauma registry for 1990–1999. Among 81,923 incidents, they were only 42 sport-related renal injuries (a total of 4.2 per year), none of which required nephrectomy.

Johnson et al.[8] had similar findings in an analysis of the US national paediatric trauma registry for the period 1995–2001. Of the 49,651 cases listed, 813 involved kidney injuries; 92 of these were associated with cycling and only 88 with participation in various types of sport. Based upon census reports for US children in 2000, the incidence of renal injuries for cycling and sports participation were approximately eight and seven incidents per million children-years, respectively, agreeing quite well with the estimates of Wan et al.[26] Moreover, only four of the sports injuries reported by Johnson et al. required a nephrectomy.[8] A further study, based upon data from the San Diego paediatric trauma registry,[25] examined 14,763 incidents occurring between 1984 and 2000. The population involved was not specified, but there were a total of 113 sports-related renal injuries in this sample, a total of seven per year. None resulted in nephrectomy and none involved individuals with a solitary kidney.

The US National Athletic Trainers' Association high school injury survey[7] analysed data on 23,666 incidents among some 4 million athletic exposures from 1995 to 1997. This series included only 18 renal injuries, and none of these resulted in nephrectomy or any other known loss of renal function. The risk of any degree of renal injury for high-school students was set at 2.3 injuries per million exposures in male basketball players, and 2.6 per million exposures in male soccer players, with corresponding figures for girls of 2.5 and 6.0 injuries per million exposures. These risks were a striking two orders lower than those observed for serious incidents of head and spinal injury.

A 30-year survey from Skaraborg County, Sweden[22] showed a similar experience to that in the US. There were approximately eight sport-related renal injuries per million person-years, although the authors commented that the incidence of such events appeared to be rising over the study period (1950–1979), perhaps because of the growing popularity of active recreation. Only two nephrectomies and one heminephrectomy had been required over the course of this Swedish survey.

Additional evidence on the relative safety of sport participation comes from the American Organ Procurement and Transplantation Network. In December of 2011, 96,000 patients were awaiting a renal transplant for various reasons, but not one of them had suffered a kidney injury during sports participation.[7] It is plain that the risk of any type of renal injury during sports participation is low, and that most of the injuries are minor in nature. One small study specifically examined the severity of injuries; it found that only one of eight sport-related incidents was severe (Grade IV or V), but that five of six bicycle-related injuries fell into the severe category.[23]

Factors modifying the inherent risk of sports-related renal injury

Factors potentially modifying the risk of renal injury during sport and active recreation include the individual's initial renal health, age, the presence of a solitary kidney, the wearing of effective protective equipment, patterns of play and the degree of supervision of the activities that are undertaken.

Initial renal health

A person with two healthy kidneys usually has a substantial renal reserve, and normal function is quite well maintained even after nephrectomy. However, the functional margin is inevitably smaller for a person who begins with a single kidney, and the initial health of the kidney then becomes a significant issue.[29] A much more cautious attitude to sport participation is required if one or both kidneys are ectopic, multicystic or for any reason show poor performance on tests of renal function.

Age

The kidneys are relatively larger in children than in adults, and they sometimes retain foetal lobulation. Both of these factors cause them to protrude below the rib cage, making them more vulnerable to blunt trauma.[30] Vulnerability is further increased in children because the rib cage is less rigid than in an adult, and there is less soft tissue support of the kidneys.[21]

Solitary kidney

A solitary kidney may hypertrophy until it is 50% larger than paired kidneys. It then faces a greater potential exposure to external trauma just because of its greater size and its protrusion below the rib cage, although statistics do not always reveal any consequence of this greater susceptibility, perhaps because only a small proportion of those with solitary kidneys are allowed to participate in vigorous activities. A solitary kidney also has a more than normal vulnerability to irreversible damage from heat stress, and the temperature limits that are set for prolonged bouts of endurance exercise should be observed particularly carefully in those with a single kidney.

Protective equipment

The US National Kidney Foundation and the Kidney and Urology Foundation of America have each advocated the use of protective padding as a means of protecting a solitary kidney from trauma. The equipment is custom-made, and the cost can be high (commonly more than US$350). Moreover, although the use of such equipment may appear logical, there is as yet no good evidence to show the extent to which it is effective in reducing renal injury.[10]

Patterns of play and degree of supervision

The risk of most types of physical injury, including damage to the kidneys, is influenced by the level of competition, the individual's playing position, and the degree of supervision of a game. The simple precautions of close supervision by a coach or parent and the firm enforcement of rules of play are likely to reduce the risks of renal injury. In general, the prevalence of injuries is greater for unsupervised play than for organized sport. The practical lesson is that the incidence of renal trauma can be reduced by a rigid enforcement of rules and a careful supervision of free play.

Conclusions

When assessing the risks of sport, account should be taken of initial renal health, the child' age, the absence of one kidney, the availability and efficacy of protective equipment, the playing position, the level of competition and the supervision of play by officials and parents. Particular care is needed for those with a solitary kidney, since this is more vulnerable to heat stress, and its hypertrophy places it at a greater risk of physical injury.

Sports and physical activities with the greatest risk of renal injury

Many physicians have considered contact sports as particularly dangerous from the viewpoint of renal injury, and available statistics show that they are responsible for a substantial proportion of injuries relative to other types of active pursuit (Table 5.3). However, because the total number of renal injuries is small and there are national and regional differences in the popularity of various sports and leisure pursuits, relative risks vary substantially from one report to another. Moreover, the data are often hard to interpret, since the reported injury percentages commonly exclude incidents that have arisen when cycling, operating all-terrain vehicles or engaging in playground recreation.

In an 18-year review of statistics for the US National Football League, Brophy et al.[31] found that the overall risk averaged 2.7 incidents of renal trauma per season. Further, all of the affected individuals were subsequently able to return to play with both kidneys intact. About a third of these patients

Table 5.3 Relative risk of sports and other active pursuits as seen in ten reports

Study	1	2	3	4	5	6	7	8	9	10
Total # of activity-related renal injuries	13,006	59	14	465	18	85	98	15	42	115
Country and date	US 2002–2010	Sweden 1950–1979	2 US trauma centres, pre-2002	11 published papers	US high schools 1995–1997	US 1995–2001	California 1984–2000	US 1993–2000	US 1990–1999	US 2000–2005
Sports										
Football	16.6%		7.1%	8.6%	66.7%	23.5%	6.1%	33.3%	61.9%	10.4%
Ice-hockey		13.6%	21.4%			3.5%		13.4%	7.1%	
Soccer	4.9%	57.6%		7.3%	18.7%	2.4%			4.8%	
Other sports	17.8%	11.8%		44.1%	18.7%	41.2%	49.0%*	20.0%	26.2%	49.6%
Other active pursuits										
Horse-riding	7.3%	8.5%					3.0%	6.7%		3.5%
Skiing	11.8%	8.5%		19.6%		8.2%		13.0%		4.3%
Snowboard						8.2%		6.7%		3.5%
Sledge			14.2%			12.9%				
Cycling	17.8%		57.1%	20.4%			27.6%	6.7%	17.4%	17.4%
Motor-cycle and ATVs	26.2%						14.3%			11.3%

Note: * Including skate-boarding, roller-blading, use of playground equipment and miscellaneous falls

Source: Studies 1–10: Bagga et al.;[32] Berqvist et al.;[22] Gerstenbluth et al.;[23] Grinsell et al.;[8] Johnson et al.;[7] McAleer et al.;[25] Wan et al.;[26, 27] Wu et al.[33]

required hospitalization, but none underwent any form of surgery. Incidents were ten times more prevalent during actual games (0.000005 per exposure) than during practices, but nevertheless the authors of this report argued that it may be safe for individuals with only one functioning kidney to play in the NFL. This verdict was accepted by 61% of NFL physicians, although a lower percentage of clinicians gave their assent to the idea that students with a single kidney could participate in high school (45%) or college (50%) games. A six-year study of Australian Rules football found that 13 cases of renal trauma had been admitted to one hospital, with 2 requiring nephrectomy;[34] however, the level of risk cannot be assessed in this report, since there is no indication of the corresponding number of exposures.

Somewhat in contrast with North American experience, a study from Sweden[22] found a predominance of renal injuries among soccer players, particularly at the start of the playing season, when they were presumably in poorer physical condition.

A survey of North American high-school students found most of the renal injuries were in football (boys) or in soccer (girls),[24] and two surveys of trauma-centre statistics found a concentration of renal injuries among football players.[26, 27]

A series of 14 activity-related renal injuries in Ohio[23] included data on cycling. This report demonstrated that the bicycle was a dangerous machine for youth; it was responsible for five of the six high-grade renal injuries (grade IV or V) seen in the study. McAleer et al.[25] also concluded that cycling and the use of all-terrain vehicles were major causes of renal injuries. This verdict was further substantiated in a survey of 116 renal injuries from blunt trauma.[33] The commonest source of injury in this last series was a motor vehicle collision (33 cases), with other causes including cycling (20 cases), use of all-terrain vehicles (13 cases), limited contact sports (20 cases), contact sports (12 cases), alpine sports (9 cases) and horseback riding (4 cases). The use of all-terrain vehicles was to blame for the most severe injuries that required nephrectomy. Interestingly, 2 of the 116 cases in this series were individuals with unilateral kidneys, and 3 other patients had abnormally positioned kidneys.[33] Among football players, the greatest risk was in pick-up games, when no protective equipment was worn.[33] One report where American football appeared more dangerous than cycling was from western New York State; possibly, cycling was not a common pursuit in this region. Johnson et al.[8] included specific data for cycling injuries in their survey, and they also found a substantial proportion of incidents were attributable to American football. However, none of the injuries needing nephrectomy were associated with contact sports; injuries requiring renal surgery were from sledding (two cases), downhill skiing (one case) and roller-blading (one case).

Perhaps the most satisfactory evidence on risk levels comes from the large surveys of Bagga et al.[32] and Grinsell et al.[24]. Bagga et al.[32] underlined the importance of cycling and use of sports vehicles, which together accounted for 44% of all physical activity-related renal trauma. Nevertheless, American football and soccer together were also responsible for more than a fifth of renal injuries. Grinsell et al.[24] put together data on 465 renal injuries from a survey of 11 articles; this analysis also found that a substantial proportion of renal injuries were due to American football and soccer, although the totals for these sports were outweighed by the risks of cycling and skiing. In this last report, the 14 incidents requiring nephrectomy were attributed to downhill skiing (five), cycling (four), horse-back riding (two), soccer (two) and American football (one).

A number of articles have looked at the risks involved in specific forms of active recreation, including the operation of all-terrain vehicles, cycling, alpine activities and horse-back riding, although unfortunately in most of these reports the lack of exposure rates does not allow a calculation of the incidence of renal injuries. Nevertheless, it does appear that risks are greater for some personal leisure pursuits than for most forms of organized sport.

All-terrain vehicles

Consensus groups in both Canada and the US have concluded that the operation of all-terrain vehicles by young and inexperienced children with inadequate protection is particularly dangerous in terms of renal trauma.[35, 36] Wu et al.[33] emphasized that dirt bikes and all-terrain vehicles were the most important sources of serious recreational injuries to the kidneys.

Cycling

The use of a bicycle by a child or a mountain bike by a young adult is another cause of concern. A study of 107 serious cycling accidents found 30 head and neck injuries, and 18 that involved the abdomen; the 3 renal injuries in this series were caused by impact of the ends of the handlebars on the abdomen.[37] Current handlebar designs are quite dangerous. In a second report, 5 of 30 handlebar injuries involved the kidneys, and in 3 of these nephrectomy or hemi-nephrectomy was required.[38] A further study found 40 handlebar injuries among 134,116 children admitted to a Swiss hospital; 1 of the 40 children concerned had sustained a renal rupture.[39] Another analysis of 1990 patients who had been injured when riding various types of vehicles found that 236 of these incidents (including 151 abdominal injuries) were due to the handlebars; 29 of these required a major operation (although usually for small bowel perforation or pancreatic trauma rather than renal injury).[40]

When a child loses control of a bicycle, he or she typically falls onto the end of the handlebars as the wheel rotates through 90 degrees. Possibly, the risk of major injury could be diminished by lessening the maximum potential rotation of the front wheel of the bicycle, altering the shape of the handlebars, and either padding the ends of the handlebars or making them compressible.[41-43] Other avoidable risk factors are use of an inappropriate size of bicycle by a child and the operation of stunt bicycles.

Alpine activities

Winter sports such as skiing, snowboarding and sledding are other likely causes of abdominal trauma. The incidence of skiing injuries in Austria is about one per visitor-year, with 2% of these injuries affecting the kidneys.[30] The Urology Department of an Innsbruck hospital treated 254 children for renal trauma over a 26-year period, mostly due to skiing incidents. In about a third of these patients, the renal injury was severe, but only four nephrectomies were needed.[30] The risk of abdominal injuries is higher for snowboarding than for skiing;[44, 45] the abdomen accounted for 0.7% of injuries in skiers and 1.2% in snowboarders, with renal injury accounting for 29.7% of all abdominal trauma in skiers and 68.4% in snowboarders.[44] Most of the skiing injuries were sustained in the afternoons, possibly because of a deterioration in snow conditions or fatigue of the skier. Problems were also more frequent in children, adolescents and those with low skill levels, suggesting the value of lessons that embrace safety precautions.[44–46] In many skiers, other adverse factors were defective bindings and the use of rented equipment.[46]

Sledding is a fairly frequent source of renal injury. Factors increasing risk for sledders include towing by a vehicle such as a snowmobile, sledding near to a road and collision with a stationary object such as a tree.[47] Five of 25 sledders who were admitted to a paediatric trauma centre had abdominal injuries, with 2 involving the kidneys; however, 11 of the same group had sustained head injuries.[47]

Horseback riding

As in other active pursuits, the head of the horseback rider is at greater risk than the abdomen. About 8% of the injuries sustained during horseback riding are abdominal (for instance, trampling by another rider after falling), whereas 38% affect the face and head. Many other injuries occur while grooming or walking beside a horse.[48] A study of 315 injuries involving horses found that eight involved the kidneys.[49] Children should ride a mount that is well-matched to their size and abilities, wear boots with heels (to minimize dragging after a fall) and stand clear of the horse's hooves when dismounted.[50]

Martial arts

Renal contusion can occur in sports such as jujitsu, judo and aikido. De Meersman et al.[51] found that 85% of judoka who had fallen 100 times on a 2.5 cm thickness mat developed significant haematuria (>50 red cells per high-powered field), and this was considered evidence of renal trauma. However, the *reported* rate of renal injuries for martial arts is quite low, 1 of 5700 injuries sustained in 24,027 training years.[52] Safety in the martial arts can be enhanced by increasing the thickness of matting, and possibly by the use of spring-loaded mats.[53]

Other sports causing renal injury

Case reports have identified other occasional incidents of renal trauma during many recreational activities, including a haematoma induced under the renal capsule by exposure to paint-gun pellets.[54]

Conclusions

Physical activities presenting a higher than average risk of renal injury appear to include operation of all-terrain vehicles, cycling, alpine sports, horseback riding and martial arts. Individuals with single kidneys should preferably choose alternative pursuits, and particular care should be observed if they continue to be involved in such activities.

Managing risks of renal trauma for the active child

Practical management issues include the advice that clinicians should give to parents on the proportion of sport-related renal injuries that are likely to require nephrectomy, on the duration of restricted activity that should be observed following less severe renal injury, on the likelihood of a permanent impairment of renal function following renal trauma, and on the restriction of sports participation for children with a solitary kidney.

Proportion of activity-related renal injuries requiring nephrectomy

Although the overall risk of renal trauma during physical activity is low, the likelihood of adverse long-term consequences is further attenuated because injuries are often quite minor and can be managed conservatively. One report found that 6% of injuries required abdominal exploration and no more than 2% underwent only nephrectomy.[55] Many of those who sustain a renal injury can return to their chosen form of physical activity after as little as two weeks of rest, although severe lacerations may require several months away from competition.[31, 56] Minor injuries are often assessed in terms of continuing haematuria, although this does not always provide a reliable guide to the extent of renal injury.[12, 30, 57]

In weighing the relative risks of various types of physical activity, it is important to look at not only the total incidence of renal trauma, but also the typical severity of injuries associated with a given type of activity. Several non-contact sports such as cycling, skiing and snowboarding seem particularly prone to cause severe injuries, with a greater chance that nephrectomy will be required following injury.

Duration of restricted physical activity following injury

The typical duration of restricted activity for minor renal trauma is two to six weeks. However, vigorous physical activity should be limited until haematuria has ceased.[6, 56]

Risk of permanent renal damage

The immediate recovery of the kidney from blunt trauma is usually quite rapid and relatively complete. However, there are sometimes long-term sequelae (usually from subcapsular bleeding and pressure necrosis[58]). The resulting impairment of renal function is particularly troubling for the individual with a solitary kidney.

A review of 157 patients with renal agenesis found that even in the absence of any known trauma, as adults they were at increased risk of hypertension, proteinuria and renal insufficiency.[59] A three-year follow-up of 13 children with high-grade renal injuries found no signs of hypertension or other renal abnormalities.[60] However, technetium-99m-dimercaptosuccinic acid renal scans have indicated that severe (Grade 5) renal trauma can ultimately cause renal scarring and a loss of kidney tissue that impairs renal function.[61] Further information is needed on the extent of this risk.

Advice to parents

Health professionals have the responsibility of communicating the level of risk associated with sport participation to the parents of a child with a single kidney. While the need to use all possible tactics to minimize dangers should be underlined, it is also important to the overall development of a child that an excess of caution does not remove safe and interesting options for involvement in health-promoting physical activity.

Although the risk of renal injury is very low in most types of physical activity, it is not non-existent. One way of explaining the level of risk to an anxious parent is to compare the incidence of kidney and head injuries. Most types of physical activity carry at least a five times greater risk of head injury than of renal trauma.[9, 10] And despite a growing public concern about concussion in American football and ice hockey, the potential risk of a head injury is not usually considered a sufficient reason to prohibit children from participating in these sports.

At the same time, there are simple precautions that can greatly reduce the risk of renal injury, as discussed above, and it is particularly important that these precautions be communicated to the parents, particularly if a child has only a single kidney.

Areas for further research

There remain many gaps in current knowledge concerning the dangers of an active lifestyle for the individual with a single kidney. Risks remain poorly defined because most available statistics lack critical information on the number of hours of exposure to a given type of physical activity per year. Moreover, some analyses of overall risk appear to exclude exposure to informal but relatively risky activities such as schoolyard play, cycling and the operation of all-terrain vehicles. A greater risk of injury might be anticipated for those with a hyper-trophied single kidney, but this is not apparent in the available data. Possibly, this is because many children with a single kidney lead severely restricted lives. The use of haematuria as a means of detecting persistent renal injury seems to be unreliable, and a simple but effective tool is needed to monitor recovery follow-ing renal trauma. More information is also needed on the immediate vulnerability to heat stress and the long-term incidence of hypertension in those sustaining serious renal injuries. Finally, there is a need for more precise evaluation of the efficacy of equipment intended to protect against renal injury.

Practical implications and conclusions

Many health professionals still seem overly cautious about recommending sport participation for children with single kidneys, although sometimes permitting more dangerous pursuits such as cycling. Risks and benefits need to be weighed carefully, with recognition that there are dangers to physical, social and mental development if the life of a child with a solitary kidney is unduly restricted. Empirical evidence shows that the absolute risk of renal injury during most types of physical activity is very low, although not non-existent. For instance, there are 2.6 incidents per million exposures in male soccer players. Many of the renal injuries incurred during physical activity are minor in nature and only a small proportion require nephrectomy. Contact sports account for perhaps a fifth of physical activity-related renal injuries. The operation of all-terrain vehicles, cycling, alpine sports and horseback riding are more common sources of renal trauma, and cycle handlebars should be redesigned to make them safer. Possible factors modifying inherent risks include initial renal health, the individual's age (children being more vulnerable than adults), careful supervision of play, choice of playing position and level of competition, and the wearing of effective protective equipment. Minor renal injuries may require only two to six weeks of restricted physical activity. Often, there are no long-term consequences to blunt renal trauma, although subcapsular haematomas can cause pressure necrosis, with later risks of hypertension, proteinuria and renal insufficiency. Health profes-sionals should emphasize that sport participation carries greater dangers for the head than for the kidneys, and that serious renal injury is more likely from motor traffic than from participation in most sports. Moreover, they should underline the importance of continued regular physical activity to the overall health and development of the child. Nevertheless, those with a solitary kidney should probably avoid sports that involve contact or have a high risk of collisions.

References

1. Bernard C. *Leçons sur les phenomènes de la vie*. Paris, France: Baillière, 1876.
2. Singer-Polignac. F. *Les concepts de Claude Bernard sur le milieu interieur, par Roger Heim et al.* [The concepts of Claude Bernard on the internal environment, by Roger Heim and associates]. Paris, France: Masson 1967.

3. Bernard C. *Introduction à l'étude de la médicine expérimentale.* [Introduction to experimental medicine]. New Brunswick, NJ: Transaction Publishers, 1999.
4. Ibrahim H, Foley R, Tan L, et al. Long-term consequences of kidney donation. *N Engl J Med* 2009; 360(5): 459–469.
5. Anderson CR. Solitary kidney and sports participation. *Arch Fam Med* 1995; 4(10): 885–888.
6. Bernard JJ. Renal trauma: evaluation, management and return to play. *Curr Sports Med Rep* 2009; 8(2): 98–103.
7. Grinsell MM, Showalter S, Gordon KA, et al. Single kidney and sports participation: perception versus reality. *Pediatrics* 2006; 118(3): 1019–1027.
8. Johnson B, Christensen C, Dirusso S, et al. A need for reevaluation of sports participation recommendations for children with a solitary kidney. *J Urol* 2005; 174(2): 686–689.
9. Psooy K. Sports and the solitary kidney: what parents of a young child with a solitary kidney should know. *Can Urol Assoc J* 2009; 3(1): 67–68.
10. Psooy K. Sports and the solitary kidney: how to counsel parents. *Can J Urol* 2006; 13(3): 3120–3126.
11. Psooy K. Sports and the solitary kidney: what parents of a young child with a solitary kidney should know. *Can Urol Assoc J* 2014; 8(7–8): 233–235.
12. Patel DR, Torres AD, Greydanus DE. Kidney and sports. *Adolesc Med Clin* 2005; 16: 111–1119.
13. Washington RL, American Academy of Pediatrics. Medical conditions affecting sports participation. *Pediatrics* 2001; 107(5): 1205–1209.
14. Risser WL, American Academy of Pediatrics Committee on Sports Medicine and Fitness. Medical conditions affecting sport participation. *Pediatrics* 1994; 94(5): 757–760.
15. Dyment PG, Committee on Sports Medicine. Recommendations for participation in competitive sport. *Pediatrics* 1988; 81(5): 737–739.
16. Sharp DS, Ross JH, Kay R. Attitudes of pediatric urologists regarding sports participation by children with a solitary kidney. *J Urol* 2002; 168(4 Pt 2): 1811–1814.
17. Spreafico F, Ternenziani M, van den Heuvel-Eibrink MM, et al. Why should survivors of childhood renal tumor and others with only one kidney be denied the chance to play contact sports? *Expert Rev Anticancer Ther* 2014; 14(4): 363–366.
18. MacAuley D, Best T. *Evidence-based sports medicine.* Chichester, UK: John Wiley, 2008.
19. Rice SG, American Academy of Pediatrics Committee on Sports Medicine and Fitness. Medical conditions affecting sports participation. *Pediatrics* 2008; 121: 841–848.
20. Sacco E, Marangi F, Pinto F, et al. Sports and genitourinary traumas. *Urologia* 2010; 77(2): 112–115.
21. Styn NR, Wan J. Urological sports injuries in children. *Curr Urol Rep* 2010; 11(2): 114–121.
22. Bergqvist D, Hedelin H, Karlsson G, et al. Abdominal injury from sporting activities. *Br J Sports Med* 1982; 16(2): 76–79.
23. Gerstenbluth RE, Spirnak JP, Elder JS. Sports participation and high grade renal injuries in children. *J Urol* 2002; 168 (6): 2575–2578.
24. Grinsell MM, Butz K, Gurka MJ, et al. Sport related kidney injury among high school athletes. *Pediatrics* 2012; 130: e40–e55.

25. McAleer IM, Kaplan GW, LoSasso BE. Renal and testis injuries in team sports. *J Urol* 2002; 168: 1805–1807.
26. Wan J, Corvino TF, Greenfield SP, et al. The incidence of recreational genitourinary and abdominal injuries in the western New York pediatric population. *J Urol* 2003; 170(4 part 2): 1526–1527.
27. Wan J, Corvino TF, Greenfield SP, et al. Kidney and testicle injuries in team and individual sports: data from the national pediatric trauma registry. *J Urol* 2003; 170(4 Part 2): 1528–1532.
28. Voelzke BB, Leddy L. The epidemiology of renal trauma. *Transl Androl Urol* 2014; 3(2): 143–149.
29. Mandell J, Cromie WJ, Caldamone AA, et al. Sports-related genitourinary injuries in children. *Clin Sports Med* 1982; 1: 483–493.
30. Radmayr C, Oswald J, Müller E, et al. Blunt renal trauma in children: 26 years clinical experience. *Eur Urol* 2002; 42(3): 297–300.
31. Brophy RH, Gamradt SC, Barnes RP, et al. Kidney injuries in professional American football. Implications for management of an athlete with 1 functioning kidney. *Am J Sports Med* 2008; 36(1): 85–90.
32. Bagga HS, Fisher PB, Taslan GE, et al. Sports-related genitourinary injuries presenting to United States emergency departments. *Urology* 2015; 85(1): 239–245.
33. Wu H-Y, Gaines BA. Dirt bikes and all-terrain vehicles: the real threat to pediatric kidneys. *J Urol* 2007; 178(4 Part 2): 1672–1674.
34. Lee S, Thavaseelan J, Low V. Renal trauma in Australian Rules football: an institutional experience. *Austr NZ J Surg* 2004; 74(9): 766–768.
35. Yanchar T. Canadian Association of Pediatric Surgeons' position statement on the use of all-terrain vehicles by children and youth. *J Pediatr Surg* 2008; 43(5): 938–939.
36. Burd R, American Pediatric Surgical Association Trauma Committee. Position statement on the use of all-terrain vehicles by children and youth. *J Pediatr Surg* 2009; 44(8): 1638–1639.
37. Winston FK, Shaw KN, Kreshak AA, et al. Hidden spears: handlebars as injury hazards to children. *Pediatrics* 1998;102(3): 596–601.
38. Sparnon AL, Ford WDA. Bicycle handlebar injuries in children. *J Pediatr Surg* 1986; 21(2): 118–119.
39. Klimek PM, Lutz T, Stranzinger E et al. Handlebar injuries in children. *Pediatr Surg Internat* 2013; 29(3): 269–273.
40. Nataraja RM, Palmer CS, Arul GS, et al. The full spectrum of handlebar injuries in children: A decade of experience. *Injury* 2014; 45(4): 684–689.
41. Acton CH, Thomas S, Clark R, et al. Bicycle incidents in children: abdominal trauma and handlebars. *Med J Austr* 1994; 160(6): 344–346.
42. Clarnette TD, Beasley SW. Handlebar injuries in children: patterns and prevention. *Austr NZ J Surg* 1997; 67(6): 338–339.
43. Kubiak R, Slongo T. Unpowered scooter injuries in children. *Acta Paedr* 2003; 92(1): 50–54.
44. Machida T, Hanazaki K, Ishizaka K, et al. Snowboarding injuries of the abdomen: comparison with skiing injuries. *Injury* 1999; 30(1): 47–49.
45. Sulheim S, Holme I, Rødven A, et al. Risk factors for injuries in alpine skiing, telemark skiing and snowboarding – case-control study. *Br J Sports Med* 2011; 45(16): 1303–1309.
46. Goulet C, Regnier G, Grimard G, et al. Risk factors associated with alpine skiing injuries in children. A case-control study. *Am J Sports Med* 1999; 27(5): 644–650.

47. Shorter NA, Mooney DP, Harmon BJ. Childhood sledding injuries. *Am J Emerg Med* 1999; 17(1): 32–34.
48. Eckert V, Lockemann U, Püschel K, et al. Equestrian injuries caused by horse kicks: First results of a prospective multicenter study. *Clin J Sports Med* 2011; 21(4): 353–355.
49. Ghosh A, DiScala C, Drew C, et al. Horse-related injuries in pediatric patients. *J Pediatr Surg* 2000; 35(12): 1766–1770.
50. Jagodzinski T, DeMuri GP. Horse-related injuries in children: a review. *Wisc Med J* 2005; 104(2): 50–54.
51. De Meersman RB, Wilkerson JE. Judo nephropathy: trauma versus non-trauma. *J Trauma* 1982; 22: 150–152.
52. Birrer RB. Trauma epidemiology in the martial arts: the results of an eighteen year international survey. *Am J Sports Med* 1996; 24(6 Suppl.): S72–S79.
53. Itagaki MW, Knight NB. Kidney trauma in martial arts. A case report of kidney contusion in jujitsu. *Am J Sports Med* 2004; 32(2): 522–524.
54. Guerrero MA, Zhouy W, El Sayed HF, et al. Subcapsular hematoma of the kidney secondary to paintball pellet injuries. *J Emerg Med* 2009; 36(3): 300–301.
55. Buckley JC, McAninch J. Revision of current American Association for the Surgery of Trauma Renal Injury grading system. *J Trauma* 2011; 70(1): 35–37.
56. Holmes FC, Hunt JJ, Sevier TL. Renal injury in sport. *Curr Sports Med Rep* 2003; 2: 103–109.
57. Santucci R, McAninch J. Diagnosis and management of renal trauma: past, present, and future. *J Am Coll Surg* 2000; 191: 433–451.
58. Banowsky LH, Wolfel DA, Lackner LH. Considerations in diagnosis and management of renal trauma. *J Trauma* 1970; 10(7): 587–597.
59. Argueso LR, Ritchey ML, Boyle ET, et al. Prognosis of patients with unilateral renal agenesis. *Pediatr Nephrol* 1992; 6(5): 412–416.
60. El-Shirbiny MT, Aboul-Ghar ME, Hafez AT, et al. Late renal functional and morphological evaluation after non-operative treatment of high-grade renal injuries in children. *BJU Int* 2004; 93(7): 1053–1056.
61. Keller MD, Coln CE, Garza JJ, et al. Functional outcomes of nonoperatively managed renal injuries in children. *J Trauma Inj Infect Crit Care* 2004; 57(1): 108–110.

6 Bladder function in health and disease

Physical activity and bladder control, haematuria and bladder cancer

Introduction

This chapter explores the interaction between impaired bladder control and various types of physical activity, looking at whether particular types of sport are likely to cause problems of incontinence, and examining the possible role of exercise programmes in improving bladder control. It also adds to the information on haematuria presented in Chapter 4, and it explores whether habitual physical activity has any role in the prevention or treatment of bladder cancers.

The problem of urinary incontinence

Urinary incontinence is defined by the International Continence Society as a "complaint of any involuntary leakage of urine".[1] Clinicians commonly distinguish a form of urinary leakage termed stress urinary incontinence, which is precipitated by physical exertion, sneezing or coughing, and is of particular concern to the athlete. However, some authors maintain that other types of incontinence can also be precipitated by repeated bouts of strenuous physical activity.

Risk factors for urinary incontinence include old age, parity (particularly if instrumentally aided delivery of a baby has been necessary), obesity, diabetes mellitus, stroke, smoking, depression, overall functional impairment, oestrogen deficiency, genitourinary surgery and the use of medications such as psychotropic agents, angiotensin converting enzyme (ACE) inhibitors and diuretics.[2-4] Incontinence is also associated with eating disorders, possibly because an inadequate intake of nutrients leads to muscle weakness;[5, 6] this factor could contribute to incontinence in gymnasts, where anorexia is sometimes a problem. Most studies of stress incontinence in athletes have been based on nulliparous individuals, although exercise is particularly likely to induce incontinence in the first few months following pregnancy.[7]

Prevalence, economic impact and clinical evaluation of urinary incontinence

Urinary leakage varies greatly in volume and frequency, and because the affected individuals are often embarrassed by their condition, the problem tends to be under-reported. In the general population, 25–40% of women have some urinary leakage at least once per year, and in 10% incontinence occurs as often as once per week.[8, 9] Leakage is less frequently in men. Incontinence is often thought as affecting mainly elderly people. However, Sandvik and associates[10, 11] summarized 13 studies of women, finding urinary leakage of unspecified severity in 20–30% of young women, rising to 30–40% in middle-age and 30–50% in the elderly. Certainly, occasional incontinence is to be expected in at least 15–30% of older community-dwelling older adults, as well as 50% of nursing home residents.[4, 5, 12]

Stress incontinence is usually a social inconvenience rather than a major health issue, but it can cause medical problems such as urinary tract and perineal infections, pressure ulcers and sleep disturbances. It also reduces the individual's quality of life[13] and discourages participation in both physical activity[14, 15] and other forms of social interaction. In 1996, the estimated costs of urinary incontinence to the US economy were $11.2 billion within the community and $5.2 billion in nursing homes.[12]

Many pathologies can be at play in those with urinary incontinence, and a careful clinical examination is required, particularly if the condition is of recent onset. Issues to be reviewed are summarized in Table 6.1.

Urinary incontinence in athletes

Stress incontinence can affect not only the elderly, but also much younger individuals, particularly those involved in vigorous athletic pursuits.[16] The prevalence of urinary leakage is influenced by the type and level of competition.[17] One review published in 2011 found 22 articles on stress incontinence in athletes,[18] and a second review from 2010 located 49 papers;[19] in 2014, a further PubMed search increased this total to 61 articles linking stress incontinence and sport participation[20] (Table 11.2). A review by Goldstick and Constatini[21] suggested that 28–80% of athletes had such complaints, with the highest prevalence among those who engaged in high-impact activities (trampolinists, gymnasts, hockey players and ballet dancers), and the lowest prevalence among those engaged in physically less demanding sports such as golf.[22] Jumping activities such as basketball and volleyball predispose to leakage, imposing ground reaction forces as much as four times body mass.[23]

Many investigators have relied on questionnaires or postal surveys to assess urinary incontinence. It has not always been clear from the responses to such instruments how frequent or serious the problem was, and whether the issue was stress incontinence or some other form of urinary leakage. A few observers have assessed incontinence more directly, measuring urinary leakage in a weighed sanitary pad[24–27] or recording the escape of fluid as a telemetrically recorded change in the electrical resistance of the pad.[28] The correlation between questionnaire responses and objective data is only moderate (a kappa coefficient of 0.45[25]). Hermieu et al.[26] commented that many women where urinary leakage

Table 6.1 Issues to be considered when examining a person who reports the onset of urinary incontinence

History:

- Onset of incontinence
- Associated urinary symptoms
- Frequency, volume and timing of leakage
- Precipitating factors
- Normality of bowel function
- Normality of sexual function
- Risk factors (parity, obesity, diabetes, stroke, smoking, depression, functional impairment, oestrogen deficiency, genitourinary surgery)
- Use of medications (psychotropic agents, angiotensin-converting enzyme inhibitors and diuretics)

Physical examination:

- Abdomen
- Cardiovascular system (signs of volume overload?)
- Physical mobility
- Neurological examination
- Genital examination (atrophy, inflammation, presence of a pelvic mass, pelvic floor weakness, urethral hypermobility, sphincter tone and adequacy of pelvic floor muscle function)

Additional measures:

- Urinalysis
- Diary of urinary voiding
- Determination of post-voiding bladder volume

was indicated by an increase in the weight of a sanitary pad had not admitted to any incontinence when completing a questionnaire. In the study of Eliasson et al., there was an average leakage of 28 g of urine during 15 minutes of activity on the trampoline,[24] and Stach-Lachinen et al.[27] reported an average loss of 26 g over 24 hours in women with active leisure pursuits. Bourcier[29] classed the problem as severe if there was continuous leakage when exercising, moderate if leakage occurred with heavy lifting or running, and mild if it only occurred with jumping.

Only 6 of some 30 studies have made direct comparisons of the prevalence of stress incontinence between athletes and sedentary individuals from the same population,[5, 25, 32, 37, 42, 44] and even then the data have not always been controlled for important covariates (Table 6.2). Nevertheless, the uncontrolled values cited for various classes of athlete remain convincing because the prevalence of stress incontinence in such individuals far exceeds the expected prevalence of leakage in young sedentary nulliparous women.

The pattern of exercise causing problems typically involves a high impact activity such as jumping or running, often with sudden and repeated increases of intra-abdominal pressure.[37] Interestingly, problems seem more prevalent during training than during competition, possibly because the catecholamine secretion of competition acts on urethral α-adrenergic receptors, facilitating closure of the

Table 6.2 Reports of urinary incontinence among athletes, former athletes and other active individuals

Author	Sample	Survey type	Incidence	Comments
Abitteboul et al.[30]	517 female amateur marathon runners aged 41 years	Cross-sectional questionnaire	30.7% had urinary incontinence, 16% during run	Usually seen towards end of the event, 7.5% at least 1/week
Alanee et al.[31]	Equestrians (31 M, 173 F) and swimmers (79 M, 102 F)	Mail and hand-distributed questionnaires	Multivariate analysis showed no association of horseback riding with urinary symptoms	No impact upon sexual dysfunction
Almeida et al.[32]	67 female athletes vs. 96 non-athletes	Questionnaire	Odds ratio of incontinence 2.9 for athletes	Mainly in artistic gymnasts and trampoline
Barreto et al.[33]	47 active women, age 32 yr, average 2.2 children attending 2 gyms	Questionnaire	72% reported urinary incontinence	Jumping 52.9%, squatting with weight 52.9%, leg press 29.4%, running 23.5%, walking 11.8%
Benjamin & Hearon[34]	25 women aviators	Questionnaire	High g force does not cause incontinence even in women with predisposition to incontinence	
Bø & Sundgot-Borden[5]	660 elite female athletes, 766 controls, aged 15–39 years	Cross-sectional case-control postal survey	Similar prevalence in athletes and in controls (41%, 39%; social problem in 15%, 16%)	Parity less frequent in athletes than in controls
Bø et al.[35]	Fitness instructors (yoga and Pilates); 152 men, 685 women	Online survey	Incontinence in 3/152 men; in women 21.4% >1/week, 3.2% 2/week, 1.7% >1/day	Bother score 4.6
Bourcier[29]	30 female athletes age 22 years	Observation during feedback sessions	7% severe, 24% moderate, 33% mild urinary incontinence	Severe = continuous drip when exercising, moderate = with heavy lift or run, mild = with jumping

Table 6.2 continued

Author	Sample	Survey type	Incidence	Comments
Carls[36]	85 female athletes aged 14–21 yr	Cross-sectional Bristol questionnaire	>25% had slight incontinence, 2–4 times/wk to 2–4 times/month. 16% negative effect on social life, 8% avoided exercise	Low response (86/550); 90% had never reported problem or heard of Kegel exercises
Caylet et al.[37]	157 elite female athletes, 426 controls aged 18–35 yr	Cross-sectional questionnaire	Stress incontinence in 28% of athletes, 9.8% of controls	Even a small loss of urine regarded as embarrassing
David[38]	132 nulliparous female athletes, age 19.5 years	Cross-sectional questionnaire	30% reported incontinence in daily life	
Da Roza et al.[39]	22 national-level female nulliparous trampolinists	Cross-sectional questionnaire	Urinary incontinence in 72.7% during practices	Risk of incontinence related to training volume
Davis & Goodman[40]	9 nulliparous female airborne trainees with stress incontinence	Self-administered questionnaire	6 weeks of rigorous airborne infantry training induced severe incontinence	Minimal incontinence before training
dos Santos et al.[41]	58 of 95 female physical education students aged 21.4 yr	Cross-sectional questionnaire	12/58 (20.7%) reported involuntary urine loss, mainly during sports activities	Seriousness of problem on 0–10 scale 2.3 (range 0–6)
Eliasson et al.[24]	35 female national level trampolinists, aged 15 yr	Cross-sectional postal survey, pad test on trampoline, measures of pelvic floor strength	100% on survey, 51.2% on pad test, 28.6% on pelvic floor strength	Leak averaged 28 g (9–56 g); no leak with laughs, coughs or sneezes
Eliasson et al.[17]	305 female trampolinists, aged 21 years, 85 competitive, 220 recreational level	Questionnaire	Prevalence of stress incontinence greater in ex-competitive (76%) than in recreational trampolinists (48%)	Other risk factors: inability to interrupt urine flow and constipation

Table 6.2 continued

Author	Sample	Survey type	Incidence	Comments
Elleuch et al.[2]	105 female athletes, 105 non-athletes, aged 21.5 yr	Cross-sectional questionnaire	Stress incontinence in 62.8% of athletes, 34% in non-athletes	60% of athletes affected on daily basis
Fernandes et al.[25]	39 female adolescent soccer players, age 15.6 yr, 24 controls	Pad test and questionnaire	Incontinence in 62.8% of athletes, vs. 25% in controls	Moderate reliability between pad test and questionnaire (kappa = 0.45)
Fischer & Berg[43]	274 female US aircrew, sometimes exposed to 9 g while flying	Anonymous questionnaire	Prevalence 26.3%, much as in general population	Only 13 of 72 incidents occurred while flying
Fozzatti et al.[44]	244 nulliparous women attending gyms and performing high-impact exercise vs. 244 controls	International incontinence questionnaire	Questionnaire scores 1.68 vs. 1.02 in controls	
Hermieu et al.[26]	188 female runners	Pad test	Incontinence: 28.1% during 15 km walk, 51% for 10 km run, 60% for half-marathon, 75% for marathon	Many of women had not admitted to urinary incontinence on questionnaire
Jacome et al.[45]	105 female athletes (athletics, basketball and football)	Questionnaire and focus group	Urinary incontinence in 41.5%, no difference between sports	Associated with lower body mass and BMI, avoided by preventive urination
Larsen & Yavorek[46]	116 women, 37 involved in paratroop training	Questionnaire and pelvic examination	24/116 had incontinence, unrelated to paratroop training	Paratroop training increased likelihood of pelvic prolapse
Nygaard et al.[22]	Female nulliparous university athletes (156, aged 19.9 yr)	Cross-sectional postal survey	28% experienced at least one episode while practising sport	Gymnastics 67%; tennis 50%; basketball 44%; field hockey 32%; track 26%; other sports <10%

Table 6.2 continued

Author	Sample	Survey type	Incidence	Comments
Nygaard[47]	Former US female Olympic athletes (age 44 yr)	Retrospective postal survey	35.8% experienced incontinence; while competing: (swimmers 4.5%, gym/track 35%); now (swimmers 0%, gym/track 41%)	Significant differences while competing, p <0.005
Poswiata et al.[48]	International or national female runners (55) and cross-country skiers (57)	Anonymous questionnaire	45.5% leakage with sneezing or coughing	No difference between runners and skiers; 42.9% slightly bothered, 18.8% moderately othered, 8% significantly bothered, 0.9% heavily bothered
Salvatore et al.[49]	Non-competitive Italian sportswomen	Cross-sectional questionnaire	Urinary incontinence in 101 (14.9%), 32/101 during sport, 48/101 in daily life, 21/101 in both	Highest for basketball, athletics and tennis or squash. BMI and parity also risk factors
Schettino et al.[50]	105 female volleyball players	Questionnaire	29.5% reported stress incontinence	65.7% had at least one symptom of stress incontinence
Simeone et al.[51]	623 casual female athletes 18–56 yr, 12 sports	Anonymous questionnaire	30% had urinary incontinence	Most frequent in football. Risk factors long training, competitive practices, high impact
Stach-Lempinen et al.[27]	82 women with urinary incompetence	Urodynamics, pad test and diary	Leakage greatest in women with greatest leisure activity	Questionnaire and Caltrac accelerometer
Thyssen et al.[52]	8 national-level Danish sport clubs; 397 women, aged 23 yr, 8.6% of group parous	Cross-sectional postal survey	Gymnastics, 56%, ballet 43%, aerobics 40%, badminton 31%, volleyball 30%, athletics 25%, handball 21%, basketball 17%	51.9% had incontinence in sport or daily life

urethral sphincter.[39, 52] The level of competition is also a significant variable; the prevalence of stress incontinence was low in a survey of non-competitive athletes,[49] and no effects were seen from horseback riding at an equestrian club,[31] among walkers[33] or in aviators with occasional exposure to high g forces.[34, 43]

The problem of stress incontinence can be sufficiently embarrassing as to preclude participation in sport or physical activity.[15, 53] A survey of 41,000 Australian women found a negative cross-sectional association between urinary leakage and habitual physical activity. About 15% of younger individuals reported such leakage when they engaged in sport or exercise, and 7% of younger women, a third of middle-aged women and a quarter of older women claimed to be avoiding sporting activities because of problems of urinary leakage.[54] Likewise, questionnaire responses from 3364 women in the US found incontinence was perceived as a moderate or substantial barrier to exercise in 9.8% of the sample;[15, 55] one in seven women experienced leakage during physical activity, and this was more likely in highly active than in less active individuals (15.9% vs. 11.8%). Among 101 non-competitive Italian sportswomen with urinary incontinence, 10.4% abandoned their favourite sport and a further 20% were obliged to alter their manner of play.[49] One survey of 82 women with urinary incontinence found that their physical activity was less than that of the general population, but exercise habits were not increased by successful treatment of their problem.[27]

Habitual physical activity and incontinence

There have as yet been no randomized controlled trials examining the impact of habitual physical activity upon urinary incontinence. In cross-sectional studies, it has been somewhat unclear whether urinary incontinence limited subsequent physical activity or whether sedentary behaviour increased the risk of incontinence (Table 6.3).

Bø et al.[14] found a much higher incidence of stress incontinence in physical education than in nutrition students, and Hygaard et all.[56] also found that very strenuous activity as a teenager increased the risk of future incontinence. However, among older individuals, incontinence was seen less frequently in the more active members of the group,[57–61] unless high-impact activities were practiced.[59] A large prospective study of middle-aged nurses showed that in those who were initially free of urinary leakage, the subsequent incidence of incontinence was less in the more active members of the sample;[61] the benefit associated with regular physical activity was reduced by co-varying for body mass index, suggesting that exercise may have reduced the risk in part by helping the active individuals to regulate their body mass. Certainly, there is a strong association between obesity and urinary incontinence.[63, 64] However, eating disorders in some categories of very active individuals such as gymnasts are also associated with an increased risk of urinary incontinence.

The strength and functional capacity of the pelvic floor can be assessed by a variety of methods, including vaginal palpation, electromyography, manometry, dynamic ultrasound and magnetic resonance imaging.[65] However, the influence of regular physical activity upon pelvic floor function remains unclear. Several reports have suggested that the pelvic floor muscles can be strengthened by appropriate training exercises (see section on treatment, below), but others maintain that excessive high-impact exercise, heavy lifting or a persistent cough can overload, stretch and weaken the ligaments and muscles of the pelvic floor, with a permanent increase in the risk of incontinence.[66, 67] The situation is further complicated by the observation that incontinence in a group of physical education students was unrelated to the strength of their pelvic floor muscles.[68] Borin et al.[69] compared the pressure developed by the pelvic floor when lying supine in 30 athletes and 10 controls. Volleyball and basketball players both developed significantly lower pressures than the non-athletes. Moreover, urinary leakage was negatively correlated with the extent of athletic involvement, suggesting that repeated exposure to high-impact stress may have had an adverse effect on the pelvic floor muscles. Another small-scale study compared seven former high-impact athletes with seven controls, finding a lesser pubo-visceral muscle thickness and a lesser ability to develop maximal voluntary pelvic muscle contractions in former athletes than in controls.[70] Eliasson et al.[17] noted that a high incidence of incontinence persisted in competitive trampolinists for five to ten years after ceasing competition, although Nygaard and associates[47] found no difference of urinary leakage between high- and low-impact athletes 20 years subsequent to their involvement in competition. Certainly, if there is continued leakage, this implies that the pelvic floor muscles are not contracting appropriately to prevent unwanted urinary flow.[22, 24, 52]

An occupational comparison between Danish nurses, who engaged in frequent bouts of heavy lifting, and the general population of Denmark found that the odds ratio of requiring an operation for genital prolapse was 1.6 in the nurses.[71] Unfortunately, no data on the extent of urinary incontinence were provided, and it is possible that the nurses may have had more frequent complaints because they had a greater knowledge of problems and/or greater access to genito-urinary surgery than the general public. Further, the study was not controlled for possible differences of parity between the nurses and the controls.

Patho-physiology and the treatment of urinary incontinence

Patho-physiology

The pelvic floor muscles normally maintain some tone, except when a person is voiding. This group of muscles can contract simultaneously, causing an inward lift and squeeze around the urethra, vagina and anus, countering a sudden rise of intra-abdominal pressure.[72] The pelvic floor muscles are "stiffer," and have a more cranial position in nulliparous women and in the continent than in those who present with urinary incontinence.[73, 74]

The preventive value of habitual physical activity remains unclear, with some investigators arguing that regular exercise strengthens the pelvic floor muscles,

Table 6.3 Influence of habitual physical activity upon urinary incontinence

Author	Sample	Survey type	Findings	Comments
Bø et al.[14]	Physical education students vs. nutrition students	Questionnaire	Urinary leakage in 26% of phys. ed. and 19% of nutrition students	Most active phys. ed. students vs. sedentary nutrition students: 31% vs. 10%
Bradley et al.[57]	297 women aged 68 yr	Questionnaire	Urinary urgency less prevalent in women exercising at least 1/week (23.8% vs. 35.2%)	High body mass index a risk factor
Danforth et al.[58]	Nurses/health study, initial age 66 yr	Biennial reporting of physical activity, self-reports of incident leakage of urine (2355 cases)	Odds ratio of leaking urine 0.81 (highest vs. lowest physical activity quintile)	Greater benefit for stress than for urge incontinence; most of activity undertaken was moderate, e.g. walking
Eliasson et al.[62]	665 women before and after birth of first child	Questionnaire at 36th week, 1 year post-partum	High impact exercise before pregnancy risk factor for urinary leakage, low-impact exercise protective	Urinary leakage before pregnancy usually persisted 1 year post-partum
Hannestad et al.[59]	27,936 Norwegian women	Questionnaire	Low-impact physical activity reduces risk, but not high-impact activity	Strong association with BMI, weak association with smoking
Kikuchi et al.[60]	Elderly aged > 70 yr (507 not incontinent, 169 incontinent)	Questionnaire	Odds ratio of incontinence 0.71 (middle), 0.58 (high) physical activity	Prevalence 34% in women, 16% in men
Nygaard et al.[56]	Case/control moderate or severe incontinence vs. mild or none, women aged 39–65 yr	Incontinence severity index scores relative to physical activity questionnaire	Incontinence increased slightly with lifetime activity (odds ratio 1.20), but not with lifetime strenuous activity	Strenuous activity as a teen increased incontinence
Townsend et al.[61]	116,671 female nurses, 4081 incident cases of urinary incontinence	Questionnaire, prospective study	Stress and urge incontinence relative risk 0.75 top vs. bottom physical activity quintile	Relative risk attenuated by adjustment for BMI-benefit partly due to weight maintenance?

and others maintaining that excessive physical activity has a weakening effect.[66] Even the importance of the thickness of the pelvic muscle floor is debated. One small study found that at the level of the mid-vagina, the pubo-visceral muscles were actually thicker in female football players who showed incontinence than in those who did not.[75] Leakage typically occurs in the latter part of competition or training sessions,[37, 62] suggesting that cumulative fatigue may be a factor, and it seems likely that the onset of such fatigue could be delayed by a strengthening of the pelvic musculature.

Ree et al.[76] examined the effects of strenuous physical activity (90 minutes of interval training relative to 90 minutes of rest) in 12 nulliparous young women with mild stress incontinence. An intra-vaginal balloon catheter demonstrated a 20% reduction in mean contraction pressures immediately after exercise, suggesting a short-term fatigue of the pelvic floor muscles. Nevertheless, it remains uncertain if chronic participation in high-impact competitive athletics has an adverse effect upon pelvic floor function. Kruger et al.[77] used two- and three-dimensional trans-labial ultrasound to underline that there was a larger hiatal area and a greater bladder neck descent during the Valsalva manouvre in 24 competitors than in 22 controls; however, these same studies demonstrated a progressive increase in the average cross-sectional area and thickness of the levator ani and pubo-rectalis muscles among participants in high-impact sports.[77, 78] This could reflect a local adaptation to repeated high impacts, but other possibilities include a selective retention in the study of individuals with an initially strong pelvic musculature or a training-induced development of the foot arches that reduced the effect of impacts upon the pelvis.[79] Bø and Sundgot-Borgen[5] found no difference in the prevalence of urinary incontinence among high- and low-impact former Olympians from the period 1970–1976 when they were examined 20–30 years after competition, but some investigators still suggest that the very high physical demands of current Olympic participation may have long-term adverse effects on genito-urinary function.

Treatment of urinary incontinence

Possible treatments of stress incontinence include bladder training, pelvic floor exercises with or without resistance, the insertion of intra-vaginal cones, bio-feedback, electrical stimulation of the pelvic muscles, drug treatment and surgery (Table 6.4). It remains difficult to choose among this wide range of possible options because none has as yet been evaluated in double-blind fashion, and none has received unanimous clinical endorsement.

Stress incontinence can apparently be reduced if the affected individual develops the ability to make a quick and strong contraction of the pelvic floor muscles when a rise of intra-abdominal pressure is anticipated.[87, 88] This technique is not always included specifically in rehabilitation programmes, but it may be that many athletes make such a contraction instinctively when they are exercising.[89] Specific exercises to increase the strength of the pelvic floor muscles were first advocated by Kegel,[90] who claimed that 84% of cases of incontinence could be cured by such a programme. Details of the approaches adopted by various authors have been reviewed by Bø.[91] Pelvic muscle exercises are certainly the simplest approach and are probably the most appropriate initial recommendation for athletes with small amounts of urinary leakage.[92] However, it takes a few weeks to learn the correct technique, and adherence to the training programme is important to the success of treatment. Moreover, because the intra-abdominal pressure levels of the athlete can be higher than in sedentary individuals, there is probably a need for greater rigour in the training programme for those who engage in high-impact sports.[66] A typical routine involves sustaining maximal efforts for 6–8 seconds,[91] possibly with 3–4 sets of 8–12 slow-velocity supervised contractions practiced three times per week, for as long as six months. There have been many demonstrations of benefit from pelvic muscle exercises in the general population,[91] with self-assessed cure rates of 32–84%, and several uncontrolled studies have also found this approach to be helpful in elite athletes. Bø et al.[93] found that after pelvic floor muscle training, 17 of 23 women reported improvements during jumping and running, and 15 noted improvements during lifting; this was confirmed by a decrease of pad leakage from an average of 28 g to 7.1 g. Mørkved et al.[94] reported a 67% cure rate with biofeedback assisted pelvic muscle training. Da Roza et al.[95] also arranged pelvic muscle training for 16 young sports students who had complained of sporadic urinary incontinence. Unfortunately, perhaps because of the time demanded by this training (60 minutes per session), only seven of the group completed the eight-week programme; in these seven individuals, the pelvic floor muscle strength was increased, and the frequency and amount of incontinence was reduced. Rivalta et al.[96] treated three nulliparous female athletes with a programme that combined pelvic floor muscle training with biofeedback, electrical stimulation and intra-vaginal cones; the three-month rehabilitation programme abolished the previous incontinence in all of this small sample.

Yoga and Pilates classes also have their advocates as a means of treating urinary incontinence,[97] but they do not seem to have any specific effect in activating the pelvic floor muscles;[98] nor do they offer any advantage relative to more specific forms of pelvic floor muscle training.[83] Many of the treatments using biofeedback have been made in the supine position, but Boursier[29] carried out training with the athletes standing in positions typical of their sport. Other investigators have used electrical or mechanical stimulation of the perineal muscles.[99]

Another simple treatment option is the insertion of an intra-vaginal tampon. One investigation found total dryness throughout 30 minutes of aerobic exercise when such a device was used by six women who had complained of stress incontinence.[100]

Medications such as the anti-depressant imipramine and the serotonin and norepinephrine uptake inhibitor duoxetine have improved the quality of life for some people with incontinence[101] but these drugs have not been tested in athletes,[102] and one recent Cochrane review found that their effect on urinary incontinence was only slightly greater than that of a placebo.[103] Anticholinergic

Table 6.4 Methods for the treatment of urinary stress incontinence

Author	Sample	Treatment	Findings	Comments
Bø et al.[80]	52 women aged 45.9 years with stress incontinence	8–12 pelvic floor max contractions, 3/day for 6 months, half of group also made sustained contractions 1/week	60% of intensive exercise, 17% of of home exercise group almost continent after 6 months of treatment	Exercises much more effective if supervised. Associated gains of pelvic floor strength
Bø et al.[81]	107 women with stress incontinence, aged 49.5 years	Pelvic floor exercises (25), electrical stimulation (25), vaginal cone (27), control (30)	Pelvic floor exercises superior to alternatives in terms of both strength and leakage	Exercises decreased average urinary leakage from 30 g to 17 g
Bourcier[29]	68 young nulliparous women: 30 athletes, 38 active women, aged 22 years	Applied biofeedback while in athletic posture, 2/week for 3 weeks, 1/week for 4 weeks	Both groups improved, but athletes not completely cured by treatment	Focus on ability to control pelvic diaphragm
Castro et al.[82]	108 women with stress incontinence	Comparison of pelvic floor exercises (31), electrical stimulation (30), vaginal cones (27) vs. controls	Patients reporting satisfaction: 58, 55, 54 and 21% respectively	3 treatment options seem equally effective
Culligan et al.[83]	62 women with little pelvic floor dysfunction	Pilates vs. pelvic floor muscle exercises	Equal increase of pelvic floor strength by perineotomy	No discussion of incontinence
Fitz et al.[84]	Stress incontinence, 16 women given biofeedback, 16 comparison group, aged 58 years	3 sets of slow contractions, 3–4 fast pelvic floor contractions 2/week for 6 weeks	Adding biofeedback improved function, reduced urinary symptoms and improved quality of life	
Mørkved et al.[85]	94 women with stress incontinence	Pelvic floor muscle training, half of group with biofeedback	Cure (2g leakage or less) in 60% of group with biofeedback, 50% in comparison group	Effect of biofeedback not statistically significant

Table 6.4 continued

Author	Sample	Treatment	Findings	Comments
Nygaard et al.[86]	71 women with urinary incontinence	3 months pelvic muscle training	Stress incontinence decreased from 2.5 to 1.4 times/day among those completing treatment (56% of enrollees)	No additional benefit from audio-tape

drugs may also offer come benefit, but they are not recommended for athletes because of the concomitant reduction of sweating. Surgical interventions such as pubo-vaginal sling procedures, retropubic suspension and periurethral injections can be offered to older patients, but they are inappropriate for young athletes who only experience incontinence when they are engaged in high-intensity sport.[104]

Physical activity and haematuria

The issue of micro-haematuria was discussed in Chapter 4. An overt red colouration of the urine in an athlete can reflect the presence of more substantial quantities of either haemoglobin or myoglobin. A strenuous bout of exercise may occasionally lead to gross haematuria. Runners are the most vulnerable, although almost any athlete can develop visible urinary bleeding after a period of intensive physical activity. Overt haematuria may be precipitated by trauma to the bladder, dehydration or the breakdown of red blood cells that occurs with sustained aerobic exercise. Resolution is usually rapid, but a detailed clinical examination for more serious causes of bleeding is required if the haematuria does not stop within 72 hours. Other potential causes of haematuria that the clinician should consider are summarized in Table 6.5.

Physical activity and bladder cancer

Bladder cancer is the sixth most common type of neoplasm in Canada, with a ten-year survival rate of about 76%.[105] There is at present no evidence that the risk of developing bladder cancer is directly related to physical inactivity, although there may be a weak indirect association because one potent cause of such tumours (cigarette smoking) is linked to various facets of a poor overall lifestyle, including physical inactivity. Physical activity could also boost ant-oxidant mechanisms, thus countering the free radical production that is associated with exposure to arsenic compounds, another recognized cause of bladder cancer.[106]

The treatment of bladder cancer may include surgery or local irradiation, and local or general chemotherapy. Commonly, survivors of such treatment face sexual and/or urinary dysfunction. Following successful suppression of the tumour, the physical activity of many patients falls below the minimum recommended for health. Encouragement of physical activity can help to correct the resulting limitations of aerobic power, muscular strength and range of motion, enhancing functional capacity and decreasing co-morbidity. Partly for this reason, Karvinen et al.[105] noted that the quality of life among survivors (particularly in the physical and functional domains) was positively related to their level of physical activity. The more active individuals showed less fatigue, had a better self-image and better erectile function. Exercisers also have a better long-term survival rate than those who remain sedentary.[106]

It might be asked whether those with a poor quality of life were the least active members of the sample because they were older, more severely affected by the tumour or had more complications during subsequent treatment, although Karvinen et al.[105] did not observe any relationship between the quality of life and age, body mass index, the invasiveness of the tumour or the type of treatment that had been implemented. Further studies are warranted to test the causal nature of this relationship. However, the information that is currently available already points to a need to encourage greater physical activity following the treatment of a bladder cancer.

Table 6.5 Potential causes of haematuria

- **Urinary tract infections.** Urinary tract infections usually cause a persistent urge to urinate, a burning pain with urination and strong-smelling urine, but occasionally the only sign of illness may be a persistent haematuria.

- **Renal infections.** Renal infections (pyelonephritis) can occur via the blood stream or the urethra. The signs and symptoms are often similar to those seen with infection of the bladder and lower urinary tract, but there may also be fever and pain in the loin.

- **Bladder or renal calculi.** Bladder and renal calculi often remain dormant for long periods, but can cause various degrees of urinary bleeding, intense pain and even urinary blockage as they are being passed.

- **Prostate enlargement.** The prostate enlargement of middle and old age compresses the urethra, partially blocking urine flow, and causing an urgent need to urinate, often with associated urinary bleeding. Infection of the prostate gland can cause similar signs and symptoms.

- **Renal disease.** Renal disease (glomerulonephritis) affecting the small glomerular capillaries can cause microscopic haematuria.

- **Cancers of the urinary tract.** Urinary bleeding can be a harbinger of advanced kidney, bladder or prostate cancer.

- **Sickle cell anaemia.** Sickle cell anemia can cause episodic haematuria.

- **Renal trauma.** A physical injury to the kidneys can cause a substantial haematuria.

- **Adverse drug reactions.** Urinary bleeding can result from adverse reactions to drugs, particularly anticoagulants such as heparin, ibuprofen and other non-steroidal anti-inflammatory drugs.

- **Menstrual contamination.** In women, urine samples may be contaminated by menstrual bleeding.

Areas for further research

Perhaps the most fundamental requirement in future research is an objective evaluation of the extent of urinary leakage. The correlation between questionnaire responses and objective weighed pad data (kappa value 0.45) is disturbingly low. Reasons for the discrepancy between subjective and objective data such as embarrassment when responding to questionnaires should be clarified. At present, we do not know the minimum frequency and volume of urinary leakage that is likely to cause a person to seek treatment. Whereas some have argued that regular physical activity strengthens the pelvic floor muscles, others have maintained that excessive exercise has a weakening effect. Further observations are thus required to decide whether habitual physical activity increases or reduces the risk of urinary leakage, and whether there is a useful ceiling of training, beyond which more strenuous effort impairs pelvic floor function.

It remains difficult to choose among possible options for the management of stress incontinence because none has as yet been evaluated in double-blind fashion. More controlled and blinded trials are needed to evaluate the various treatment possibilities, and to examine the impact of successful treatment upon subsequent exercise participation. There is also a need to clarify the reasons predisposing to severe haematuria following heavy endurance exercise.

Practical implications and conclusions

Stress incontinence has a high prevalence in young nulliparous female athletes involved in high-impact sports. Although leakage during competition is typically small (around 25 g), social embarrassment can cause under-reporting of the problem, impaired physical performance and unwillingness to engage in active pursuits. Physicians and coaches should monitor athletes closely for this problem. Problems can be eased by changing from a high- to a low-impact sport, but this is obviously not a practical solution for elite competitors. Some have argued that high-intensity sport and heavy lifting can cause chronic strain of the pelvic floor, but urinary leakage can probably be reduced through a combination of pelvic floor muscle exercises and development of the arches of the feet to reduce impact forces. If leakage is small, the competitor should be advised that this is a common phenomenon with no serious health consequence. It can usually be managed by using absorbent pads.

Gross haematuria can sometimes follow endurance activity; usually there are no serious consequences to such a manifestation, but a thorough genito-urinary investigation is required if bleeding persist for more than 72 hours.

Physical activity apparently has no direct influence on the risk of bladder cancer. However, following successful treatment, habitual physical activity is often less than the minimum recommended for good health. Counselling may be needed to suggest methods of continuing regular exercise in the face of urinary or faecal incontinence. Greater physical activity can enhance the quality of life, and by reducing the risk of various chronic diseases, it also increases overall survival.

References

1. Abrams P, Cardozo L, Fall M, et al. The standardization of terminology of lower urinary tract function: report from the standardisation sub-committee of the International Continence Society. *Neurourol Urodyn* 2002; 21: 167–178.
2. Abrams P, Cardozo L, Khoury S, et al. *Incontinence* (4th ed). Plymouth, Devon, UK: Plymbridge Distributors, 2009.
3. Bump R, Norton P. Epidemiology and natural history of pelvic floor dysfunction. *Obstet Gynecol Clin North Am* 1998; 25(4): 723–746.
4. Hunskaar S, Burgio K, Diokno A, et al. Epidemiology and natural history of urinary incontinence (UI). In: Abrams P. Cardozo L, Khoury S, et al. (eds) *Incontinence* (4th ed). Plymouth, Devon, UK: Plymbridge Distributors. 2002, pp. 155–201.
5. Bø K, Sundgot Borgen J. Prevalence of stress and urge urinary incontinence in elite athletes and controls. *Med Sci Sports Exerc* 2001; 33: 1797–1802.
6. de Araujo MP, de Oliveira E, Zuchi EVM, et al. Relação entre incontinência urinária em mulheres atletas corredoras de longa distância e distúrbio alimentar. [The relationship between urinary incontinence and eating disorders in female long-distance runners]. *Rev Assoc Med Bras* 2008; 54(2): 146–149.
7. Wilson PD, Herbison RM, Herbison GP. Obstetric practice and the prevalence of urinary incontinence three months after delivery. *Br J Obstet Gynaecol* 1996; 103: 154–161.
8. Buckley BS, Lapitan MC. Epidemiology Committee of the Fourth International Consultation on Incontinence, Paris, 2008. Prevalence of urinary incontinence in men, women and children – current evidence: findings of the Fourth International Consultation on Incontinence. *Urology* 2010; 76: 265–270.
9. Tennstedt SL, Link CL, Steers WD, et al. Prevalence of and risk factors for urine leakage in a racially and ethnically diverse population of adults: the Boston Area Community Health (BACH) Survey. *Am J Epidemiol* 2008; 167: 390–399.
10. Sandvik H. Female urinary incontinence: studies of epidemiology and management in general practice. Doctoral thesis. Dept of Public Health & Primary Care, University of Bergen. Bergen, Norway: 1984.
11. Hannestad YS, Rortveit G, Sandvik H, et al. A community-based epidemiologic survey of female urinary incontinence: the Norwegian EPINCONT study. *J Clin Epidemiol* 2000; 53: 1150–1157.
12. Fantl JA, Newman DK, Colling J, et al. Urinary incontinence in women with SUI demonstrated total dryness when adults: acute and chronic management. 2, update [96-0682]. Rockville, MD: US Department of Health and Human Services. Public Health Service, Agency for Health Care and Policy Research, 1996.
13. Coyne KS, Sexton CC, Irwin DE, et al. The impact of overactive bladder, incontinence and other lower urinary tract symptoms on quality of life, work productivity, sexuality and emotional well-being in men and women: results from the EPIC study. *BJU Int* 2008; 101: 1388–1395.
14. Bø K, Maehlum S, Oseid S, et al. Prevalence of stress urinary incontinence among physically active and sedentary female students. *Scand J Sports Sci* 1989; 11(3): 113–116.
15. Nygaard I, DeLancey JO, Arnsdorf L, et al. Exercise and incontinence. *Obstet Gynecol* 1990; 75: 848–851.
16. Caetano AS, Tavares MCGCF, Lopes MHBdaM. Urinary incontinence and physical activity practice. *Rev Bras Med Esporte* 2007; 13(4): 245e–248e.

17. Eliasson K, Edner A, Mattson E. Urinary incontinence in very young and mostly nulliparous women with a history of regular organised high-impact trampoline training: occurrence and risk factors. *Int Urogynecol J* 2008; 19: 687–696.
18. Popova-Dobreva D. Urinary incontinence among athletes. *Bull Transilvania* 2011; 4(53): 1.
19. Jean-Baptiste J, Hermieu J-F. Fuites urinaires et sport chez la femme. [Sport and urinary incontinence in women]. *Progrès Urol* 2010; 20: 483–490.
20. Lousquy R, Jean-Baptiste J, Barranger E, et al. Incontinence urinaire chez la femme sportive. [Sport and urinary incontinence in women]. *Gynécol Obstét Fertil* 2014; 42: 597–603.
21. Goldstick O, Constatini N. Urinary incontinence in physically active women and female athletes. *Br J Sports Med* 2014; 48: 296–298.
22. Nygaard I, Thompson FL, Svengalis SL, et al. Urinary incontinence in elite nulliparous athletes. *Obstet Gynecol* 1994; 84: 183–187.
23. Groothausen J, Siemer H, Kemper HCG, et al. Influence of peak strain on lumbar bone mineral density: An analysis of 15-year physical activity in young males and females. *Pediatr Exerc Sci* 1997; 9: 159–173.
24. Eliasson K, Larsson T, Mattson E. Prevalence of stress incontinence in nulliparous elite trampolinists. *Scand J Med Sci Sports* 2002; 12: 106–110.
25. Fernandes A, Fitz F, Silva A, et al. Evaluation of the prevalence of urinary incontinence symptoms in adolescent female soccer players and their impact on quality of life. *Occup Environ Med* 2014; 71: A59–A60.
26. Hermieu J-F, Fatton B, Souffir J, et al. Pad test chez la femme pratiquent la course à pied: évaluation de la fréquence et de l'importance de l'incontinence urinaire. [Pad test in women runners: evaluation of the frequency and extent of urinary incompetence]. Cited by L Mouly, Incontinence urinaire chez les coureuses participant au marathon de Toulouse 2012. [Urinary incontinence in female runners participating in the 2012 Toulouse marathon.] Docotral thesis in Medicine, University of Toulouse, Toulouse, France, 2013.
27. Stach-Lampinen B, Nygård C-H, Laippala P, et al. Is physical activity influenced by urinary incontinence? *BJOG* 2004; 111: 475–480.
28. Less R. Incontinence in elite female athletes. Undergraduate research paper, University of Minnesota Digital Conservancy, 2010, http://conservancy.umn.edu/handle/11299/97985
29. Bourcier A. Conservative treatment of stress incontinence in sportswomen. *Neurol Urodyn* 1990; 9: 232–234.
30. Abitteboul Y, Leonard F, Mouly L, et al. Incontinence urinaire chez des coureuses de loisir de marathon. [Urinary incontinence in non-professional female marathon runners]. *Progrès Urol* 2015; 25(11): 636–641.
31. Alanee S, Heiner J, Liu N, et al. Horseback riding: impact on sexual dysfunction and lower urinary tract symptoms in men and women. *Urology* 2009; 73: 109–114.
32. Almeida MBA, Barra AA, Saltlel F, et al. Urinary incontinence and other pelvic floor dysfunctions in female athletes in Brazil: a cross-sectional study. *Scand J Med Sci Sports* Sep 15; doi: 101111/sms12546, 2015.
33. Barreto E, Filoni E, Fitz FF. Symptoms of lower urinary tract in women who practice physical exercise regularly. *MTP Rehab J* 2014; 12: 372–378.
34. Benjamin CR, Hearon CM. Urinary continence in women during centrifuge exposure to high +Gz. *Aviat Space Environ Med* 2000; 71(2): 131–136.
35. Bø K, Bratland-Sanda S, Sundgot-Borgen J. Urinary incontinence among group

fitness instructors including yoga and Pilates teachers. *Neurourol Urodyn* 2011; 30: 370–373.

36. Carls C. The prevalence of stress urinary incontinence in high-school and college-age female athletes in the midwest: Implications for education and prevention. *Urol Nursing* 2007; 27(1): 21–25.

37. Caylet N, Fabbro-Peray P, Marès P, et al. Prevalence and occurrence of stress urinary incontinence in elite women athletes. *Can J Urol* 2006; 13(4): 3174–3179.

38. David H. Le sport au féminin (conséquences périnéales chez la nullipare). [Female sport (perineal consequences in the nulliparous)]. Doctoral thesis, School of Midwifery, Université de Marseilles, Marseilles, France, 1993.

39. Da Roza T, Brandão S, Mascarenhas T, et al. Volume of training and the ranking level are associated with the leakage of urine in young female trampolinists. *Clin J Sports Med* 2015; 25: 270–275.

40. Davis GD, Goodman M. Stress urinary incontinence in nulliparous female soldiers in airborne infantry training. *J Pelvic Surg* 1996; 2(2): 68–71.

41. do Santos ES, Caetano AS, Tavares MdaC, et al. Incontinência urinária entre estudantes de educação física [Urinary incontinence among physical education students]. *Rev Esc Enferm USP* 2009; 43(2): 307–312.

42. Elleuch MH, Ghattassi I, Guermazi M, et al. L'incontinence urinaire chez la femme sportive nullipare. Enquête épidémiologique. A propos de 105 cas. [Urinary incontinence in the nulliparous female athlete. Epidemiological study of 105 cases]. *Ann Réadapation Méd Phys* 1998; 41: 479–484.

43. Fischer JR, Berg PH. Urinary incontinence in United States Air Force female aircrew. *Obstet Gynecol* 1999; 84(4): 532–536.

44. Fozzatti C, Riccetto C, Hermann V, et al. Prevalence study of stress urinary incontinence in women who perform high-impact exercises. *Int Urogynecol J* 2012; 23: 1687–1691.

45. Jacome C, Oliveira D, Marques A, et al. Prevalence and impact of urinary incontinence among female athletes. *Int J Gynecol Obstet* 2011; 114: 60–63.

46. Larsen WL, Yavorek T. Pelvic prolapse and urinary incontinence in nulliparous-college women in relation to paratrooper training. *Int J Urogynecol* 2007; 18: 769–771.

47. Nygaard I. Does prolonged high-impact activity contribute to later urinary incontinence? A retrospective cohort study of female Olympians. *Obstet Gynecol* 1997; 90: 718–722.

48. Poświata A, Socha T, Opara J. Prevalence of stress incontinence in elite female endurance athletes. *J Hum Kinetics* 2014; 44: 91–96.

49. Salvatore S, Serati M, Laterza R, et al. The impact of urinary stress incontinence in young and middle-age women practising recreational sports activity: an epidemiological study. *Br J Sports Med* 2009 43: 1115–1118.

50. Schettino MT, Mainini G, Ercolano S, et al. Risk of pelvic floor dysfunctions in young athletes. *Clin Exp Obstet Gynecol* 2014; 41(6): 671–676.

51. Simeone C, Moroni A, Pettenò A, et al. Occurrence rates and predictors of lower urinary tract symptoms and incontinence in female athletes. *Urologia* 2010; 77(2): 139–146.

52. Thyssen HH, Clevin L, Olesen S, et al. Urinary incontinence in female elite female athletes and dancers. *Int Urogynecol J Pelvic Floor Dysfunct* 2002; 13: 15–17.

53. Norton C. The effects of urinary incontinence in women. *Int Rehabil Med* 1982; 4: 9–14.

54. Brown W, Miller YD. Too wet to exercise? Leaking urine as a barrier to physical activity in women. *J Sci Med Sport* 2001; 4(4): 373–378.
55. Nygaard I, Girts T, Fultz NH, et al. Is urinary incontinence a barrier to exercise in women? *Obstet Gynecol* 2005; 106: 307–314.
56. Nygaard I, Shaw JM, Bardsley T, et al. Lifetime physical activity and female stress urinary incontinence. *Am J Obstet Gynec* 2015; 213: 40.e1–e10.
57. Bradley CS, Kennedy CM, Nygaard IE. Pelvic floor symptoms and lifestyle factors in older women. *J Women's Health* 2005; 14(2): 128–136.
58. Danforth KN, Shah AD, Townsend MK, et al. Physical activity and urinary incontinence among healthy, older women. *Obstet Gynecol* 2007; 109: 721–727.
59. Hannestad YS, Rotveit G, Daltveit AK, et al. Are smoking and other lifestyle factors associated with female urinary incontinence? The Norwegian EPINCONT Study. *BJOG* 2003; 110: 247–254.
60. Kikuchi A, Niu K, Ikeda Y, et al. Association between physical activity and urinary incontinence in a community-based elderly population aged 70 years and older. *Eur Urol* 2007; 52: 868–875.
61. Townsend MK, Danforth KN, Rosner B, et al. Physical activity and incident urinary incontinence in middle-aged women. *J Urol* 2008; 179(3): 1012–1017.
62. Eliasson K, Nordlander I, Larson B, et al. Influence of physical activity on urinary leakage in primiparous women. *Scand J Med Sci Sports* 2005; 15: 87–94.
63. Burgio KL, Matthews KA, Engel BT. Prevalence, incidence and correlates of urinary incontinence in healthy, middle-aged women. *J Urol* 1991; 146(5): 1255–1259.
64. Subak LL, Wing R, West DS, et al. Weight loss to treat urinary incontinence in overweight and obese women. *N Engl J Med* 2009; 360: 481–490.
65. Raizada V, Bhargava V, Jung SA, et al. Dynamic assessment of the vaginal high pressure zone using high definition manometry, 3-dimensional ultrasound, and magnetic resonance imaging for the pelvic floor muscles. *Am J Obstet Gynec* 2010; 203(2):172: e1–e8.
66. Bø K. Urinary incontinence, pelvic floor dysfunction, exercise and sport. *Sports Med* 2004; 34(7): 451–464.
67. Nichols DH, Milley PS. Functional pelvic anatomy: the soft tissue supports and spaces of the female pelvic organs. In: Nygaard I, Glowaski C and Saltzman L (eds) *The human vagina*. Amsterdam, Netherlands: Elsevier/North Holland, 1978, pp. 21–37.
68. Bø K, Stien R, Kulseng-Hanssen S. Clinical and urodynamic assessment of nulliparous young women with and without stress incontinence symptoms: a case-control study. *Obstet Gynecol* 1994; 84: 1028–1032.
69. Borin LCMdS, Nunes FR, Guirro ECdO. Assessment of pelvic floor muscle pressure in female athletes. *PM R* 2013; 5: 189–193.
70. Brandão S, Da Roza T, Mascarenhas T, et al. Do asymptomatic former high impact sports practitioners maintain the ability to contract the pelvic floor muscles? *J Sports Med Phys Fitness* 2015; 55: 1272–1276.
71. Jørgensen S, Hein HO, Gyntelberg F. Heavy lifting at work and risk of genital prolapse and herniated lumbar disc in assistant nurses. *Occup Med* 1994; 44: 47–49.
72. DeLancey J. Anatomy and physiology of urinary continence. *Clin Obstet Gynecol* 1990; 33(2): 298–307.
73. Haderer J, Pannu H, Genadry R, et al. Controversies in female urethral anatomy and their significance for understanding urinary continence: observations and literature review. *Int Urogynecol J Pelvic Floor Dysfunct* 2002; 13: 15–17.

74. Peschers U, Schaer G, Anthuber C, et al. Changes in vesical neck mobility following vaginal delivery. *Obstet Gynecol* 1996; 88: 1001–1006.

75. Da Roza T, Brandão S, Oliveira D, et al. Football practice and urinary incontinence: Relation between morphology, function and biomechanics. *J Biomech* 2015; 48: 1587–1592.

76. Ree ML, Nygaard I, Bø K. Muscular fatigue in the pelvic floor muscles after strenuous physical activity. *Acta Obstet Gynec* 2007; 86: 870–876.

77. Kruger JA, Dietz HP, Murphy BA. Pelvic floor function in nulliparous athletes *Ultrasound Obstet Gynecol* 2007; 30: 81–85.

78. Kruger JA, Murphy BA, Heap SW. Alterations in levator ani morphology in elite nulliparous athletes: a pilot study. *Aust NZ J Obstet Gynec* 2005; 45: 42–47.

79. Nygaard I, Giowacki C, Saltzman CL. Relationship between foot flexibility and urinary incontinence. *Obset Gynec* 1996; 87: 1049–1051.

80. Bø K, Hagen RH, Jørgensen J, et al. Pelvic floor muscle exercise for the treatment of female stress urinary incontinence: III. Effects of two different degrees of pelvic floor muscle exercises. *Neuriourol Urodyn* 1990; 9: 489–502.

81. Bø K, Talseth T, Holme I. Single blind, randomised controlled trial of pelvic floor exercises, electrical stimulation, vaginal cones, and no treatment in management of genuine stress incontinence in women. *BMJ* 1999; 318: 487–493.

82. Castro RA, Arruda RM, Zanetti MRD, et al. Single-blind randomized, controlled trial of pelvic floor muscle training, electrical stimulation, vaginal cones, and no active treatment in the management of stress urinary incontinence. *Clinics* 2008; 64: 465–472.

83. Culligan PJ, Scherer J, Dyer K, et al. A randomized clinical trial comparing pelvic floor muscle training to a Pilates exercise program for improving pelvic muscle strength. *Int Urogynecol J* 2010; 21: 401–408.

84. Fitz FF, Resende APM, Stüpp L, et al. Efeito da adição do biofeedback ao treinamento dos músculos do assoalho pélvico para tratamento da incontinência urinária de esforço [Effect of the adding of biofeedback to the training of the pelvic floor muscles to treatment of stress urinary incontinence]. *Rev Bras Ginecol Obstet* 2012; 34(11): 505–510.

85. Mørkved S, Bø K, Fjørtoft T. Effect of adding biofeedback to pelvic floor muscle training to treat uroidynamic stress incontinence. *Obstetr Gynec* 2002; 100(4): 730–739.

86. Nygaard I, Kreder KJ, Lepic MM, et al. Efficacy of pelvic floor muscle exercises in urge, and mixed urinary incontinence. *Am J Obstet Gynec* 1996; 174: 120–125.

87. Bourcier AP. Incontinence during sports and fitness activities. In: Baessler K, Schussler B, Burgio KL, et al. (eds) *Pelvic floor re-education: principles and practice*. London, UK: Springer Verlag, 2008, pp. 267–270.

88. Miller JM, Ashton-Miller JA, Delancey JO. A pelvic muscle precontraction can reduce cough-related urine loss in selected women with mild SUI. *J Am Geriatr Soc* 1998; 46: 870–874.

89. Constantinou CE, Govan DE. Contribution and timing of transmitted and generated pressure components in the female urethra. *Prog Clin Biol Res* 78; 113–120.

90. Kegel A. Physiologic therapy for urinary stress incontinence. *JAMA* 1951; 146: 915–917.

91. Bø K. Physical activity, fitness and bladder control. In: Bouchard C, Shephard RJ, Stephens T (eds) *Physical activity, fitness and health*. Champaign, IL: Human Kinetics, 1994, pp. 774–796.

92. Hay-Smith E, Bø K, Berghmans L, et al. *Pelvic floor muscle training for urinary incontinence in women*. The Cochrane Collaboration; issue 3. 2001.

93. Bø K, Hagen R, Kvarstein B, et al. Female stress urinary incontinence and participation in different sport and social activities. *Scand J Sports Sci* 1989; 11(3): 117–121.

94. Mørkved S, Bø K, Fjørtoft T. Is there any additional effect of adding biofeedback to pelvic floor muscle training? A single-blind randomized controlled trial. *Obstet Gynecol* 2002; 100(4): 730–739.

95. Da Roza T, de Araujo MP, Viana R, et al. Pelvic floor muscle training to improve urinary incontinence in young nulliparous sport students: a pilot study. *Int Urogynecol J* 2012; 23(8): 1069–1073.

96. Rivalta M, Sighinolfi MC, Micali S, et al. Urinary incontinence and sport: first and preliminary experience with a combined pelvic floor rehabilitation program in three female athletes. *Health Care Women Intern* 2010; 31: 435–443.

97. Huang WH, Kuo WY, Chen JJ, et al. Pilates may have better fitness promotion effect than fitness exercise for stress urinary incontinence in women. *Med Sci Sports Exerc* 2011; 43(Suppl. 1): 577.

98. Baessler K, Junginger B. Gymnastics for urinary incontinence: destroying the myth. *Neurouro Urodyn* 2010; 29: 1052–1053.

99. Lauper M, Kuhn A, Gerber R, et al.. Pelvic floor stimulation: what are the good vibrations? *Neurourol Urodyn* 2009; 28: 405–410.

100. Glavind K. Use of a vaginal sponge during aerobic exercises in patients with stress urinary incontinence. *Int Urogynecol J Pelvic Floor Dysfunc* 1997; 8: 351–353.

101. Cardozo L, Lange R, Beardsworth SVA, et al. Short- and long-term efficacy and safety of duloxetine in women with predominant stress urinary incontinence. *Curr Med Res Opin* 2010; 26(2): 253–261.

102. Corcos J, Gajewski J, Hertitz D, et al. Canadian Urological Association guidelines on urinary incontinence. *Can J Urol* 2006; 13: 3127–3138.

103. Mariappan P, Alhasso AA, Grant A, et al. Serotonin and noradrenaline reuptake inhibitors (SNRI) for stress urinary incontinence in adults. *Cochrane Database Syst Rev* 2005; (3): CD004742. 2005.

104. Bø K. Pelvic floor physical therapy in elite athletes. In: Bø K, Berghmans B, Mørkved S, et al. (eds) *Evidence-based physical therapy for the pelvic floor*. Oxford, UK: Butterworth-Heinmann Elsevier, 2007, pp. 369–378.

105. Karvinen KH, Courneya KS, North S, et al. Associations between exercise and quality of life in bladder cancer survivors: A population-based study. *Cancer Epidemiol Biomarkers Prev* 2007; 16(5): 984–990.

106. International Agency for Research on Cancer. Arsenic, metals, fibres and dusts. *IARC Monogr Eval Carcinog Risks Hum* 2012; 100: 11–465.

7 Physiology of the spleen at rest and during exercise

Introduction

In this chapter, we will explore the anatomy and physiology of the spleen in both humans and animals, looking at reactions to physical activity and other stressors. We will consider also mechanisms underlying changes in dimensions of the spleen and their practical significance in terms of changes in oxygen transport, blood clotting and the immune response. The clinical issues of athlete management in infectious mononucleosis and Sickling disease are considered in subsequent chapters (Chapters 8 and 9).

The spleen was well known to the ancient Greeks. Erasistratus maintained that it served only to maintain the symmetry of the abdomen, but Plato suggested that its responsibility was to keep the liver "bright and shining", and Hippocrates argued that its primary function was to produce black bile, one of the four basic humours in his understanding of human physiology.[1] Galen called the spleen "mysterii organon", claiming that humours unsuitable for its nutriment were discharged by a canal that emptied from the spleen into the stomach.

The biological importance of the spleen seems to vary substantially from one species to another. The English cardiovascular physiologist Sir Joseph Barcroft and his colleagues first drew attention to the contribution of the spleen to running ability in the dog and cat.[2, 3] In these animals the haemoglobin concentration and haematocrit were about 50% higher for the splenic pulp than for the general circulation. Moreover, vigorous treadmill exercise caused the volume of the spleen to shrink to a half or even a third of its resting value, thus increasing the animal's blood volume and potential oxygen carrying capacity by 6–15%. Furthermore, this seemed to be an active, neurally regulated response to exercise which was lost if the nerve supply to the spleen was sectioned. In the same era, Scheunert and Krywanek[4] demonstrated that the increased hamatocrit and haemoglobin that developed in experimental animals during vigorous exercise was abolished if the spleen was removed surgically. Granaat[5] pointed out that the spleen contained relatively large amounts of the hormone norepinephrine, and that the release of this substance or some other pressor hormone into the circulation could influence performance, contributing to the rise of blood pressure observed at the onset of exercise.

The practical importance of the spleen to the human exercise response for long remained open to debate. Certainly, people have lived for many years following splenectomy, with no apparent difficulty in exercising, although with an increased risk increase of death from some medical conditions. A 28-year follow-up of 740 American World War II veterans who had undergone splenectomy found that relative to control subjects who had been treated for an acute inflammation of the nose and throat, there was a 4.6-fold increase in deaths from pneumonia and a 1.35-fold increase in deaths from ischaemic heart disease, but apparently no other adverse effects.[6] The pneumonia was attributed to some reduction of immune function, and the increased incidence of ischaemic heart disease was thought to reflect either a loss of the normal splenic function of sequestering and eliminating aging and injured red cells, or to an increase in platelet counts (which often persists for a long time after splenectomy).

Ebert and Stead[7] argued strongly against a reservoir function for the spleen in humans. Their research appeared to confirm earlier observations that exercise-[8] and epinephrine-induced[9] changes of haematocrit were identical in normal and splenectomized subjects, and they attributed the contrary results of some investigators to technical errors. Despite a careful marshalling of evidence by Stewart and McKenzie,[10] the view thus persisted that in humans, the main functions of the spleen were the breakdown of senescent erythrocytes, the synthesis of antibodies and the storage of monocytes, iron and viable red cells.[11] As recently as 2012, a highly respected respiratory physiologist (John West) affirmed that stress did not lead to any expulsion of red cells from the human spleen.[12]

The present chapter makes a critical examination of the contribution of the spleen to the human exercise response. After summarizing the classical findings in experimental animals, it looks at the anatomy of the spleen and methods of determining its volume. It then considers findings during exercise and other forms of stress, and evaluates the practical role of this organ in oxygen transport, blood clotting and immune function both at rest and during physical activity. Finally, it examines likely mechanisms causing any changes in splenic dimensions.

Physical activity and the spleen in experimental animals

In some species, the spleen is a large organ, containing a substantial fraction of the body's red blood cells. For example, in a 350 kg Weddell seal, the spleen contains some 20 L of red cells[13, 14] or as much as 50% of the animal's total red cell volume. Comparable figures are 54% of the total blood volume for the horse, 26% for the sheep and 20% for the dog, compared with less than 10% of the total blood volume in humans.[15]

Dating from the classical observations of Sir Joseph Barcroft,[2, 3] there has been strong evidence that the splenic store of red cells has an important reservoir function in many animals, and that this store is called upon during vigorous physical activity and other forms of stress (Table 7.1). The extent of the splenic contribution has been demonstrated by direct observation of changes in dimensions of an exteriorized spleen, by data showing an increased red blood cell count and haematocrit during vigorous exercise, by finding an increased proportion of large (spleen-derived) red cells in the circulation, and by ultrasonic measurements showing decreases in spleen area or volume. The practical contribution of the infused blood to endurance performance has been reflected by temporary increases in maximal oxygen intake, a response analogous to that obtained through the banned practice of athletic "blood doping". Changes are abolished by splenectomy, both in horses[22] and in dogs.[16, 28, 30]

The reservoir function of the spleen has been demonstrated for a substantial range of experimental animals (Table 7.1), including thoroughbred- and race-horses,[26, 29, 31–34] greyhounds, foxhounds and other types of dog,[18, 19, 21, 23–25, 28] sheep,[20] guinea pigs[17] and diving seals.[13, 27, 35, 36] Horses show a 65–75% increase of haematocrit during exercise,[31, 37] and in the diving seal a reduction of splenic volume from 24 to 4 L augments the red cell volume by 20 L, increasing oxygen stores by enough to allow the animal to sustain an underwater dive for an additional eight minutes.[14]

Anatomy of the human spleen

If the human spleen can contract in response to the circulatory needs of vigorous physical activity, one would anticipate finding smooth muscle in its capsule and/or trabeculae. Early investigators failed to demonstrate any smooth muscle in the human spleen.[11] However, tests using antigens that react to smooth muscle myosin have now shown significant if small amounts of smooth muscle in both the collagenous walls of the splenic capsule and its trabeculae.[38] Contraction of the smooth muscle appears to be mediated by α-adrenoreceptors, since α-adrenergic stimulation increases blood reticulocyte counts, with an associated decrease in size of the spleen. In contrast, the stimulation of β-adrenoreceptors has the opposite effect, leading to a drop in reticulocyte count, apparently with an increase in the dimensions of the spleen.[39]

The precise volume of the human spleen has yet to be clearly established. Rushmer[40] suggested that under resting conditions it contained 200–250 mL of blood. Ayers et al.[41] found that the average mass of 30 isolated spleens was 212 g, and autopsy records for 539 spleens found an average mass of 168 g[42]. However, these figures probably underestimated the normal volume, since blood tends to leak from the spleen during autopsy. In vivo estimates[43–46] range from 130 to 360 mL,[43, 46] depending in part on methodology. Scintigraphic data tend to yield high values, and these figures may have been biased upwards by failure to allow for counts coming from radiographically tagged red cells in overlapping organs such as the heart and kidney rather than from the spleen itself.

The practical implication of current estimates is that even if vigorous physical activity were to cause a 50% emptying of the human spleen, it could contribute no more than 100–120 mL to a total blood volume of 5 L (at most, an increase of 2.0–2.4%).

Table 7.1 Response of the spleen to physical activity and other stimuli, as seen in experimental animals

Author	Species	Stimulus	Effect	Comments
Barcroft & Florey[3]	2 dogs with exteriorized spleens	17 seconds of running in laboratory and to and fro on laboratory roof	Volume of spleen decreased to 40% of resting size	Effects persisted 20 min after ceasing exercise
Barcroft & Stephens[3]	2 dogs with exteriorized spleens. Some observations also on cats	Running and swimming; even larger response with severe haemorrhage	Spleen reduced to a half or a third of initial volume, increasing blood volume by up to 20%	Response depends on integrity of splenic nerve supply
Dane et al.[16]	6 adult foxhounds	Treadmill running at 60–80% of maximal oxygen intake	Splenectomy eliminated exercise polycythaemia	Splenectomy caused a 30% reduction in maximal oxygen intake
Digges et al.[17]	Guinea pigs		Alpha-type adrenoreceptors demonstrated in splenic capsule	
Gunteroth et al.[18]	30 dogs	Epinephrine injection	Within 15 seconds of injection, 45–50% increase of haematocrit	Similar response to fright
Gunteroth & Mullins[19]	37 dogs with barium titanate crystals sewn to spleen, ultrasound and impedance data	Treadmill exercise 6.4 km/h, 5% grade	Half of dogs initially showed splenic contraction	Effect lessened with habituation to exercise
Hodgetts[20]	13 Merino sheep	Injection of epinephrine	Increase in haematocrit from 31% to 40%	
Horvath et al.[21]	50 greyhounds	Racing on track	Increase in reticulocyte count immediately after the race, normalized after 1–2 hours	Probably due to catecholamine-mediated splenic contraction
Hurford et al.[13]	5 Wedell seals	Diving or injection of epinephrine	Ultrasonography shows 30% change in spleen size with dive; haematocrit increased from 44% to 55%	Equivalent to infusion of 20 L blood

Table 7.1 continued

Author	Species	Stimulus	Effect	Comments
Kunugiyama et al.[22]	6 thoroughbred horses	Treadmill running	Total erythrocyte volume, measured by ^{51}Cr, increased by exercise	Effect of running abolished by splenectomy
Longhurst et al.[23]	Dogs	Treadmill running	Alpha-adrenergic blockade (by phentolamine) reduced maximal oxygen intake 16.7%, splenectomy reduced 12.6%	
Neuhaus et al.[24]	6 greyhounds	704 m race	Haematocrit increased from 48% to 67%	
Rovira et al.[25]	15 dogs	100 second agility exercise	12% increase of blood volume, 21% increase of red cell volume, 4% increase of packed cell volume	
Thomas & Fregin[26]	5 sedentary horses	Treadmill exercise to 90% of maximal heart rate	Haematocrit increased from 33% to 47% (50% increase in circulating red cells)	
Thornton et al.[27]	Seal pups	Magnetic resonance imaging of spleen	Rapid contraction of spleen to 16% of original volume during forced dives	Blood transferred to hepatic sinus with splenic contraction
Vatner et al.[28]	6 unrestrained dogs	Running 3.2 km behind recording van at up to 40 km/h	Haematocrit increased from 40% to 49%	Effect of running abolished by splenectomy
Wagner et al.[29]	6 thoroughbred horses (3 with splenectomy)	Treadmill running	Splenectomy reduced maximal oxygen intake by 31%	Decrease in maximal oxygen intake restored by transfusion

Physical activity and changes in volume of the human spleen

Issues of methodology

Except in rare circumstances,[41] the human spleen cannot be exteriorized in the manner adopted in some animal experiments. Methods to determine changes in volume of the human spleen include haemoglobin and haematocrit determinations, ultrasonography, magnetic resonance imaging and most frequently recording of changes in the emissions of previously injected ^{99}Technetium-labelled red cells and 11-Indium labelled granulocytes and platelets from the region of the spleen (Table 7.2).

Each of these approaches has its limitations. Haemoglobin and haematocrit-based estimates of changes in splenic volume depend on a knowledge of associated exercise-related changes in plasma volume. Ultrasound or radio-nuclide measurements commonly assume that the changes of splenic dimensions are uniform and can be visualized in a single plane, and some radionuclide data have been compromised by failure to exclude emissions from the presence of radioisotopes in adjacent organs such as the kidneys and the lungs.

Experimental findings

Two early studies[7, 8] based on changes in haemoglobin and serum protein concentrations found no evidence that physical activity affected the splenic volume of human subjects. Although vigorous physical activity increased haemoglobin and haematocrit levels, similar responses were observed after splenectomy, suggesting that the spleen was not responsible (Table 7.2).

Wolski[46] scanned both anterior and posterior views of the spleen following the radionuclide labelling of red cells. She found that exercising for 30 minutes at a load increasing from 25 to 50 and then 75% of maximal oxygen intake led to a 7–9% increase in the total circulating red cell volume under both normoxic and hypoxic conditions; she suggested that filtration of fluid through the walls of the blood vessels explained 68–78% of the changes in haematocrit that were seen during exercise.

Twelve more recent cycle ergometer or treadmill studies[43, 44, 46–55] have found the splenic contents making a significant contribution to the red cell count during physical activity, with recovery of pre-exercise values over a recovery period of 10–20 minutes (Table 7.2).

One study was based on 21 patients with thalassaemia, 10 of whom had undergone splenectomy. Changes in haematocrit and plasma protein concentrations were measured.[47] Maximal voluntary cycle ergometer exercise induced small increases of both haemoglobin (1.0 g/dL in those with intact spleens, 0.4 g/dL in splenectomized patients) and haematocrit (3.3%, 1.4%), with larger increases in the concentration of serum proteins (4–5 g/L) due to extravasation of fluid from the circulation.

Other observers, using the more precise technologies of technetium scintigraphy or ultrasound, found that physical activity induced decreases in splenic

Table 7.2 Volume changes of the human spleen in response to an acute bout of exercise

Author	Methodology	Participants	Exercise stimulus	Findings
Negative findings				
Dill et al.[8]	Changes in haemoglobin and serum protein concentrations	10 healthy men, 2 splenectomized individuals	20 minute treadmill run at 9.3 km/h	Changes in haemoglobin parallel changes in serum protein concentrations; similar response seen in splenectomized individuals
Ebert & Stead[7]	Changes in haemoglobin, haematocrit and serum protein, dye estimate of plasma volume	6 healthy men, 2 with splenectomy	Cycle ergometer test to exhaustion in 3–5 min; splenectomized subjects did not exercise to exhaustion	Increase of haemoglobin and haematocrit with exercise similar in normal and splenectomized individuals
Positive findings				
Haemoglobin-based estimates				
Agostoni et al.[47]	Changes in haemoglobin and plasma protein concentrations	α-thalassaemia patients (10 splenectomized, 11 not)	Peak effort on cycle ergometer	Exercise-induced haemo-concentration greater in patients with intact spleens (but small effect, 1.0 vs. 0.4 g/dL)
Technetium-based estimates				
Allsop et al.[43]	99Technetium labelling of erythrocytes, 111Indium labelling of platelets and granulocytes	10 normal healthy individuals (5 for technetium, 5 for Indium studies)	4 minutes of supra-maximal exercise on cycle ergometer (110–120% of steady-state maximal value)	Rapid 54% drop of splenic volume (technetium) radioactivity, with rapid recovery post-exercise. Much slower changes in platelets and granulocytes
Flamm et al.[48]	99Technetium labelling of erythrocytes	10 men 4 women	Cycle ergometry at 0%, 50%, 75% and 100% of maximal oxygen intake	46% decrease of blood volume in spleen, 4.3% increase of haematocrit

Table 7.2 continued

Author	Methodology	Participants	Exercise stimulus	Findings
Froelich et al.[49]	[99]Technetium labelling of erythrocytes	7 women, 3 men	Graded cycle ergometer exercise to voluntary exhaustion	39% decrease of splenic volume (compared with 14% decrease in liver)
Laub et al.[44]	[99]Technetium labelling of erythrocytes and changes in haematocrit	4 men, 1 woman	Graded cycle ergometry to maximal effort	Progressive decrease of spleen volume to 34% initial value, 3.4% increase of haematocrit
Otto et al.[50]	[99]Technetium labelling of erythrocytes	20 healthy men, 10 controls	Modified Bruce treadmill protocol	21.5% decrease of spleen volume (279 to 219 mL) with exercise, no change in controls
Sandler et al.[51]	[99]Technetium labelling of erythrocytes	10 patients undergoing radionuclide ventriculography	Supine symptom-limited cycle ergometer exercise	45% reduction of spleen radioactivity immediately post-exercise, largely recovered 10 min post-exercise. Related changes in red cell count
Stewart et al.[52]	[99]Technetium labelling of erythrocytes	9 healthy men	Cycle ergometer exercise at 60% of maximal oxygen intake for 5, 10 or 15 min, followed by ride to exhaustion	Submaximal exercise reduced splenic volume 28, 30 and 36%, ride to exhaustion gave 56% decrease in splenic volume, recovery over 20 min

Ultra-sound based estimates

Author	Methodology	Participants	Exercise stimulus	Findings
Engan et al.[53]	Ultrasound and capillary haemoglobin concentration	1 woman, 7 men	Cycling at 100 W at altitudes of 0, 1370 metres	Decreases of spleen volumes: 213 to 186, 186 to 112 mL with exercise
Frances et al.[54]	Ultrasound data	7 women, 1 man	1 min isometric andgrip at 40% max. voluntary contraction	13% decrease of spleen volume

Table 7.2 continued

Author	Methodology	Participants	Exercise stimulus	Findings
Lodin-Sundström et al.[55]	Ultrasound	11 healthy lowlanders (5 women, 6 men)	Modified Harvard step test at altitudes of 1370, 3700 and 4200 m	Decreases of spleen volumes: 250 to 207, 230 to 173 and 221 to 158 mL, respectively
Multiple techniques				
Wolski[46]	[51]Cr red cell volume, ^{125}I plasma volume, [99]technetium, haematocrit	6 trained, 6 untrained subjects, 4 splenectomized	Maximal exercise and 30 min exercise at 25 rising to 50 and 75% of maximal oxygen intake in normoxia and 16% oxygen	142–187 mL of red cells released by spleen (7–9% of total red cell volume). Increase of haematocrit not seen in splenectomized subjects. Response similar in normoxia and hypoxia

volumes of 11–66% (average 34%), with a corresponding increase in circulating red blood cell volumes. In most studies, the activity undertaken was aerobic, but one investigation looked at the effects of a maximal isometric handgrip exercise;[54] this form of activity produced a smaller splenic response than that seen in most of the aerobic exercise tests.

Four studies compared healthy individuals and small numbers of patients who had undergone splenectomy.[7, 8, 46, 47] In two of these four investigations, the anticipated effects of physical activity were absent in those who had undergone splenectomy.

Two studies examined the effects of adding hypoxia to the stress of vigorous physical activity.[53, 55] The effects seemed additive, with a larger decrease of splenic volume in response to the combined stimuli.

Circulatory impact of changes in splenic dimensions during physical activity

Any expulsion of red cells from the spleen increases the oxygen carrying capacity of the blood. The process is analogous to the banned practice of blood doping, detected in some endurance athletes such as the long-distance cyclist Lance Armstrong.[1] Although unit volume of a person's blood has a greater oxygen-carrying capacity after splenic emptying, this advantage must be set against the negative effects of an associated increase in blood viscosity, and thus a potential reduction in maximal cardiac output. The adverse effect of greater viscosity is compounded by any decrease of plasma volume, particularly when an athlete is exercising in a hot environment.

Observations on rats[56, 57] compared the treadmill running endurance of splenectomized and sham-operated animals after 120 days of recovery from surgery. Somewhat surprisingly, although the two groups of female animals showed no substantial differences in physical endurance, the splenectomized males were able to maintain exhausting exercise at a speed of 24 m/min on a 12% slope for a longer period than the control animals with normal spleens (10.2 vs. 6.7 min). However, in other animal studies splenectomy has adversely affected the exercise response. Studies in horses have suggested that blood viscosity may rise by as much as 50% during exercise, whether running at speeds of 6–9 or 13–16 m/s.[37] Splenectomy decreased the rise of mean arterial pressure normally seen during treadmill running, and this was attributed to a reduced preloading of the ventricle.[34, 58] In the seal, a sphincter on the hepatic sinus appears to buffer the release of red cells into the blood stream during diving or vigorous physical activity, thus reducing immediate adverse changes in blood viscosity.[27] A second important function of the spleen, particularly in animals such as the horse, may be to reduce the resting red cell count and thus the viscosity of the blood when the cardiac output is low.[59, 60]

What are the implications of a 40% decrease in splenic volume for the human circulation? Assuming a resting splenic volume of 200 mL, the total blood volume would increase by some 80 mL or 1.6%. In addition to increased ventricular loading, there would be a small increase of haematocrit, supplementing the effects of exercise-induced dehydration on the oxygen-carrying capacity of the blood. Various observers have suggested that exercise and other stressors can increase the oxygen carrying capacity of unit volume of blood by 3.4%,[44] 6.5%[61] or 7–9%,[46] but that emptying of the spleen accounts for only a part of this response. Nevertheless, contraction of the spleen could influence the outcome of a closely competed endurance event, even if the circulatory functions of the human spleen are of much less practical importance than in animals such as the horse and the seal.

Response of the spleen to stressors other than physical activity

When a person faces actual or simulated stressors, including injection of epinephrine, splenic nerve stimulation, exposure to hypoxia, performance of the Valsalva manoeuvre, breath-holding and breath-hold diving, the responses of the spleen seem rather similar to those seen during vigorous to maximal exercise (Table 7.3). Decreases of splenic volume are accompanied by increases of haemoglobin and haematocrit values, and these responses are generally absent in individuals who have undergone splenectomy.[61, 62]

The common mediating factor for physical activity and other stressors is probably a contraction of the splenic capsule in response to epinephrine and/or adrenergic nerve stimulation. A combination of hypoxia with physical activity

Table 7.3 Response of human spleen to stressors other than physical activity

Author	Methodology	Participants	Stressor	Findings
Nerve stimulation, catecholamines				
Ayers et al.[41]	Volume recorded directly on dynograph	13 isolated perfused spleens obtained at operation	Splanchnic nerve stimulation and infusion of catecholamines	Decreases in volume of 0.3 mL 6 mL and 8 mL at stimulation frequencies of 3, 7 and 10 Hz, respectively; changes of 11–13 mL with catecholamines
Bakovic et al.[65]	Ultrasound	13 healthy men	Intravenous epinephrine (slow infusion of low doses)	Early 30% decrease of splenic volume; associated decrease of blood pressure and activation of sympathetic nerves to muscles
Knecht et al.[66]	Ultrasound	10 healthy, 5 splenectomized men	Subcutaneous epinephrine, 0.5 mg/m²	Splenic contraction 34.8%, 36.4% increase of granulocyte and 13.2% increase of platelet counts. Changes not seen after splenectomy
Valsalva manoeuvre				
Frances et al.[54]	Ultrasound data	7 women, 1 man	Lower body negative pressure, Valsalva manoeuvre	Respective decreases of spleen volume of 9%, 8%
Inoue et al.[67]	Magnetic resonance imaging	6 men, 6 women	Valsalva manoeuvre	13.3% decrease of splenic volume on volume of 173 mL
Hypoxia				
Engan et al.[53]	Ultrasound and capillary haemoglobin concentration	1 woman, 7 men	5 min cycling at 100 W at altitudes of 0, 1370 m	Decreases of spleen volumes: 213 to 186 and 186 to 112 mL respectively
Haffner et al.[68]	Ratio of spleen weight to body weight	42 cases of drowning vs. 42 cases of hanging or strangulation		Spleen weight 18% lower in drowning, possibly related to stresses of hypoxia and cooling

Table 7.3 continued

Author	Methodology	Participants	Stressor	Findings
Lodin-Sundström and Schagatay[69]	Ultrasound (splenic diameter)	5 women, 4 men	20 min breathing 14.2% oxygen	Arterial oxygen saturation 87%, Spleen volume decreased 16%
Lodin-Sundström et al.[55]	Ultrasound	11 healthy lowlanders (5 women, 6 men)	Modified Harvard step test at altitudes of 1370, 3700 and 4200 m	Greater decrease of spleen volumes with hypoxia 250 to 207, 230 to 173 and 221 to 158 mL, respectively
Richardson et al.[70]	Ultrasound, haemoglobin, haematocrit	4 men, 1 woman	20 min breathing 12.8% oxygen	18% reduction of spleen volume, 2.1% increase of haemoglobin and haematocrit
Wolski[46]	^{51}Cr red cell volume, ^{125}I plasma volume, ^{99}technetium, haematocrit	6 trained, 6 untrained subjects, 4 splenectomized	Maximal exercise and 30 min exercise at 25 rising to 50 and 75% of maximal oxygen intake in normoxia and 16% oxygen	142–187 mL of red cells released by spleen (7–9% of total red cell volume). Increase of haematocrit not seen in splenectomized subjects. Response similar in normoxia and hypoxia

Breath-holding & breath-hold diving

Author	Methodology	Participants	Stressor	Findings
Bakovic et al.[71]	Ultrasound	10 breath-hold divers, 17 others (7 post-splenectomy)	5 maximal breath-holds with face immersed in cold water	20% decrease in spleen volume after first dive, partial recovery 60 min after final dive
Bakovic et al.[62]	Changes of red and white cell counts, plasma protein concentrations	18 breath-hold divers, 21 others, 6 post-splenectomy	5 maximal breath-holds with face immersed in cold water	Total red cell volume increased 4.9% in divers, 1.7% in non-divers, no change after splenectomy. Plasma protein. 5.8, 2.2, 9%. White cells +14.9%, +7.2%, no change
Engan et al.[53]	Ultrasound and capillary haemoglobin concentration	1 woman, 7 men	Maximum breath-holds, before and after Mt Everest climb	Decreases of spleen volumes: 213 to 184, 206 to 132 mL

Table 7.3 continued

Author	Methodology	Participants	Stressor	Findings
Espersen et al.[64]	[99]Technetium and ultrasound	10 divers, 12 non-divers	30 s and maximum breath-holds	Splenic contractions of 10, 30–40%
Hurford et al.[63]	Ultrasound, hamatocrit and haemoglobin	Pearl divers (10 women, 3 men)	Repeated breath-hold dives to 6 m	Splenic volume decreased 19.5%. 9.5% increase of haemoglobin, 10.5% increase of haematocrit
Inoue et al.[67]	Magnetic resonance imaging	6 men, 6 women	30 s expiratory or inspiratory breath-hold	10.2% decrease of splenic volume on volume of 173 mL
Lodin-Sundström and Schagatay[69]	Ultrasound (splenic diameter)	5 women, 4 men	2 min breath-holds	Arterial oxygen saturation 89%. Spleen volume decreased 34%
Palada et al.[72]	Ultrasound	7 trained divers	15–20 s breath-holds	Decrease of splenic volume within 3 s, 20% at full inspiration, 10% at small lung volume, accentuated by cold forehead
Prommer et al.[73]	Ultrasound, blood volumes by CO rebreathing	10 breath-hold divers (3 . women) 7 male scuba divers	5 dives to 3 m depth	25% reduction of spleen size in breath-hold divers, no significant change in scuba group
Richardson et al.[74]	Haemoglobin levels	78 volunteers, divers, skiers and untrained	3 maximal breath-holds, separated by 2 min rest	Increase of haemoglobin in all groups, especially divers (2.7%)
Schagatay et al.[61]	Haemoglobin, haematocrit, plasma protein	20 subjects (10 splenectomized)	5 maximal breath-holds separated by 2 min intervals	Haemoglobin +3.3%, haematocrit + 6.4%, no change in splenectomized
Schagatay et al.[75]	Haemoglobin, haematocrit, ultrasound	5 men, 5 women with varied diving experience	3 maximal breath-holds separated by 2 min intervals	All subjects showed splenic contraction, average 18%, haemoglobin + 2.4%, haematocrit + 2.2%

augments the extent of such contraction.[53, 55] Hurford et al.[63] found a different response in trained breath-hold divers, suggesting that training can increase the splenic response to breath-holding, and possibly to other stressors. However, Espersen et al.[64] did not find any difference in the resting size of the spleen or its contractility between divers and control subjects.

Impact of physical activity upon splenic functions other than red cell storage

The spleen provides a reservoir, not only of red cells, but also of white cells and thrombocytes. Thus, this organ is important to immune responses and mechanisms of blood clotting, and physical activity-induced emptying or partial emptying of the spleen has an impact upon both of these processes.

The importance of the spleen to the immune response became apparent in the early part of the 20th century. Morris and Bullock[76] noted the role of the spleen in offering an adequate resistance to infections. In 1926, O'Donnell had reported a case of acute septicaemia in a six-year-old boy, apparently a sequel to a splenectomy that had been performed two years earlier. His father had also undergone splenectomy, and had died of a septic pneumonia. Perla and Marmoston[77] and King and Shumacker[78] also presented case reports showing a reduced resistance to infection following splenectomy.

It is now thought that the white pulp of the spleen provides a reservoir of lymphocytes, initiates the humoral (antibody) response to infections and synthesizes antibodies. The red pulp of the spleen acts as a filter that removes aging red cells while conserving their iron content, and it provides a reservoir of thrombocytes and immature red cells.

The spleen contains around 40% of the body's white blood cells[79] and as many as a third of the body's platelets.[80] In stressful situations, including vigorous physical activity, these elements are liberated into the general circulation as a part of the general "fight or flight" reaction. However, the timing of their release differs from that of the red cells. Most of the red cells have left the spleen within 60 seconds of commencing a bout of physical activity, whereas the release of granulocytes and platelets occurs over a period of about ten minutes of sustained exercise. This suggests that the movement of the leucocytes is mediated by the progressive, exercise-related decrease in visceral blood flow rather than an active contraction of the splenic capsule.[43] The release of leucocytes is exacerbated by the administration of adrenergic agonists; adrenergic mechanisms modify the expression of adhesion molecules that normally attach leucocytes to the vessel walls in reservoir sites such as the spleen, the lungs and Peyer's patches.[81–83]

The administration of either epinephrine or norepinephrine increases circulating lymphocyte and granulocyte counts. There is a biphasic response, with a lymphocytosis predominating in the first 30 minutes, followed later by a granulocytosis and a decrease in lymphocyte numbers. The largest response is an α-adrenergic effect upon the release of natural killer cell and granulocytes, with lesser β-adrenergic effects upon T and B lymphocyte numbers.[84] A blockage of both alpha and beta-adrenergic nerve pathways is needed to prevent all leucocytic responses to either physical activity[85] or the infusion of catecholamines.[86] However, the blockade of β-adrenergic receptors suppresses much of the exercise-induced leucocytosis,[87] particularly the natural killer cell component.[88] In contrast, increased granulocyte count are α-adrenergic receptor dependent[84] and selective α-adrenergic agonists such as salbutamol augment overall lymphocyte counts.[89]

The possible contribution of splenic contraction to these changes remains a matter of dispute. Frey[90] demonstrated that the catecholamine-induced lympho-cytosis was absent in rabbits following splenectomy and Nielsen et al. had similar findings in human subjects.[91] Schaffner et al.[92] measured splenic size sonograph-ically. In their study of 13 human subjects, the increase of granulocyte count with epinephrine injection was closely correlated with splenic contraction. Ojiri et al.[93] further noted that in dogs, the lymphocytic effect of epinephrine was abolished by isolating the spleen from the rest of the circulation. However, several authors have found a persistence of exercise-and catecholamine-induced leucocytosis, even in recently splenectomized individuals.[94-97] Schedlowski et al.[98] further reported that epinephrine infusion induced equal increases of natural killer cell counts in both normal and splenectomized individuals, and the response to norepinephrine was actually increased after splenectomy. Early human studies indicated that although catecholamines did not induce a lymphocytosis imme-diately after splenectomy, other mechanisms apparently restored this function over the following weeks.[90, 99]

The spleen contains about a third of the body's platelets, including a high proportion of the large platelets that are active in coagulation. The expulsion of these large platelets into the general circulation in response to physical activity or stress is presumably an attempt to protect against haemorrhage during a fight, but it could also predispose to thrombosis, particularly if arteries that are narrowed by arteriosclerosis.[80, 100]

Influence of splenic contraction upon calculations of changes in plasma volume

The traditional method for examining changes of plasma volume during exercise relies upon haematocrit readings. How far is this widely used calculation threat-ened by the effects of splenic contraction?

Some authors have attributed the increases of red cell count during physical activity entirely to the changes in plasma volume that result from increases in blood pressure, changes of osmotic pressure within the muscles, changes in permeability of the blood vessel walls and fluid losses in sweating.[12, 101] Certainly, substantial amounts of fluid can be lost from the blood through such mechanisms.

Stewart used radio-isotope labelled serum albumin to assess plasma volume changes during a bout of exhausting exercise.[15] There was no change in total red cell volume, but the splenic component of the plasma volume decreased from 3.8% to 1.6%. It was thus argued that there had been splenic infusion of blood with a high concentration of red cells, and that this could account for 25% of the increase in haematocrit observed during physical activity. Such a response would be enough to introduce a substantial error into the traditional Dill and Costill calculation of changes in plasma volume[102]. These authors had assumed that a constant circulating red cell volume would serve as a marker to detect changes of plasma volume. Plainly, their assumption would become invalid if splenic contraction boosted the circulating red cell concentration by up to 10%.[44, 46] However, Agostoni et al.[47] found similar changes of plasma protein and red cell volume during exercise, arguing that most of the increase in red cell count was due to extravasation of fluid from the circulation. Accepting these findings, a splenic boosting of haematocrit would not be large enough to cause a major error in the time-honoured method of evaluating exercise-induced changes in plasma volumes.

Mechanism of changes in splenic volume

The splenic nerve comprises 98% sympathetic fibres, and there are α-adrenergic receptors in the wall of the spleen.[103] Moreover, the capsule of the spleen contains at least some myosin. Further, both sympathetic nerve activity and venous catecholamine concentrations have been shown to increase in parallel with splenic constriction.[52, 62, 104] The volume of the isolated human spleen also decreases in response to stimulation of the splanchnic nerves[41] or the infusion of small doses of epinephrine.[65, 66] It is thus tempting to attribute the decrease of splenic volume during exercise or environmental stress as a response to an increase in sympathetic nerve activity, although one objection to this explanation is that the time course of the exercise response is not closely related to the increase in catecholamine concentrations.[44]

It remains important to underline that even if sympathetic nerves are involved in the process, the decrease of splenic volume could still reflect either an active contraction of the splenic capsule or an effect of the sympathetic nerves in restricting the local arterial in-flow.[43] One argument against a circulatory explanation is that the changes of splenic volume follow a differing time course to changes in heart rate or mean systemic arterial blood pressure. Specifically, the onset of splenic contraction is more rapid than the exercise-induced increase in sympathetic nerve activity observed in the leg vessels. Nevertheless, the sympathetic innervation of the visceral blood vessels could proceed more rapidly than that of the leg vasculature, since a differential activation of lumbar and renal sympathetic nerves has been demonstrated, at least in rabbits.[105] The recovery of resting splenic dimensions also occurs more slower than restoration of the resting heart rate, taking as long as 2 minutes following a single maximal breath-hold,[64] 8–9 minutes following serial breath-holds,[75] around 10 minutes after the cessation of breathing low oxygen mixtures[70] and as much as 20 minutes following a bout of maximal exercise.[52]

By relating changes in splenic volume to the duration of exercise, it may be possible to determine whether changes in splenic volume are a passive response to a reduction of the local arterial blood supply or a consequence of active contraction of the splenic capsule. A reduction of the local blood supply would likely induce a progressive change, proportional to the duration of exercise, whereas an active contraction would probably be relatively rapid and independent of the duration of activity. Stewart[115] compared changes of spleen volume in response to constant intensity exercise of varying duration. The decrements of spleen volume were similar (28–36%) with 5, 10 and 15 minute bouts of activity at 60% of maximal oxygen intake, supporting the hypothesis of an intensity-dependent contraction.[152] After exercise to exhaustion, there was a 59% decrease of splenic volume, with recovery over the following 20 minutes. The decrease in splenic volume bore a semi-logarithmic relationship to catecholamine concentrations, although the correlation coefficients of 0.67 and 0.46 for epinephrine and norepinephrine respectively suggest that factors other than catecholamines also contributed to the change in splenic dimensions.

Areas for further research

The most convincing demonstration of the importance of the spleen to exercise performance is to compare responses between healthy individuals and those who have undergone splenectomy. Human research of this type has been limited to date, and there is scope for further observations, including data on maximal oxygen intake and endurance at known fractions of peak effort. There is also a need for more studies of additive responses, examining how typical responses to physical activity are modified by combination with such stimuli as hypoxia or competitive stress. Finally, there is a need for clarification of the contribution of splenic contraction to the changes of leucocyte numbers seen during physical activity and other forms of stress.

Practical implications and conclusions

In some animals, an active contraction of the spleen can make a substantial contribution to red cell count and total blood volume, boosting performance during vigorous physical activity. Because the human spleen is relatively small (~200 mL volume), a 30–40% emptying early during vigorous activity has only a small effect on blood volume (<5%) and haamatocrit (<10%). Nevertheless, the infusion of red cells from the spleen may cause some errors in the traditional method for calculating changes of plasma volume during exercise and could affect the outcome of a closely competed race. Similar responses are seen with the injection of epinephrine or the presentation of other stressful stimuli such as a maximal breath-hold or the breathing of a hypoxic gas mixture. Emptying seems an active response, mediated by alpha-adrenergic fibres in the splenic nerve, although it remains to be clarified how far this reflects a contraction of smooth muscle in the splenic capsule and how far it is attributable to a reduction of local arterial blood flow.

The spleen is also is an important component of the body's immune system, contributing leukocytes and platelets to the general circulation as part of the "fight or flight" reaction. The mobilization of leukocytes proceeds more slowly than that of the red cells; it depends not only upon an active contraction of the spleen, but also upon a catecholamine-mediated modulation of leucocyte adhesion molecules.

Splenectomy impairs exercise performance in horses. However, data on the responses of humans following splenectomy are sparse. Patients can live many years after removal of their spleens, although there may be some impairment of immune responses and a loss of blood boosting during vigorous exercise.

References

1. Shephard RJ. *An illustrated history of health and fitness, from prehistory to our post-modern world.* Cham, Switzerland: Springer, 2015.
2. Barcroft J, Stephens JG. Observations on the size of the spleen. *J Physiol* 1927; 64: 1–22.
3. Barcroft J, Florey H. The effects of exercise on the vascular conditions in the spleen and the colon. *J Physiol* 1929; 68(2): 181–189.
4. Scheunert A, Krzywanek FW. Über reflektorisch geregelte Schwankungen der Blutkörperchemenge [About reflexly controlled variations in body blood content]. *Pflüg Archiv* 1926; 212: 477–485.
5. Granaat D. The spleen in the regulation of the arterial blood pressure. *J Physiol* 1953; 122: 209–219.
6. Robinette DC, Fraumeni J. Splenectomy and subsequent mortality in veterans of the 1939–1945 war. *Lancet* 1977; 310(8029): 127–129.
7. Ebert RV, Stead EA. Demonstration that in normal man no reserves of blood are mobilized by exercise, epinephrine and hemorrhage. *Am J Med Sci* 1941; 201: 655–664.
8. Dill DB, Talbott JH, Edwards HT. Studies in muscular activity. VI. Response of several individuals to a fixed task. *J Physiol* 1930; 69: 267–305.
9. Lucia SP, Aggeler PM, Husser GD, et al. Adrenalin effect on blood count and hematocrit values. *Proc Soc Exp Biol Med* 1937; 36: 582–584.
10. Stewart IB, McKenzie DC. The human spleen during physiological stress. *Sports Med* 2002; 32(6): 361–369.
11. Weiss L. The spleen. In: Weiss L (ed.) *Cell and tissue biology; a textbook of histology* (6th ed). Baltimore, MD: Urban & Schwarzenberg, 1988, pp. 515–538.
12. West JB. *Respiratory physiology: the essentials* (9th ed). Baltimore, MD: Lippincott, Williams and Wilkins, 2012.
13. Hurford WE, Hochachka PW, Schneider RC, et al. Splenic contraction, catecholamine release, and blood volume redistribution during diving in the Weddell seal. *J Appl Physiol* 1996; 80: 298–306.
14. Qvist J, Hill RD, Schneider RC, et al. Hemoglobin concentrations and blood gas tensions of free-diving Weddell seals. *J Appl Physiol* 1986; 61: 1560–1569.
15. Stewart IB. Splenic contraction, catecholamine release, and blood volume redistribution during exercise in man. Ph.D. Thesis, School of Human Kinetics. Vancouver, BC: University of British Columbia, 2002.
16. Dane DM, Hsia CCW, Wu EY, et al. Splenectomy impairs diffusive oxygen transport in the lung of dogs. *J Appl Physiol* 2006; 101: 289–297.
17. Digges KG, McPherson GA, Summers RJ. Pharmacological investigation of alpha-receptors in guinea-pig splenic capsule. *J Autonom Pharmacol* 1981; 1: 313–20.

18. Guntheroth WG, McGough GA, Mullins GL. Continuous recording of splenic diameter, vein flow, and hematocrit in intact dogs. *Am J Physiol* 1967; 213: 690–694.

19. Guntheroth WG, Mullins GL. Liver and spleen as venous reservoirs. *Am J Physiol* 1963; 204: 35–41.

20. Hodgetts VE. The dynamic red cell storage function of the spleen in sheep. III. Relationship to determination of blood volume, total red cell volume, and plasma volume. *Austr J Exp Biol Med Sci* 1961; 39: 187–195.

21. Horvath SJ, Couto CG, Yant K, et al. Effect of racing on reticulocyte concentrations in greyhounds. *Vet Clin Pathol* 2014; 43(1): 15–23.

22. Kunugiyama I, Ito N, Narizuka M, et al. Measurement of erythrocyte volumes in splenectomized horses and sham-operated horses at rest and during maximal exercise. *J Vet Med Sci* 1997; 59(9): 733–737.

23. Longhurst JC, Musch TI,Ordway G. O$_2$ consumption during exercise in dogs: roles of splenic contraction and α-adrenergic vasoconstriction. *Am J Physiol* 1986; 251: H502–H509.

24. Neuhaus D, Fedde MR, Gaehtgens P. Changes in haemorheology in the racing greyhound as related to oxygen delivery. *Eur J Appl Physiol* 1992; 65(3): 278–285.

25. Rovira S, Muñoz A, Benito M. Fluid and electrolyte shifts during and after agility competitions in dogs. *J Vet Med Sci* 2007; 69(1): 31–35.

26. Thomas DP, Fregin GF. Cardiorespiratory and metabolic responses to treadmill exercise in the horse. *J Appl Physiol* 1981; 50: 864–868.

27. Thornton SJ, Spielman DC, Pelc NL, et al. Effects of forced diving on the spleen and hepatic sinus in northern elephant seal pups. *Proc Nat Acad Sci USA* 2001; 98: 9413–9418.

28. Vatner SF, Higgins CB, Millard RW, et al. Role of the spleen in peripheral vascular response to severe exercise in untethered dogs. *Cardiovasc Res* 1974; 8: 276–282.

29. Wagner P, Erickson BH, Kubo K, et al. Maxium oxygen transport and utilisation before and after splenectomy. *Equine Vet J* 1995; 18 (Suppl.): 82–89.

30. Hsia CC, Johnson RL, Dane DM, et al. The canine spleen in oxygen transport: gas exchange and hemodynamic responses to splenectomy. *J Appl Physiol* 1985; 103(5): 1496–1505.

31. Boucher JH, Connes P. Hemorheopathy in exercising horses. *Clin Hemorheol Microcirc* 2008; 40: 73–75.

32. Hinchcliff KW, Kaneps AJ, Geor RJ. *Equine exercise physiology: the science of exercise in the athletic horse.* Edinburgh, Scotland: Saunders/Elsevier, 2008.

33. Persson SGB, Funkquist P, Nyman G. Total blood volume in the normally performing standardbred trotter: age and sex variations. *J Vet Med* 1996; 43: 57–64.

34. Persson SGB, Ekman L, Lydin G, et al. Circulatory effects of splenectomy in the horse. 1. Effect of the red cell distribution and variability of hematocrit in peripheral blood. *Zentralblatt Veterinarmed* 1973; 20: 441–445.

35. Hochachka PW, Liggins GC, Guyton GP, et al. Hormonal regulatory adjustments during voluntary diving in seals. *Comp Biochem Physiol* 1995; 112B(2): 361–375.

36. Snyder GK. Respiratory adaptations in diving mammals. *Resp Physiol* 1983; 54(3): 269–294.

37. Catalini G, Dottavio ME, Rasia M. Acute training in race horses at two different levels of effort: A haemorheological analysis. *Clin Hemorheol Microcirc* 2007; 37: 245–252.

204 Physiology of the spleen

38. Pinkus GS, Warhol MJ, O'Connor EM, et al. Immunohistochemical localization of smooth muscle myosin in human spleen, lymph node, and other lymphoid tissues. *Am J Pathol* 1986; 123: 440–453.

39. Freden K, Lundborg P, Vilén, L, et al. The peripheral platelet count in response to adrenergic alpha-and beta-1-receptor stimulation. *Scand J Haematol* 1978; 21: 427–432.

40. Rushmer RF. *Structure and function of the cardiovascular system.* Philadelphia, PA: W.B. Saunders, 1972.

41. Ayers AB, Davies BN, Withrington PG. Responses of the isolated, perfused human spleen to sympathetic nerve stimulation, catecholamines and polypeptides. *Br J Pharmacol* 1972; 44: 17–30.

42. Sprogoe-Jakobsen S, Sprogoe-Jakobsen U. The weight of the normal spleen. *Forensic Sci Internat* 1997; 88: 215–223.

43. Allsop P, Peters AM, Arnoit RN, et al. Intrasplenic blood cell kinetics in man before and after brief maximal exercise. *Clin Sci* 1992; 93: 47–54.

44. Laub M, Hvid-Jacobsen K, Hovind P, et al. Spleen emptying and venous hematocrit in humans during exercise. *J Appl Physiol* 1993; 74: 1024–1026.

45. Wadenvik H, Kutti J. The spleen and pooling of blood cells. *Eur J Haematol* 1988; 41: 1–5.

46. Wolski LA. The impact of splenic release of red cells on hematocrit changes during exercise. Ph.D. thesis, School of Human Kinetics, University of British Columbia, Vancouver, BC, 1998.

47. Agostoni P, Wasserman K, Guazzi M, et al. Exercise-induced hemoconcentration in heart failure due to dilated cardiomyopathy. *Am J Cardiol* 1999; 83(2): 278–280.

48. Flamm SD, Taki J, Moore R, et al. Redistribution of regional and organ blood volume and effect on cardiac function in relation to upright exercise intensity in healthy human subjects. *Circulation* 1990; 81: 1550–1559.

49. Froelich JW, Strauss HW, Moore RH, et al. Redistribution of visceral blood volume in upright exercise in healthy volunteers. *J Nucl Med* 1988; 29: 1714–1718.

50. Otto AC, Rona du Toit DJ, Pretorius PH, et al. The effect of exercise on normal splenic volume measured with SPECT. *Clin Nucl Med* 1995; 20(10): 884–887.

51. Sandler MP, Kronenberg MW, Forman MB, et al. Dynamic fluctuations in blood and spleen radioactivity: splenic contraction and relation to clinical radionuclide volume calculations. *J Am Coll Cardiol* 1984; 3(5): 1205–1211.

52. Stewart IB, Warburton DER, Hodges ANH, et al. Cardiovascular and splenic responses to exercise in humans. *J Appl Physiol* 2003; 94: 1619–1626.

53. Engan HK, Lodin-Sundström A, Schagatay F, et al. The effect of climbing Mount Everest on spleen contraction and increase in hemoglobin concentration during breath holding and exercise. *High Alt Med Biol* 2014; 15(1): 52–57.

54. Frances MF, Dujic Z, Shoemaker JK. Splenic constriction during isometric handgrip exercise in humans. *Appl Physiol Nutr Metab* 2008; 33(5): 990–996.

55. Lodin-Sundström A, Lunde A, Palm O, et al. *Blood boosting by splenic contraction during exercise at various altitudes.* Xth World Congress on High Altitude Medicine and Physiology & Mountain Emergency Medicine, International Society of Mountain Medicine (ISMM), Bolzano, Italy, 25–31 May 2014.

56. Alberti LR, Petroianu A, Riocha RF, et al. Efeito da esplenectomia no desempenho físico de rato [Effect of splenectomy on rat physical performance]. *Bras Méd* 2009; 46(1): 17–22.

57. Caldeira DAM, Rocha RF, Alberti LR, et al. Influência da esplenectomia na capacidade física em ratos [Influence of splenectomy on the physical performance in rats]. *Rev Bras Hematol Hemoter* 2005; 27(3): 197–200.

58. McKeever KH, Hinchcliff KW, Reed SM, et al. Splenectomy alters blood pressure response to incremental treadmill exercise in horses. *Am J Physiol* 1993; 265: R409–R13.

59. Elsner R, Meiselman HJ. Splenic oxygen storage and blood viscosity in seals. *Marine Mam Sci* 1995; 11: 93–96.

60. Fedde MR, Wood SC. Rheological characteristics of horse blood: significance during exercise. *Resp Physiol* 1993; 94: 323–325.

61. Schagatay E, Andersson JP, Hallen M, et al. Selected contribution: Role of spleen emptying in prolonging apneas in humans. *J Appl Physiol* 2001; 90: 1623–1629.

62. Baković D, Eterović D, Saratlija-Novaković Z, et al. Effect of human splenic contraction on variation in circulating blood cell counts. *Clin Exp Pharmacol Physiol* 2005; 32(11): 944–951.

63. Hurford WE, Hong SK, Park YS, et al. Splenic contraction during breath-hold diving in the Korean Ama. *J Appl Physiol* 1990; 69: 932–936.

64. Espersen K, Frandsen H, Lorentzen T, et al. The human spleen as an erythrocyte reservoir in diving-related interventions. *J Appl Physiol* 2001; 92: 2071–2079.

65. Baković D, Pivac N, Zubin Maslov P, et al. Spleen volume changes during adrenergic stimulation with low doses of epinephrine. *J Physiol Pharmacol* 2013; 64(5): 649–655.

66. Knecht H, Jost R, Gmür J, et al. Functional hyposplenia after allogeneic bone marrow transplantation is detected by epinephrine stimulation test and splenic ultrasonography. *Eur J Haematol* 1988; 41(4): 382–387.

67. Inoue Y, Nakajima A, Mizukami S, et al. Effect of breath holding on spleen volume measured by magnetic resonance imaging. *PLoS One* 2013; 8(6): e68670.

68. Haffner HT, Graw M, Erdelkamp J. Spleen findings in drowning. *Forensic Sci Internat* 1994; 66: 93–104.

69. Lodin-Sundström A, Schagatay E. Spleen contraction during 20 min normobaric hypoxia and 2 min apnea in humans. *Aviat Space Environ Med* 2010; 81(6): 545–549.

70. Richardson MX, Lodin A, Reimers J, et al.. Short term effects of normobaric hypoxia on the human spleen. *Eur J Appl Physiol* 2008; 104: 395–399.

71. Baković D, Valic Z, Eterovic D, et al. Spleen volume and blood flow response to repeated breath-hold apneas. *J Appl Physiol* 2003; 95: 1460–1466.

72. Palada I, Eterović D, Obad A, et al. Spleen and cardiovascular function during short apneas in divers. *J Appl Physiol* 2007;103: 1958–1963.

73. Prommer N, Ehrmann U, Schmidt W, et al. Total haemoglobin mass and spleen contraction: a study on competitive apnea divers, non-diving athletes and untrained control subjects. *Eur J Appl Physiol* 2007; 101: 753–759.

74. Richardson M, de Bruijn R, Holmberg HC, et al. Increase of hemoglobin concentration after maximal apneas in divers, skiers, and untrained humans. *Can J Appl Physiol* 2005; 30(3): 276–281.

75. Schagatay E, Haughey H, Reimers J. Speed of spleen volume changes evoked by serial apneas. *Eur J Appl Physiol* 2005; 93: 447–452.

76. Morris DH, Bullock FD. The importance of the spleen in resistance to infection. *Ann Surg* 1919; 70: 513–521.

77. Perla D, Marmorston J. *The spleen and resistance.* London,UK: Baliière, Tindall and Cox, 1935.

78. King H, Shumacker HB. Splenic studies 1. Susceptibility to infection after splenectomy performed in infancy. *Ann Surg* 1952; 136: 239–242.

79. Bierman HR, Byron RL, Kelly KH. The role of the spleen in the leukocytosis following intra-arterial administration of epinephrine. *Blood* 1953; 8: 153–164.

80. Bakovic D, Eterovic D, Palada I, et al. Does breath-holding increase the risk of a thrombotic event? *Platelets* 2008; 19: 314–315.

81. Krüger K, Mooren FC. T cell homing and exercise. *Exerc Immunol Rev* 2007; 13: 37–54.

82. Shephard RJ. Adhesion molecules, catecholamines and leucocyte redistribution during and following exercise. *Sports Med* 2003; 33(4): 261–284.

83. Shephard RJ, Gannon G, Hay JB, et al. Adhesion molecule expression in acute and chronic exercise. *Crit Rev Immunol* 2000; 20(3): 245–266.

84. Benschop RJ, Rodriguez-Feuerhahn M, Schedlowski M. Catecholamine-induced leukocytosis: Early observations, current research, and future directions. *Brain Behav Immun* 1996; 10: 77–91.

85. Krüger K, Lechtermann A, Fobker M, et al. Exercise-induced redistribution of T lymphocytes is regulated by adrenergic mechanisms. *Brain Behav Immun* 2008; 22(3): 324–338.

86. French EB, Street CM, Aitchison WRC. Studies on adrenaline-induced leucocytosis in normal man. II. The effects of alpha and beta blocking agents. *Br J Haematol* 1971; 21: 423–428.

87. Ahlborg B, Ahlborg G. Exercise leukocytosis with and without beta-adrenergic blockade. *Acta Med Scand* 1970; 187: 241–246.

88. Murray DR, Irwin M, Rearden CA, et al. Sympathetic and immune reactions during dynamic exercise. Mediation of a beta2-adrenergic-dependent mechanism. *Circulation* 1992; 86: 203–213.

89. Gader AMA, Cash JD. The effect of adrenaline, noradrenaline, isoprenaline and salbutamol on the resting levels of white blood cells in man. *Scand J Haematol* 1975; 14: 5–10.

90. Frey W. Zur Frage der funktionellen Milzdiagnostik mittels Adrenalin [On the question of functional diagnosis of the spleen by adrenaline]. *Z Ges Exp Med* 1914; 3: 416–440.

91. Nielsen HB, Secher NH, Kristensen JH, et al. Splenectomy impairs lymphocytosis during maximal exercise. *Am J Physiol* 1997; 272(6 Pt. 2): R1847–R52.

92. Schaffner A, Augustiny N, Otto RC, et al. The hypersplenic spleen: a contractile reservoir of granulocytes and platelets. *Arch Int Med* 1985; 145: 651–654.

93. Ojiri Y, Noguchi K, Shiroma N, et al. Uneven changes in circulating blood cell counts with adrenergic stimulation to the canine spleen. *Clin Exp Pharmacol Physiol* 2002; 29: 53–59.

94. Baum M, Gertner T, Liesen H. Role of the spleen in the leucocytosis of exercise; consequences for physiology and pathophysiology. *Int J Sports Med* 1996; 17(8): 604–607.

95. Hess O. Suprarenin und weißes Blutbild [The suprarenals and white cell concentration]. *Dtsch Arch Klin Med* 1921; 141: 151–164.

96. Iversen PO, Arvesen BL, Benestad HB. No mandatory role for the spleen in the exercise-induced leucocytosis in man. *Clin Sci* 1994; 86: 505–510.

97. Patek AJ, Daland GA. The effect of adrenalin injection on the blood of patients with and without spleens. *Am J Med Sci* 1935; 190: 14–22.

98. Schedlowski M, Hosch W, Oberbeck R, et al. Catecholamines modulate human natural killer (NK) cell circulation and function via spleen-independent beta-2-adrenergic mechanisms. *J Immunol* 1996; 156: 93–99.
99. Schenk P. Die Adrenalinwirkung auf das Blut des Menschen und ihre Beziehung zur Milzfunktion [The effect of adrenaline on human blood and its relationship to splenic function]. *Med Klin* 1920; 16: 279–282.
100. Bakovic D, Pivac N, Eterovic D, et al. Changes in platelet size and spleen volume in response to selective and non-selective beta-adrenoceptor blockade in hypertensive patients. *Clin Exp Pharmacol Physiol* 2009; 36(4): 441–446.
101. Johnson RL, Heigenhauser GJF, Hsia CCW, et al. Determination of gas exchange and acid-base balance during exercise. In: Rowell LB, Shepherd JT (eds) *Handbook of physiology, section 12. Exercise: regulation and integration of multiple systems.* New York, NY: Oxford University Press, 1996, pp. 515–584.
102. Dill DB, Costill DL. Calculation of percentage changes in volumes of blood, plasma, and red cells in dehydration. *J Appl Physiol* 1974; 37: 247–248.
103. Mignini F, Streccioni V, Amenta F. Autonomic innervation of immune organs and neuroimmune modulation. *Autonom Autocoid Pharmacol* 2003; 23: 1–25.
104. Shoemaker JK, Mattar. L, Kerbeci P, et al. WISE 2005: stroke volume changes contribute to the pressor response during ischemic handgrip exercise in women. *J Appl Physiol* 2007; 103: 228–233.
105. Ramchandra R, Barrett CJ, Guild SJ, et al. Evidence of differential control of renal and lumbar sympathetic nerve activity in conscious rabbits. *Am J Phsiol* 2006; 290: R701–R708.

8 Physical activity and infectious mononucleosis

Introduction

The previous chapter examined normal responses of animal and human spleens to various intensities of exercise. This chapter turns to the clinical problem of how the spleen is affected by infectious mononucleosis and the extent to which physical activity should be restricted during such infections.

Infectious mononucleosis is an infection that affects the function of the spleen and other body organs, with adverse effects upon the health of both athletes and other physically active individuals. A clinical syndrome of fever, a sore throat and swollen glands was first described in 1889 by the German physician Emil Pfeiffer (1846–1921). He termed the condition "Drüsenfieber" or glandular fever.[1, 2] The term infectious mononucleosis was coined by Sprunt and Evans in 1920.[3] They wrote an article entitled *Mononuclear leukocytosis in reaction to acute infection (infectious mononucleosis)*. A new virus was discovered by Epstein and Barr in 1968, and this was quickly linked to the development of infectious mononucleosis.[4] Estimates of the prevalence of infectious mononucleosis show substantial variation, depending upon the thoroughness of population testing and the rigour of diagnostic criteria. The annual infection rate for 253,000 US university entrants, based upon observation of a typical clinical picture, the appearance of atypical lymphocytes in blood samples and a positive heterophile antibody test was estimated at 1–3%.[5–7] There have been suggestions that the condition is more prevalent in athletes than in sedentary subjects, due to such factors as the sharing of drinking bottles, although this supposition lacks clear documentation and no differences were seen in one comparison between 202 endurance athletes and 200 controls.[8] Concerns of the sports physician include a possible rupture of the enlarged spleen during infection and a possible progression of the disease from infectious mononucleosis to the chronic fatigue syndrome if normal activity is resumed too rapidly.

Infectious mononucleosis is often transmitted in saliva and has thus been called the "kissing disease". It is particularly prevalent in young adults, and its clinical manifestations can seriously compromise both a student's athletic performance and his or her ability to study for several weeks.[10] Physical activity is normally restricted during the acute phase because of fears of rupture of the enlarged spleen and a possible subsequent progression of the disease to the chronic fatigue syndrome (CFS).[11, 12] We will here consider issues of diagnosis, methods of determining the extent of splenic enlargement and other measures of disease status, and the potential relationship of infectious mononucleosis to CFS, assessing the practical risks associated with engaging in vigorous physical activity at various points in the disease process.

Diagnosis of infectious mononucleosis

Infectious mononucleosis has a long incubation period (30–50 days). This hampers detection of disease onset and a description of its subsequent course.

Clinical signs

Clinical manifestations during the acute phase of the disease include a painful swelling of the lymph glands, particularly at the back of the neck, a general feeling of malaise and fatigue, fever, sweating, a sore throat, inflammation of the pharynx and a loss of appetite.[9, 19, 21] These complaints are relatively consistent (Table 8.1) but unfortunately they are seen also with a number of other common infectious diseases.

Laboratory tests

Laboratory tests provide more certain proof of infection. Common manifestations (Table 8.2) includes a lymphocytosis (with more than 10% of the total white cells being atypical lymphocytes) and a positive heterophile IgM antibody test.[22-24] These basic laboratory indices are relatively specific, and a positive finding can be accepted with reasonable confidence, but unfortunately they lack sensitivity, missing a substantial proportion of those who are in fact infected. Additional options include a search for Epstein-Barr nuclear antigen and IgG and IgM viral capsid antigens (VCA).[17, 24, 25] Although such tests are several times more expensive than the basic measures, they are more sensitive, particularly in the early phases of the disease. False positive results can arise from the persistence of antibodies formed during a past infection, a problem that can be addressed by

Table 8.1 Acute clinical manifestations of infectious mononucleosis, based in part on the analysis of Kinderknecht[9]

- 80–100% of cases: painful swelling of lymph gland in the neck, malaise, fatigue, sweats and a sore throat
- 50–80% of cases: inflammation of the pharynx, a loss of appetite, nausea, enlargement of the spleen, headache and chills
- 30–50% of cases: cough, a swelling around the eyes (periorbital oedema) and red spots on the palate (palatine petechiae)
- <30% of cases: enlargement of the liver, jaundice and a rash

---

Table 8.2 Sensitivity and specificity of common laboratory evidence of infectious mononucleosis relative to an accepted reference standard (the presence of a heterophile antibody or specific markers of Epstein Barr virus in the serum)

Measure	Sample	Sensitivity	Specificity	Reference standard	Author
>50% lymphocytes, >10% atypical lymphocytes	709 patients aged 16–73 yr with clinical mononucleosis	27%	100%	Heterophile antibody*	Aronson et al.[13]
>50% lymphocytes, >10% atypical lymphocytes	181 patients with clinical mononucleosis, 181 controls	27%	100%	Heterophile antibody*	Brigden et al.[14]
Heterophile antibody (latex agglutination)*	140 recent EBV infections, 40 controls	87–95%	98–100%	Heterophile antibodies* and recent EBV antibodies	Bruu et al.[15]
Heterophile antibody (latex agglutination or solid-phase based kits)*	53 serum samples from EBV infection, 47 EBV immune or healthy individuals	70–92%	96–100%	EBV specific serology	Elgh & Linderholm [16]
Heterophile antibody (latex agglutination or solid-phase based kits)*	103 patients with suspected infectious mononucleosis, aged 2–60 yr	63–84%	84–100%	EBV specific serology (VCA Ig G, IgM, EBV NA)	Linderholm et al.[17]
Polymerase chain reaction	Children, average age 9 yr; 28 with mononucleosis, 26 sero-positive, 25 sero-negative	75% at 1 week	98% at 1 week	Serology (anti VCA IgM and anti EBV nuclear antibodies)	Pitetti et al.[18]
Epstein Barr specific antibodies (EDV VCA, EBV NA)	139 patients with recent mononucleosis infection, 40 healthy controls	95–99%	84–100%	Positive heterophile antibody test and EBV antibodies typical of recent infection	Bruu et al.[15]

Notes: * Sensitivity measures the percentage of true cases detected by the test procedure; specificity measures the proportion of abnormal test results that are true indicators of infection. False negative results are found with 25% of cases in week 1, 5–10% in week 2 and 5% in week 3.[19, 20] EBV = Epstein Barr virus; VCA = viral capsid antigens; EBV NSA = Epstein Barr virus nuclear antibodies.

determining the avidity of VCA IgG for its target, or making an immunoassay with a late marker antigen such as Epstein Barr virus nuclear antibodies.[8, 26, 27] Other ancillary and less reliable laboratory evidence of infection includes abnormal liver function tests, particularly increased circulating concentrations of the hepatic enzyme alkaline phosphatase,[22] and increased concentrations of circulating pro-inflammatory cytokines.[28]

Measuring splenic enlargement

The spleen is usually enlarged during the first few weeks of infection.[29] Unfort-unately, this is not a very helpful diagnostic marker. Clinical attempts to detect an enlarged spleen are highly fallible, and even when using more sophisticated laboratory techniques, differences of methodology and the spread of normal values is such that serial measurements of spleen dimensions are needed to avoid missing pathological enlargement of what may have initially been a small spleen. Moreover, differential diagnosis must consider a multiplicity of other causes of splenic enlargement. However, laboratory evidence of a progressive decrease in splenic size is often used as an indicator of resolution of the disease.

Clinical determinations

Clinical attempts to detect an enlarged spleen by palpation and/or percussion are relatively ineffective (Table 8.3). The results of clinical examination vary widely from one observer to another. The coefficient of inter-observer agreement for abdominal palpation as measured by Cohen's kappa is 0.56–0.70[30]), and for abdominal percussion, kappa is only 0.19–0.41.[31] The reported reproducibility of the clinical information also depends on whether the study is part of a routine examination or is a deliberate and careful experimental assessment,[32] on the method of palpation or percussion that is used, on the obesity of the individuals that are assessed and on the proportion of enlarged spleens present in the sample. Tamayo et al.[38] compared three differing techniques of palpation and three techniques of percussion. The figures cited (Table 8.3) are for the most effective of each of these approaches: ballottement (palpation of the abdominal wall while applying pressure over the spleen from the back) and Castell percussion (noting the difference of tone when percussing over the seventh inter-sternal space during inspiration and expiration). One final but important objection to attempts at clinical estimates of splenomegaly is the risk that over-vigorous palpation of the abdomen could cause the rupture of an infected spleen.[40]

Laboratory determinations

Splenic dimensions are commonly determined by two- or three-dimensional ultrasonography.[41] This has an important advantage over scintigraphy in that it avoids repeated exposure to radiation. Other laboratory approaches include computed tomography (CT),[42–45] scintigraphy (detecting radiation from [99]Technetium

Table 8.3 Sensitivity and specificity of clinical attempts to detect an enlarged spleen by palpation or percussion of the abdomen, using ultrasound, scintigraphy or autopsy as the gold standard of spleen size

Author	Sample	Reference standard	Sensitivity	Specificity	Comment
Barkun et al.[30, 31]	118 patients, average spleen length = 15.4 cm	Ultrasonography	62%, 46%	72%, 97%	1–3 examiners, Traube's space percussion and palpation + percussion
Dommerby et al.[33]	29 patients with infectious mononucleosis	Ultrasonography	17%	Not stated	Method of clinical examination not stated
Halpern et al.[34]	214 patients, 92 with enlarged spleens at scintigraphy	Scintigraphy (L >12 cm, B >7 cm)	28%	69%	3 clinical examiners for most patients
Ingeberg et al.[35]	32 patients prior to splenectomy for various disorders	Scintigraphy and operation	59% (16/27)	100% (5/5)	Palpability
Rea et al.[29]	150 patients with infectious mononucleosis	None	8% have palpable spleen		
Riemen-schneider et al.[36]	47 patients	Autopsy	20%	100%	Routine clinical examinations
Sullivan et al.[37]	65 patients, 17 with enlarged spleens	Scintigraphy	70.6% (palpation), 82.4% (Castell percussion)	89.6% (palpation), 83.3% (Castell percussion)	
Tamayo[38]	27 men with suspected HIV infection, 9 with splenomegaly; values reported for most effective of 3 techniques	Ultrasonography, L >13 cm	Ballottement 0–58.3% (37.2%), Castell percussion 23.1–75.0% (39.4%)	Ballottement 50–100% (84.1%) Castell percussion 60–100% (81.0%)	Individual values and average for 8 examiners
Westin et al.[39]	99 patients	Scintigraphy	57%	100%	Palpation

sulphur colloid[46, 47] or [113]Indium-labelled granulocytes or platelets[48]) and simple radiography.[49] Measurements of splenic volume have also been made at autopsy.[50]

The volumes reported depend substantially on methodology, and it is thus inappropriate to make comparisons of dimensions between studies that have used different measuring techniques. De Odorico et al.[41] compared the results for two- or three-dimensional ultrasonography. They concluded that the 3D method was the more reliable, and gave systematically lower estimates, but in normal clinical practice where multiple determinations were needed, 2D data provided simpler and more practicable indices. Radionuclide data generally indicate larger volumes than ultrasonography, but in some instances the accuracy of scintigraphy has been compromised by a failure to exclude emissions from adjacent organs such as the kidneys and lungs. However, autopsy values tend to be smaller than ultrasonography data, perhaps because of postmortem changes in the shape of the spleen.

The spleen is irregularly shaped, and the translation of linear measurements into an estimate of volume is another source of controversy. Many formulae have been proposed to calculate splenic volumes[45, 46, 48, 51–55] (Table 8.4). Some formulae show a close correlation with the weights of resected spleens, and can thus be used to judge changes in the size of a given individual's spleen. However, it is difficult to compare absolute values between authors who have used differing formulae. Because of these problems, some investigators have simply reported percentage changes relative to their initial estimate of splenic volume.[56–58] Others have gauged splenomegaly in terms of the length rather than the volume of the organ, or have calculated an arbitrary volumetric "index".[59–61]

Dimensions of the normal, healthy spleen

Ultrasonography probably provides the best estimate of normal splenic dimensions. The length of the normal adult spleen is in the range 12–14 cm.[63–65] However, such estimates are based on small and rather heterogeneous population samples, and have not considered the likely dimensions in some classes of athlete such as basketball players with extreme body builds.

Reported values are summarized in Table 8.5. Rosenberg et al.[66] proposed age-related upper limits of length increasing from 7 cm at an age of 12 months to 12 cm in girls and 13 cm in boys aged >15 years. Using 3D ultrasonography, De Odorico et al.[41] estimated that the normal adult spleen had a length of 8.9 cm, a height of 8.6 cm and a thickness of 4.0 cm. Using an ellipsoid formula, the estimated average volume was then 164 mL. Such values were said to agree with subsequent measurements on three cadavers to within 2%. Zhang and Lewis[48] used a radionuclide technique; they set the upper limit of normal volumes at 256 mL, but they also claimed that their absolute estimates differed by only 0.2 ± 6.7% from the volumes as measured at postmortem. Other autopsy data defined 2.5–97.5% confidence limits of 61 to 364 mL in 1266 men and 63 to 310 mL in 316 women.[42] Assuming these volumes were normally distributed, they would imply a standard deviation of ± 68 mL about respective mean values of 213 and 187 mL for men and women.[67] The axial CT data of Henderson et al.[42] imply a similar SD of ± 76 mL, but the postmortem data of Myers and Segal[78] show a much smaller SD, of ± 38 mL.

Table 8.4 Formulae proposed by various authors for calculating splenic dimensions

Author	Proposed formula	Justification
Allsop et al.[56]	Percentage of initial estimate	Uncertainties inherent in absolute Technetium estimates
Downey[51]	Volumetric index [0.43 (L × B × V)]	Correlation with autopsy weight of spleen in 101 patients (r = 0.78)
Ishibashi et al.[61]	Splenic index [(L × T)]	Index correlates well with spleen weight at surgical resection (r = 0.92)
Laub et al.[57]	Percentage of initial estimate	Uncertainties inherent in absolute Technetium estimates
Pietri & Boscaini[59]	Volumetric index [(L × B × T)/27]	Recommended to use as an empirical index, able to distinguish normal from enlarged spleen
Prassopoulos et al.[53]	V = 30 + 0.58 (L × B × T)	Chosen formula shows strong correlation with summated areas as measured by computed tomography in 140 normal individuals
Rodrigues et al.[60]	Volumetric index [V = (L × B × T)]	Yields much larger volume than found at post-mortem (284 vs. 148 mL), but index shows linear relationship to post-mortem values ($r^2 = 0.94$)
Samuels[54, 62]	V = (3.14 B²L)/3	Arbitrary formula, giving somewhat lower absolute volumes than Spencer formula
Silverman et al.[46]	V = (L × B)³ᐟ²	Assumption that mass and volume are proportional; correlation with actual mass to within ± 45 mL
Spencer[55]	V = 0.257 (lateral area)¹·⁵	Formula based on theoretical relationships between lateral area and volume
Wolski[58]	Radioactivity in anterior and posterior scans, relative to unit volume of blood	Expressed as absolute values & percentage change
Yetter et al.[45]	V = 0.524 (B × T × [maximum L × cranio-caudal L]/2	Comparison of various ellipsoid formulae with "gold standard" values obtained by helical computed tomography
Zhang & Lewis[48]	V (mL) = 9.88A (cm²) – 534, where A was the area of a posterior radionuclide scan	Mean difference from volume of resected spleens as low as 0.2 ± 6.7%

Notes: L = length, B = breadth, T = thickness, V = volume of spleen

Table 8.5 Estimates of absolute splenic dimensions in healthy but (in most cases) non-athletic individuals

Author	Subjects	Methodology	Dimensions	Comment
Boyd[67]	1266 men, 316 women	Autopsy, accidental death	V = 187 mL (women), 263 mL (men)	2.5–97.5% range approximates SD of ± 68 mL
DeLand[68]	440 adults	Autopsy	V = 163 mL	Correlated with height and body mass
De Odorico et al.[41]	52 normal subjects, aged 21–58 yr	2D ultrasound	L = 9.11 cm, B = 9.55 cm, T = 4.09 cm, V = 191.5 mL	2 observers
De Odorico et al.[41]	52 normal subjects, aged 21–58 yr	3D ultrasound;	L = 8.94 cm, B = 8.55 cm, T = 4.01 cm, V = 164.2 mL	2 observers; values consistently smaller than 2D ellipsoid formulae.
Frank et al.[69]	793 adults, 17–82 yr	Ultrasound	95% of sample less than L = 11 cm, B = 7 cm, T = 5 cm	
Garby et al.[70]	1598 subjects aged >16 yr	Autopsy	V = 117 mL (F), 167 mL (M)	Volumes related to height and body mass
Henderson et al.[42]	11 normal subjects	Axial CT	V = 219 ± 76 mL	
Hoefs et al.[71]	11 normal subjects	Scintigraphy	V = 201 ± 77 mL	
Hosey et al.[72]	631 university athletes	Ultrasound	L = 10.7, B = 5.2	Men > women, 7% met current criteria for splenomegaly
Hosey et al.[73]	Longitudinal observations on 20 patients with infectious mononucleosis	Ultrasound	Peak increase in splenic length of 33.6% with infectious mononucleosis	Peak change 12 days after onset of illness
Krumbhart & Lippencott[74]	4000 adults without noteworthy disease of spleen	Autopsy	V = 151 mL	
Loftus et al.[75]	30 autopsy cases	Post-mortem and ultrasound	Sonographic L = 8.8 cm; postmortem L = 10.5 cm, V = 110 mL	? change of shape when spleen removed from body

Table 8.5 continued

Author	Subjects	Methodology	Dimensions	Comment
Markisz et al.[47]	116 children with liver or spleen trauma	Scintigraphy (Technetium 99m sulphur colloid)	Volume linearly related to body mass, V = 260 mL at 60 kg	
McCorkle et al.[76]	Tall athletes (n = 66); height = 1.92 m (M), 1.77 m (F)	2D ultrasound	L = 12.2, B = 8.9, T = 5.6 cm	Measurements not made by a registered sonographer; population mean for L = 8.9 cm
Megremis et al.[77]	512 healthy children	Ultrasound	L = 10.3 cm (F), 10.7 cm (M) at age 14–17 yr	Values strongly correlated with age, height and body mass
Meyers and Segal[78]	366 adults	Autopsy	V = 125 mL (F), 175 mL (M)	SD approximates ± 39 mL, based on 2.5–97.5% confidence limits
Prassopoulos and Cavouras[43]	87 boys, 66 girls aged 5 months to 15 yr	Computed tomography	Values peaked at 13 yr, V = 177 mL	No sex difference in volumes; no effect of age after age 13 yr
Prassopoulos et al.[53]	140 patients free of splenic disease	Computed tomography	Mean V = 214.6 mL, range 107–315 mL	No effect of height; V = 30 + 0.58 (L × B × T)
Rodrigues et al.[60]	32 normal spleens	Ultrasound and postmortem	Post-mortem V = 148 mL, ultrasound V = 284 mL	Ultrasound V = (L × B × T)
Rosenberg et al.[66]	89 boys and 141 girls, neonates to age 20 yr	2D Ultrasound	Length 7 cm at 12 months, rising to 12 cm (F) and 13 cm (M) at age >15 yr	22 patients with abnormal spleens all exceeded guidelines
Spielman et al.[79]	82 male, 47 female university students	2D ultrasound (3D testing cumbersome, and issues with complex shape of spleen)	L = 11.4 cm, B = 10.8 cm, T = 5.0 cm V = 334 mL (men), 10.3 × 9.5 × 4.2 cm, 220 mL (women)	Spleen length, width and volume correlated with standing height, lesser correlation between height and spleen thickness
Sprogøe-Jakobsen & Sprogøe-Jakobsen[50]	539 normal spleens	Autopsy	Average V = 135 mL (female), 168 mL (male)	Related to height and body mass

Table 8.5 continued

Author	Subjects	Methodology	Dimensions	Comment
Yetter et al.[45]	66 M, 51 F, average age 57 yr, including various splenic pathologies	Ultrasound and helical computed tomography	Methodological difference of 61.8 mL; computed tomography V = 512.6 mL, sonography V = 450.8 to 570.8 mL, depending on formula used	CT volume differs from ultrasonic (ellipsoid formula)
Zhang and Lewis[48]	14 patients with hematologic disorders	Scintigraphy (^{113}Indium)	Upper limit of normality V = 256 mL	Difference from actual volume at post-mortem 0.2 ± 6.7%

Notes: L = length, B= breadth, T = thickness, V = spherical volume

The spleen must often be assessed in children, adolescents and athletes with unusual body builds. In children, splenic dimensions show moderately strong relationships to standing height, body mass and age, commonly with correlation coefficients of 0.7 to 0.8. The spleen appears to reach its maximal size around the age of 13 years.[43] Some observers have also reported modest effects of height upon splenic volume in adults, particularly in tall basketball players.[50, 79] Thus, in a sample of 129 university athletes, Spielman et al.[79] found height correlations of 0.4 for men and 0.3 for women. However, significant correlations with height have been seen only if the sample included individuals with extreme body types, or both children and adults; in adults, the correlation coefficients are generally too weak ($r < 0.03$) to warrant size-specific adjustments of norms.[53, 80]

Splenic size in infectious mononucleosis

We have already emphasized challenges to the use of laboratory determinations of splenic size as a component in the diagnosis of infectious mononucleosis. Some authors have nevertheless claimed that the increase over normal dimensions is usually large enough to contribute to a confident clinical diagnosis. Thus, Dommerby et al.[33] reported that at ultrasonography, infected individuals showed a splenic enlargement of at least 25%, and that three days after appearance of the first symptoms, spleen lengths and widths were 50–60% greater than in a control group with other throat infections. In their patients, dimensions progressively returned to normal over four weeks, as the mononucleosis abated. In contrast, Hosey et al.[72] found that in healthy university athletes the lengths and breadths of the spleen as measured by ultrasound were such that 7% of these individuals would have been classed as having splenic enlargement. Although on average there was a 33.6% increase in size of the spleen with infection,[73] this was no greater than the standard deviation commonly reported for healthy adults (above). Moreover, even if incontrovertible evidence of an enlarged spleen can be adduced, the many other possible causes of such enlargement have to be considered before reaching a diagnosis of infectious mononucleosis (Table 8.6).

The splenomegaly associated with infectious mononucleosis peaks around the 12th day of infection, and substantial changes in splenic dimensions over serial measurements provide a clearer indication of that the spleen has been infected. In healthy controls, weekly intra-individual changes in spleen length are less than 10%.[73]

Management of the athlete with an enlarged spleen

The effects of the disease process upon tissue structures increase the vulnerability of the enlarged spleen to rupture,[82] and a normalization of splenic volume is often one consideration in clinical decisions as to when an athlete can with infectious mononucleosis can return to competitive activity. Dommerby et al.[33] suggested that although the initial enlargements of the liver and spleen were unrelated to abnormal hepatic enzyme levels, a parallel normalization of these two indicators occurred over the course of the following month, as the disease resolved. However, there remain uncertainties about the sensitivity of either illness severity or splenic enlargement as measures of the immediate risk of splenic rupture.[22, 83, 84]

Likelihood of splenic rupture

Splenic rupture usually occurs during the first three to four weeks of infectious mononucleosis,[22, 85] although one case has been reported seven weeks after onset

Table 8.6 Possible pathologies to be considered in the differential diagnosis of splenic enlargement

- **Trauma:** splenic haematoma or contusion
- **Infections:** bacterial, viral, fungal or parasitic infections affecting spleen
- **Haematological problems:** acute or chronic anaemia, sickle cell disease
- **Chronic inflammatory conditions:** sarcoidosis, lupus erthyematosis, rheumatoid arthritis, inflammatory bowel disease, systemic vasculitis
- **Liver conditions:** cirrhosis or hepatitis of the liver, congestive heart failure, portal hypertension
- **Metabolic diseases:** disorders of amino acid, lipid and carbohydrate metabolism, glycogen storage disease, glycoprotein disorders, mucopolysaccharoidoses
- **Malignancies and other infiltrative disease:** splenic tumours, leukaemia, lymphoma, multiple myeloma, polycythaemia, thrombocythaemia, myelofibrosis, metastases of tumours elsewhere in the body, amyloidosis, histocytosis

Source: Based in part on Turner and Garg[81]

of the illness,[85] and one recurrence of rupture was seen ten weeks after the first symptoms had developed.[86] Most such incidents are concentrated in contact sports, but damage can also follow a Valsalva manouevre[87, 88] and in some instances the injury appears to be "spontaneous".[89] Five actual and four suspected cases of atraumatic splenic rupture were found in a series of 8116 patients with infectious mononucleosis.[40] Given that symptoms are often vague, the risk of spontaneous rupture remains uncertain, but a prevalence of 0.1–0.5% has been suggested in athletes.[87, 90] Rupture should be suspected if the patient suddenly complains of acute abdominal pain.[91] The escape of blood into the peritoneum may irritate the diaphragm, with a resulting referral of pain to the shoulder.[85, 92, 93] Following rupture, radiography, ultrasonography and/or computed tomography may reveal not only an enlarged spleen, but also an accumulation of fluid in the peritoneum and a subcapsular splenic haematoma.[85, 90]

Surgical vs. expectant treatment of splenic rupture

Early splenectomy was once regarded as the safest clinical option following splenic rupture, but this reflected an overestimation of the mortality associated with expectant treatment.[92] There are occasional fatalities following a "spontaneous" rupture of the spleen[94–98] but such incidents are rare[22] and they do not warrant a hasty splenectomy. There are indeed several arguments against such surgery. Some reports have shown an immediate operative death rate as high as 1% from an overwhelming meningeal or pneumococcal septicaemia,[85, 99–101] although this risk can now be attenuated by the preoperative administration of pneumococcal and other vaccines.[102] Moreover, removal of the spleen may compromise the individual's subsequent immune responses.[103]

Many authors now regard conservative treatment as a better option, provided that the condition of the patient is stable, and that transfusion can be limited to fewer than four units of blood (in order to minimize the risks of transmitting hepatitis and/or HIV infection via the infused blood[87, 104–106]). Arguments against conservative management include a slower return to competition, the risks of repeated blood transfusion and the danger that the enlarged spleen may still contain undetected haematomas that will predispose to an early second rupture.[40, 90, 93, 98, 104, 107–109]

Overall management of infectious mononucleosis

The general management of infectious mononucleosis is largely symptomatic. There is no evidence of benefit from routine use of corticosteroids[110–112] or antiviral drugs like acyclovir.[113, 114] However, corticosteroids may be indicated if there is severe oedematous obstruction of the airway,[22] and antiviral medication may prove helpful in the late treatment of individuals who have developed chronic fatigue.[115, 116]

Following a period of modified bed rest, recovery is usually uneventful, although serious complications can develop in some 5% of patients.[117] Penman[118] collected reports of some 100 cases with fatal outcomes, including deaths attributed to neurological complications, respiratory obstruction, inflammation of the heart muscle and liver failure. For the athlete, the most serious issues are inflammation of the pharynx, enlargement of the spleen with a potential for its rupture[85] and possible progression to a variant of CFS in the later phases of the disease. However, the factors triggering such a progression and the nature of the relationship to CFS as yet remain controversial.[5, 110, 119]

One controlled study of university students noted a slightly faster recovery from infectious mononucleosis in those individuals who were permitted *ad libitum* physical activity during their illness,[120] and another study of army cadets found no complications from a return to light training as soon as the patients were afebrile.[121] However, vigorous activity seems to be unwise while the virus is still active. In addition to issues of possible splenic rupture and progression to CFS, there is a slight risk of developing myocarditis, with chest pain, ECG abnormalities and damage to the heart muscle as shown by the release of cardiac troponin.[122, 123]

Clinical decisions on a return to light, non-contact physical activity and progressive reconditioning are guided by (1) regression of symptoms, (2) normalization of splenic size[124] and (3) epidemiologic data on the likelihood of splenic rupture. Rutkow[111] somewhat arbitrarily recommended against athletic participation for as long as six months post-infection. More recently, most authors have opted for only three to four weeks of rest if the athlete is asymptomatic and ultrasound demonstrates a recovery of normal splenic dimensions.[5, 84, 109, 110, 125–128] Nevertheless, some sports physicians still advise avoiding contact sports and activities demanding the Valsalva manoeuvre for at least two months, and highly trained athletes may take as long as three months to regain their normal level of competitive performance.[22]

Shah and Richards[129] suggested that athletes with mononucleosis be protected by a customized spleen guard immediately after infection, and others have advocated wearing a flak jacket.[129, 130] However, there is as yet no objective evidence of protection against splenic rupture from either of these measures.

Potential progression to chronic fatigue syndrome

There have been suggestions that in a patient with infectious mononucleosis, premature vigorous physical activity prolongs chronic fatigue and is a risk factor for progression to CFS.[144] If true, this could be a further argument for restricting physical activity during and immediately following infection.

Complaints of persistent fatigue, daytime sleepiness and depression often follow the acute phase of infectious mononucleosis.[21] Sometimes, the characteristics of this fatigue match the American Psychological Association criteria for the diagnosis of CFS,[145] although reported relationships between infectious mononucleosis and CFS are inconsistent (Table 8.7).[119, 141, 146, 147] One major problem in resolving the risk is that CFS itself seems to be a heterogenous group of conditions.[145] The Epstein-Barr virus is not universally detected in CFS,

Table 8.7 Published information on relationship between IM and CFS

Author	Sample	Study design	Findings
Buchwald et al.[131]	150 patients with IM	6-month prospective survey	Fatigue and poor functional status in 38% of patients with IM at 2 months, 12% at 6 months
Candy et al.[132]	71 primary care patients with IM	Postal questionnaire at 1 yr (70% response rate)	Fatigue in 4% of IM patients persists >6 months. No clear precipitating factors
Crawford et al.[133]	110 university students who underwent serum conversion for EBV	3-year follow-up	EBV type I infection is associated with the 25% of students with IM who develop CFS
Feder et al.[134]	48 pediatric patients with chronic fatigue	Follow-up averaging 3.8 years	Acute illness preceded fatigue in 78% of cases of CFS
Hickie et al.[135]	253 patients with EBV or other viral infections	6-month prospective study	11% of patients with IM met APA criteria of CFS at 6 months, irrespective of infecting virus
Katz & Jason;[136] Huang et al.[137]	301 adolescents with heterophile positive IM	2-year prospective study	Criteria for CFS met in 13%, 7% and 4% of patients with IM at 6, 12 and 24 months, mainly in females
Kraus et al.[21]	178 students with IM (Hoagland criteria), matched controls with non EBV respiratory infections	1-year prospective study	IM causes greater fatigue in acute phase, persistent in 11% of patients for 100 days, 6% for 1 yr
Krilov et al.[138]	58 children aged 7–14 years with chronic fatigue	Retrospective evaluation of charts	Symptoms of CFS began with acute illness in 60% of cases
Lerner et al.[139]	58 patients with CFS, 68 controls	Testing every 6–12 weeks for 24–42 months	Serum EBV VCA IgM consistently positive in subset of 33/58 CFS patients
Marshall et al.[140]	23 children	Clinical examination, 17–40 month follow-up on 17/23	Only 3 of 23 patients had current or recent EBV infection; 6/17 had episodes of fatigue at follow-up

Table 8.7 continued

Author	Sample	Study design	Findings
Moss-Morris et al.[141]	246 cases of IM without prior history of CFS	6-month prospective study	9.4% of patients met APA criteria of CFS at 3 months, 7.8% at 6 months. Perceived stress and limitation of physical activity during IM unrelated to likelihood of developing CFS
Smith et al.[142]	15 adolescents with chronic fatigue	9-month follow-up in 6 subjects	Acute illness coincided with onset of symptoms in 11 cases; monospot positive in 7 cases
White et al.[143]	250 cases of IM or upper respiratory infections	6-month prospective cohort study	CFS at 6 months associated with positive monospot test (odds ratio 2.1) and lower physical fitness (odds ratio 0.35)

Notes: APA = American Psychogical Association; CFS = chronic fatigue syndrome; EBV = Epstein-Barr virus; IM = infectious mononucleosis

although type 1 EBV is present in a subset of cases who have previously experienced infectious mononucleosis.[133, 139] Moreover, retrospective questioning of patients with CFS often provides evidence of a prior illness resembling infectious mononucleosis,[134, 138, 142] and prospective studies of adolescents with infectious mononucleosis have found that six months later, 13% develop CFS.[137, 148] It remains unclear whether late complaints of fatigue indicate a lingering infection, as suggested by a continued elevation of pro-inflammatory cytokines,[28] or whether the initial infection is simply triggering what is essentially a psychological disorder.[136, 141, 149]

A retrospective comparison of 47 CFS cases with matched controls found a greater number of the affected individuals reporting exercise >3 times/week in the period before onset of the disease (67% vs. 40%).[144] However, the statistical significance of this observation (p <0.02) is weakened by the fact that it is but 1 of 18 *post-hoc* comparisons. A pedometer case-control study of 301 adolescents with infectious mononucleosis found that CFS was usually associated with a low rather than a high level of habitual physical activity[150–152] but, by contrast, an increase of physical activity was often associated with an immediate worsening of symptoms.[153] In a third study, Huang et al.[137] found no differences of physical activity between individuals who developed late fatigue and those who did not.

We may conclude that a small proportion of cases of infectious mononucleosis progress to CFS. More information is needed on the contribution of premature physical activity to this outcome and on exercise responses in such individuals. But as with other forms of CFS, it seems likely that excessive physical activity may worsen the patient's condition once CFS has developed.

Areas for further research

There remains scope to find a better method of determining splenic dimensions. It is also desirable to clarify the value of splenic size as a means of determining the current status of mononucleosis infections and the immediate risk of splenic rupture. The risk of spontaneous rupture in patients with infectious mononucleosis remains uncertain, and a clearer assessment of this risk would help to determine the amount of caution that should adopted with respect to sport participation during the later stages of infection. Does the wearing of a customized spleen guard offer useful protection against splenic rupture? And in the event of rupture, what are the relative merits of surgery vs. conservative treatment? Finally, is physical activity during infection likely to trigger a progression of the condition to CFS? It remains unclear whether late complaints of fatigue indicate a lingering infection, as suggested by a continued elevation of pro-inflammatory cytokines, or whether the infection has simply triggered what is essentially a psychological disorder.

Practical implications and conclusions

Infectious mononucleosis is sufficiently prevalent among young adults that the condition must be suspected if an athlete presents with fever, swollen lymph glands, a sore throat and tiredness. Although most patients recover without incident, physical activity should be moderated until the acute infection has passed and spleen size has normalized because of potential dangers of splenic rupture and progression to CFS. Careful assessment is important, as symptoms are non-specific, and a positive diagnosis may entail a substantial period of withdrawal from normal competition. Physical examination must be reinforced by laboratory tests, including demonstration of a lymphocytosis with abnormal lymphocytes, a heterophil positive slide test and the appearance of specific EBV antigens. Palpation and percussion are ineffective methods of detecting any associated splenic enlargement. Even laboratory evaluations of splenic enlargement must take account of methodology, the formulae used in calculating dimensions, and the individual's body size. Sonographic data usually demonstrate an enlarged spleen during the first few weeks of infection, but the dimensions of the spleen in any given individual may remain within what is a broad range of normality. Splenic dimensions are more useful in following the course of the disease. By three to four weeks after the onset of infection, the risks of injury from contact trauma, a Valsalva manoeuvre or spontaneous rupture of the spleen are sufficiently low to allow a graded return to physical activity. Sudden onset of abdominal pain should nevertheless arouse suspicions splenic rupture. Debate continues on the merits of surgical vs. conservative treatment of such an incident. Surgical intervention may trigger a dangerous septicaemia and compromise subsequent immune function. Conservative treatment entails a longer absence from competition, the risk of substantial blood transfusions and the possibility of a recurrent rupture. Discussion continues on the frequency with which infectious mononucleosis can progress to CFS and on possible factors that provoke prolonged fatigue. But for most athletes, infectious mononucleosis offers no more than the inconvenience of four weeks of restricted activity, with little risk to long-term health.

References

1. Godt M. *Der Wiesbadener Arzt und Entdecker des Drüsenfiebers Dr. Emil Pfeiffer (1846–1921)* [The Wiesbaden physician and discoverer of glandular fever Dr. Emil Pfeiffer (1846–1921)]. Duisburg/Köln, Germany: Verlag für Wissenschaft und Kultur, 2010.
2. Graser F. Hundert Jahre Pfeiffersches Drüsenfieber [A hundred years of Pfeiffer's Drüsenfieber]. *Klin Padiatr* 1991; 203(34): 187–190.
3. Sprunt TPV, Evans FA. Mononuclear leukocytosis in reaction to acute infection (infectious mononucleosis). *Bull Johns Hopkins Hosp* 1920; 31: 410–407.
4. Evans AS, Niedserman JC, McCollom RW. Serological studies of infectious mononucleosis with Epstein-Barr virus. *N Engl J Med* 1968; 279: 1121–1127.
5. Auwaerter PG. Infectious mononucleosis: return to play. *Clin Sports Med* 2004; 23(3): 485–497.
6. Brodsky AL, Heath CW. Infectious mononucleosis; epidemiologic patterns at United States colleges and universities. *Am J Epidemiol* 1972; 96: 87–93.
7. Chang RS, Char DFB, Jones JH, et al. Incidence of infectious mononucleosis at the universities of California and Hawaii. *J Infect Dis* 1979; 140(4): 479–486.
8. Pottgiesser T, Wolfarth B, Schumacher YO, et al. Epstein-Barr virus serostatus: no difference despite aberrant patterns in athletes and control group. *Med Sci Sports Exerc* 2006; 38(10): 1782–1791.
9. Kinderknecht JJ. Infectious mononucleosis and the spleen. *Curr Sports Med Rep* 2002; 1: 116–120.
10. Macsween KF, Higgins CD, McAulay KA, et al. Infectious mononucleosis in university students in the United Kingdom: evaluation of the clinical features and consequences of the disease. *Clin Infect Dis* 2010; 50: 699–706.
11. Rutkow IM. Rupture of the spleen in infectious mononucleosis. *Arch Surg* 1970; 113: 718–720.
12. Rawsthorne GB, Cole TP, Kyle J. Spontaneous rupture of the spleen in infectious mononucleosis. *Br J Surg* 1970; 57: 396–398.
13. Aronson MD, Komaroff AL, Pass T, et al. Heterophil antibody in adults with sore throat. Frequency and clinical presentation. *Ann Intern Med* 1982; 96(4): 505–508.
14. Brigden ML, Au S, Thompson S, et al. Infectious mononucleosis in an outpatient population: diagnostic utility of 2 automated hematology analyzers and the sensitivity and specificity of Hoagland's criteria in heterophile-positive patients. *Arch Pathol Lab Med* 1999; 123: 875–881.
15. Bruu A-L, Hjetland R and Holter E, et al. Evaluation of 12 commercial tests for detection of Epstein-Barr virus-specific and heterophilic antibodies. *Clin Diagnost Lab Immunol* 2000; 7(3): 451–456.
16. Elgh F, Linderholm M. Evaluation of six commercially available kits using purified heterophile antigen for the rapid diagnosis of infectious mononucleosis compared with Epstein-Barr virus-specific serology. *Clin Diagnost Virol* 1996; 7: 17–21.

17. Linderholm M, Boman J, Juto P, et al. Comparative evaluation of nine kits for rapid diagnosis of infectious mononucleosis and Epstein-Barr virus specific serology. *J Clin Microbiol* 1994; 32: 259–261.

18. Pitetti R, Laus S, Wadowsky R. Clinical evaluation of a quantitative real time polymerase chain reaction assay for diagnosis of primary Epstein-Barr virus infection in children. *Pediatr Infect Dis J* 2003; 22: 736–739.

19. Hoagland RJ. Infectious mononucleosis. *Primary Care* 1975; 96: 505–508.

20. Mason WR, Adams EK. Infectious mononucleosis: an analysis of 100 cases with particular attention to diagnosis, liver function tests and treatment of selected cases with prednisone. *Am J Med Sci* 1958; 236: 447–506.

21. Lambore S, McSherry J, Kraus AS. Acute and chronic symptoms of mononucleosis. *J Fam Pract* 1991; 33.1: 33–37.

22. Maki DG, Reich RM. Infectious mononucleosis in the athlete. Diagnosis, complications, and management. *Am J Sports Med* 1982; 10: 62–73.

23. Ebell MH. Epstein-Barr virus infectious mononucleosis. *Am Fam Phys* 2004; 70: 1279–1287.

24. Bell AT, Fortune B. What test is the best for diagnosing infectious mononucleosis? *J Fam Pract* 2006; 55(9): 799–802.

25. Putukian M, O'Connor FG, Stricker PR, et al. Mononucleosis and athletic participation: an evidence-based subject review. *Clin J Sports Med* 2008; 18(4): 309–315.

26. Robertson P, Beynon S, Whybin R, et al. Measurement of EBV-IgG AntiVCA avidity aids the early and reliable diagnosis of primary EBV infection. *J Med Virol* 2003; 70: 617–623.

27. Vetter V, Kreutzer L, Bauer G. Differentiation of primary from secondary anti-EBNA-1-negative cases by determination of avidity of VCA-IgG. *Clin Diagnost Virol* 1994; 2: 29–39.

28. Broderick G, Katz BZ, Rernandes H, et al. Cytokine expression profiles of immune imbalance in postmononucleosis chronic fatigue. *J Translat Med* 2012; 10: 191.

29. Rea TD, Russo JE, Kafon W, et al. Prospective study of the natural history of infectious mononucleosis caused by Epstein-Barr virus. *J Am Board Fam Pract* 2001; 14: 234–242.

30. Barkun AN, Camus M, Green L, et al. The bedside assessment of splenic enlargement. *Am J Med* 1991; 91: 512–518.

31. Barkun A, Camus M, Meagher T, et al. Splenic enlargement and Traube's space: how useful is percussion? *Am J Med Sci* 1989; 87: 562–566.

32. Grover SA, Barkun AN, Sackett DL. does this patient have splenomegaly? *JAMA* 1993; 270(18): 2218–2221.

33. Dommerby H, Stangerup SE, Stangerup M, et al. Hepatosplenomegaly in infectious mononucleosis, assessed by ultrasound scanning. *J Laryngol Otol* 1986; 100: 573–579.

34. Halpern D, Coel M, Ashburn W, et al. Correlation of liver and spleen size. Determinations by nuclear medicine studies and physical examination. *Arch Int Med* 1974; 134: 123–124.

35. Ingeberg S, Støckel M, Sørensen PJ. Prediction of spleen size by routine radioisotope scintigraphy. *Acta Haematol* 1983; 69(4): 243–248.

36. Riemenschneider PA, Whalen JP. The relative accuracy of estimation of enlargement of the liver and spleen by radiologic and clinical methods. *Am J Roentgenol Rad Ther Nucl Med* 1965; 94: 462–468.

37. Sullivan S, Williams R. Reliability of clinical techniques for detecting splenic enlargement. *BMJ* 1976; 2(6043): 1043–1044.

38. Tamayo SG, Rickman LS, Mathews WC, et al. Examiner dependence on physical diagnostic tests for the detection of splenomegaly: a prospective study with multiple observers. *J Gen Intern Med* 1993; 8: 69–75.

39. Westin J, Lanner SO, Larsson A, et al. Spleen size in polycythemia: a clinical and scintigraphic study. *Acta Med Scand* 1972; 191: 263–271.

40. Farley DR, Zietlow SP, Bannon MP, et al. Spontaneous rupture of the spleen due to infectious mononucleosis. *Mayo Clin Proc* 1992; 67: 846–853.

41. De Odorico I, Spaulding KA, Pretorius DH, et al. Normal splenic volumes estimated using three-dimensional ultrasonography. *J Ultrasound Med* 1999; 18: 231–236.

42. Henderson JM, Heymsfield SB, Horowitz J, et al. Measurement of liver and spleen volume by computed tomography. Assessment of reproducibility and changes found following a selective distal splenorenal shunt. *Radiology* 1981; 141(2): 525–527.

43. Prassopoulos P, Cavouras D. CT assessment of normal splenic size in children. *Acta Radiol* 1994; 35(2): 152–154.

44. Strauss LG, Clorius JH, Frank T, et al. Single photon emission computerized tomography (SPECT) for estimates of liver and spleen volume. *J Nucl Med* 1984; 25: 81–85.

45. Yetter E, Acosta K, Olson M. Estimating splenic volume: sonographic measurements correlated with helical CT determination. *Am J Radiol* 2003; 161: 1615–1620.

46. Silverman S, DeNardo GL, Siegel E. Determination of spleen size by scintigraphy. *Cancer, Biother Radiopharm* 1999; 14(5): 407–411.

47. Markisz JA, Treves ST, Davis RT. Normal hepatic and splenic size in children: scintigraphic determination. *Pediatr Radiol* 1987; 17: 273–276.

48. Zhang B, Lewis SM. Use of radionuclide scanning to estimate size of spleen in vivo. *J Clin Pathol* 1987; 40: 508–511.

49. Blendis LM, Williams R, Kreel L. Radiological determination of spleen size. *Gut* 1969; 10: 433–435.

50. Sprogoe-Jakobsen S, Sprogoe-Jakobsen U. The weight of the normal spleen. *Forensic Sci Internat* 1997; 88: 215–223.

51. Downey MT. Estimation of splenic weight from ultrasonographic measurements. *Can Assoc Radiol J* 1992; 43: 273–277.

52. Larson SM, Tuell SH, Moores KD, et al. Dimensions of the normal adult spleen and prediction of spleen weight. *J Nucl Med* 1971; 12: 173–226.

53. Prassopoulos P, Daskaloglannaki M, Raissaki M, et al. Determination of normal splenic volume on computed tomography in relation to age, gender and body habitus. Eur *Radiol* 1997; 7: 246–248.

54. Samuels LD. Estimation of spleen size from posterior spleen scans. *Can Assoc Radiol J* 1969; 20: 192–198.

55. Spencer RP. Relationship of surface area on roentgenograms and radioisotopic scans to organ volumes. *J Nucl Med* 1967; 8: 785–791.

56. Allsop P, Peters AM, Arnoit RN, et al. Intrasplenic blood cell kinetics in man before and after brief maximal exercise. *Clin Sci* 1992; 93: 47–54.

57. Laub M, Hvid-Jacobsen K, Hovind P, et al. Spleen emptying and venous hematocrit in humans during exercise. *J Appl Physiol* 1993; 74: 1024–1026.

58. Wolski LA. The impact of splenic release of red cells on hematocrit changes during exercise. Ph.D. thesis, School of Human Kinetics. University of British Columbia, Vancouver, BC, 1998.

59. Pietri H, Boscaini M. Determination of a splenic volumetric index by ultrasonic scanning. *Ultrasound Med* 1984; 3: 19–23.
60. Rodrigues AJ, Rodrigues CJ, Germano MA, et al. Sonographic estimate of normal spleen volume. *Clin Anat* 1995; 8: 252–255.
61. Ishibashi H, Higuchi N, Shimamura R, et al. Sonographic assessment of spleen size. *J Clin Ultrasound* 1991; 19: 21–25.
62. Samuels LD, Stewart C. Estimation of spleen size in sickle cell anemia. *J Nucl Med* 1970; 11: 12–14.
63. Ayers AB. The spleen. In: Grainger RG and Allison DJ (eds) *Diagnostic radiology: an Anglo-American textbook of imaging.* Edinburgh, Scotland Churchill Livingstone, 1992, p. 2403.
64. Meire H, Farrant P. The liver. In: Baxter GM, Allan PLP and Morley P (eds) *Clinical diagnostic ultrasound.* Oxford, UK: Blackwell Science 1999, pp. 379–380.
65. Fried AM. Retroperitoneum, pancreas, spleen, and lymph nodes. In: McGahan JP, Goldberg BB, (eds) *Diagnostic ultrasound: a logical approach.* Philadelphia, PA: Lippincott-Raven, 1998, p. 777.
66. Rosenberg HK, Markowitz RI, Kolberg H, et al. Normal splenic size in infants and children: sonographic measurements. *Am J Radiol* 1991; 157: 119–121.
67. Boyd E. Normal variability in weight of the adult human liver and spleen. *Arch Pathol* 1933; 16: 350–372.
68. Leland FH. Normal spleen size. *Radiology* 1970; 97: 5689–5692.
69. Frank K, Linhart P, Kortsik C, et al. Sonographische Milzgrößenbestimmung: Normalmaße beim milzgesunden Erwachsenen. [Sonographic determination of spleen size: normal dimensions in adults with a healthy spleen]. *Ultraschall Med* 1986; 7(3): 134–137.
70. Garby L, Lammert O, Kock KF, et al. Weights of brain, heart, liver, kidneys and spleen in healthy and apparently healthy adult Danish subjects. *Am J Hum Biol* 1993; 5: 291–296.
71. Hoefs JC, Wang FW, Lilien DL, et al. A novel, simple method of functional spleen volume calculation by liver-spleen scan. *J Nucl Med* 1999; 40(10): 1745–1755.
72. Hosey RG, Mattacola CG, Kriss V, et al. Ultrasound assessment of spleen size in collegiate athletes. *Br J Sports Med* 2006; 40: 251–254.
73. Hosey RG, Kriss V, Uhl TL, et al. Ultrasonographic evaluation of splenic enlargement in athletes with acute infectious mononucleosis. *Br J Sports Med* 2008; 42: 974–977.
74. Krumbhaar EB, Lippencott SW. The postmortem weight of the "normal" spleen at different ages. *Am J Med Sci* 1939; 197: 344–358.
75. Loftus WK, Chow LTC, Metreweli C. Sonographic measurement of splenic length; correlation with measurement at autopsy. *J Clin Ultrasound* 1999; 27: 71–74.
76. McCorkle R, Thomas B, Suffaletto H, et al. Normative spleen size in tall healthy athletes: Implications for safe return to contact sports after infectious mononucleosis. *Clin J Sports Med* 2010; 20: 413–415.
77. Megremis SD, Vlachonikolos IG, Tsilimigaki AM. Spleen length in childhood with US: normal values based on age, sex and somatometric parameters. *Radiology* 2004; 231: 129–134.
78. Myers J, Segal RJ. Weight of the spleen I. Range of normal in a non-hospital population. *Arch Pathol* 1974; 98: 33–35.
79. Spielmann AL, DeLong DM, Kliewer MA. Sonographic evaluation of spleen size in tall, healthy athletes. *Am J Radiol* 2004; 184: 45–49.

80. Niederau C, Sonnenberg A, Muller J, et al. Sonographic measurements of the normal liver, spleen, pancreas, and portal vein. *Radiology* 1983; 149: 537–540.

81. Turner J, Garg M. Splenomegaly and sports. *Curr Sports Med Rep* 2008; 7(2): 113–116.

82. Daneshbod K, Liao KT. Hyaline degeneration of splenic follicular arteries in infectious mononucleosis: histochemical and electron microscope studies. *Am J Clin Pathol* 1973; 59: 473–479.

83. Brolinson PG, McGinley S. Autoimmune hepatitis and splenomegaly: commentary. *Clin J Sports Med* 2008; 18(1): 96.

84. Waninger KN, Harcke HT. Determination of safe return to play for athletes recovering from infectious mononucleosis. A review of the literature. *Clin J Sports Med* 2005; 15: 410–416.

85. Johnson MA, Cooperberg PL, Boisvert J, et al. Spontaneous splenic rupture in infectious mononucleosis: sonographic diagnosis and followup. *Am J Roentgenol* 1981; 136: 111–114.

86. McLean ER, Diehl W, Edoga JK, et al. Failure of conservative management of splenic rupture in a patient with mononucleosis. *J Pediatr Surg* 1987; 22: 1034–1035.

87. Asgari MM, Begos DG. Spontaneous splenic rupture in infectious mononucleosis: a review. *Yale J Biol Med* 1997; 70: 175–182.

88. Sakulsky SB, Wallace RB, Silverstein MN, et al. Ruptured spleen in infectious mononucleosis. *Arch Surg* 1967; 34: 349–352.

89. King RB. Spontaneous rupture of the spleen in infectious mononucleosis. *N Engl J Med* 1941; 224: 1056–1060.

90. Khoo SG, Ullah I, Manning KP, et al. Spontaneous splenic rupture in infectious mononucleosis. *Ear, Nose Throat J* 2007; 86(5): 300–301.

91. Rotolo JE. Spontaneous splenic rupture in infectious mononucleosis. *Am J Emerg Med* 1987; 5: 383–385.

92. Rutkow IM. Rupture of the spleen in infectious mononucleosis. A critical review. *Arch Surg* 1978; 13: 718–720.

93. Safran D, Bloom GP. Spontaneous splenic rupture following infectious mono-nucleosis. *Am Surgeon* 1990; 56(10): 601–605.

94. Alberty R. Surgical implications of infectious mononucleosis. *Am J Surg* 1981; 141: 559–561.

95. Bell JS, Mason JM. Sudden death due to spomntaneous rupture of the spleen from infectious mononucleosis. *J Forensic Sci* 1980; 25: 20–24.

96. Papadakis M. Infectious mononucleosis. *West J Med* 1982; 137: 141–144.

97. Ali J. Spontaneous rupture of the spleen in patients with infectious mononucleosis. *Can J Surg* 1993; 36: 49–52.

98. Jones TJ, Pugsley WG, Grace RH. Fatal spontaneous rupture of the spleen in asymptomatic infectious mononucleosis. *J R Coll Surg Edinb* 1985; 30: 398.

99. DiCataldo A, Puleo S, LiDestri GR, et al. Splenic trauma and overwhelming postsplenectomy infection. *Br J Surg* 1987; 74: 343–345.

100. Em SH, Shandling B, Simpson JS, et al. Nonopenative management of traumatic spleen in children: how and why. *J Pediatr Surg* 1978; 113: 117–119.

101. Fleming WR. Spontaneous splenic rupture in infectious mononucleosis. *Austr NZ J Surg* 1991; 61: 389–390.

102. Stockinger ZT. Infectious mononucleosis presenting as spontaneous splenic rupture without other symptoms. *Mil Med* 2003; 168(9): 722–724.

103. Schumacher MJ. Serum immunoglobulin and transferrin levels after childhood splenectomy. *Arch Dis Childh* 1970; 45: 114–117.
104. Guth AA, Pachter HL, Jacobowietz GR. Rupture of the pathologic spleen: is there a role for nonoperative therapy? *J Trauma Inj Infect Crit Care* 1996; 41: 214–218.
105. Schuler JG, Filtzer H. Spontaneous splenic rupture. The role of nonoperative management. *Arch Surg* 1995; 130: 662–665.
106. Toorenvliet BR, Kortekaas RT, Niggebrigge AH. Conservatieve behandeling van een spontane miltruptuur bij een patiënt met de ziekte van Pfeiffer. [Conservative treatment of a spontaneous splenic rupture in a patient with infectious mononucleosis.] *Ned Tijdschr Geneeskd* 2002; 146(36): 1696–1698.
107. Ein SH, Shandling B, Simpson JS, et al. Nonoperative management of traumatic spleen in children: how and why. *J Pediatr Surg* 1978; 113: 117–119.
108. Longo WE, Baker CC, McMillen MA, et al. Nonoperative management of adult blunt splenic trauma:Criteria for successful outcome. *Ann Surg* 1989; 210: 626–629.
109. Oski FA. Management of a football player with mononucleosis. *Infect Dis J* 1994; 13: 938–939.
110. Becker JA, Smith JA. Return to play after infectious mononucleosis. *Sports Health* 2014; 6(2): 232–238.
111. Candy B, Hotop M. Steroids for symptom control in infectious mononucleosis. Cochrane Database. *2006 Syst Rev* 2006; 3: CD004402.
112. Tynell E, Aurelius E, Brandell A, et al. Acyclovir and prednisolon treatment of acute infectious mononucleosis: a multicenter, double-blind, placebo-controlled study. *J Infect Dis* 1996; 174: 324–331.
113. van der Horst C, Joncas, Ahronheim G. Lack of effect of peroral acyclovir for the treatment of acute infectious mononucleosis. *J Infect Dis* 1991; 164: 788–792.
114. Jenson HB. Virologic diagnosis, viral monitoring, and treatment of Epstein-Barr virus infectious mononucleosis. *Curr Inect Dis Rep* 2004; 6: 200–207.
115. Lerner AM, Beqaj SH, Deeter RG, et al. Valacyclovir treatment in Epstein-Barr virus subset chronic fatigue syndrome: thirty-six months follow-up. *In Vivo* 2007; 21: 707–714.
116. Watt T, Oberfoell S, Balise R, et al. Response to Valganciclovir in chronic fatigue syndrome patients with human herpesvirus 6 and Epstein-Barr virus IgG antibody titers. *J Med Virol* 2012; 84: 1967–1974.
117. Murray BJ. Medical complications of infectious mononucleosis. *Am Fam Phys* 1984; 30: 195–199.
118. Penman HG. Fatal infectious mononucleosis a critical review. *J Clin Pathol* 1970; 23: 765–771.
119. Shephard RJ. Chronic fatigue syndrome: an up-date. *Sports Med* 2001; 31: 167–194.
120. Dalrymple W. Infectious mononucleosis-2, relation of bedrest and activity to prognosis. *Postgrad Med J* 1964; 35: 345–349.
121. Welch MJ, Wheeler L. Aerobic capacity after contracting infectious mononucleosis. *J Orthop Sports Phys Ther* 1986; 8(4): 199–202.
122. Fraisse A, Paut O, Zandotti C, et al. Le virus d'Epstein-Barr. Une cause inhabituelle de myocardite aiguë sévère chez l'enfant. [Epstein-Barr virus: an unusual cause of severe acute viralmyocarditis in children.] *ArchPédiatr* 2000; 7: 752–755.
123. Lopéz SZ, Vicario JM, Lerín FJ, et al. Epstein-Barr myocarditis as the first symptom of infectious mononucleosis. *Intern Med* 2010; 49: 569–571.

124. O'Connor TE, Skinner IJ, Kiely P, et al. Return to contact sports following infectious mononucleosis: the role of serial ultrasonography. *Ear, Nose Throat J* 2011; 90(8): E21–E4.
125. Bailey DM, Davies B, Budgett R, et al. Recovery from infectious mononucleosis after altitude training in an elite middle distance runner. *Br J Sports Med* 1997; 31: 153–154.
126. Berezin SW. Management of a football player with infectious mononucleosis. *Pediatr Infect Dis J* 1994; 13(10): 938–939.
127. Hosey RG, Rodenberg RE. Training room management of medical conditions: infectious diseases. *Clin Sports Med* 2005; 24: 477–506.
128. Sevier TL. Infectious disease in athletes. *Med Clin N Am* 1994; 78: 389–412.
129. Shah N, Richards D. Facilitating sport participation with a customized spleen guard: a case of a basketball player with splenomegaly. *Clin J Sports Med* 2008; 18: 92–95.
130. Jong MD, Bytomski J. Idiopathic splenomegaly and return to play – men's soccer. *Med Sci Sports Exerc* 2005; 37 (Suppl.): 279–280.
131. Buchwald DS, Rea TD, Katon WJ, et al. Acute infectious mononucleosis: characteristics of patients who report failure to recover. *Am J Med Sci* 2000; 109: 531–537.
132. Candy B, Chalder T, Cleare AJ, et al. Predictors of fatigue following the onset of infectious mononucleosis. *Psychol Med* 2003; 33: 847–855.
133. Crawford DH, Macsween KF, Higgins CD, et al. A cohort study among university students: Identification of risk factors for Epstein-Barr virus seroconversion and infectious mononucleosis. *Clin Infect Dis* 2006; 43(1): 276–282.
134. Feder HM, Dworkin PH, Orkin C. Outcome of 48 pediatric patients with chronic fatigue. A clinical experience. *Arch Fam Med* 1994; 3(12): 1049–1055.
135. Hickie I, Davenport T, Wakefield D, et al. Post-infective and chronic fatigue syndromes precipitated by viral and non-viral pathogens: prospective cohort study. *BMJ* 2006; 333(7568): 575.
136. Katz BZ, Jason LA. Chronic fatigue syndrome following infections in adolescents. *Curr Opin Pediatr* 2013; 25(1): 95–102.
137. Huang Y, Katz BZ, Mears C, et al. Post-infectious fatigue in adolescents: The role of physical activity. *Arch Pediatr Adolesc Med* 2010; 164(9): 803–809.
138. Krilov LR, Fisher M, Friedman SB, et al. Course and outcome of chronic fatigue in children and adolescents. *Pediatrics* 1998; 102(2): 360–366.
139. Lerner AM, Beqaj SH, Deeter RG, et al. IgM serum antibodies to Epstein-Barr virus are uniquely present in a subset of patients with the chronic fatigue syndrome. *In Vivo* 2004; 18: 101–106.
140. Marshall GS, Gesser RM, Yamanishi K, et al. Chronic fatigue in children: clinical features, Epstein Barr virus and human herpesvirus 6 serology and long term follow-up. *Pediatr Infect Dis J* 1991; 10: 287–290.
141. Moss-Morris R, Spence MJ, Hou R. The pathway from glandular fever to chronic fatigue syndrome: can the cognitive behavioural model provide the map? *Psychol Med* 2011; 41: 1099–1107.
142. Smith MS, Mitchell J, Corey L, et al. Chronic fatigue in adolescents. *Pediatrics* 1991; 88(2): 195–202.
143. White PDT, Thomas JM, Kangro HO, Bruce-Jones WDA, et al. Predictions and associations of fatigue syndromes and mood disorders that occur after infectious mononucleosis. *Lancet* 2001; 358: 1946–1954.

144. MacDonald KL, Osterholm MT, LeDell KH, et al. A case-control study to assess possible triggers and cofactors in chronic fatigue syndrome. *Am J Med* 1996; 100: 548–554.

145. Vollmer-Conna U. Chronic fatigue syndrome in adolescence. Where to from here? *Arch Pediatr Adolesc Med* 2010; 164(9): 880–881.

146. Fukuda K, Straus SE, Hickie I, et al. The chronic fatigue syndrome: a comprehensive approach to its definition and study. *Ann Intern Med* 1994; 121: 953–959.

147. Sumaya CV. Serologic and virologic epidemiology of Epstein-Barr virus: relevance to chronic fatigue sydrome. *Rev Infect Dis* 1991; 13 (Suppl. 1): S19–S25.

148. Katz BZ, Shiraishi Y, Mears CJ, et al. Chronic fatigue syndrome after infectious mononucleosis in adolescents. *Pediatrics* 2009; 124(1): 189–193.

149. Carter BD, Edwards JF, Kronenberger WG, et al. Case control study of chronic fatigue in pediatric patients. *Pediatrics* 1995; 95(2): 179–186.

150. Van der Werf SP, Prins JB, Vercoulen JH, et al. Identifying physical activity patterns in chronic fatigue syndrome using actigraphic assessment. *J Psychosom Res* 2000; 49(5): 373–379.

151. Vercoulen JH, Bazelmans E, Swanink CMA, et al. Physical activity in chronic fatigue syndrome: assessment and its role in fatigue. *J Psychiatr Res* 1997; 11(6): 661–673.

152. Evering RMH, Tönis TM, Vollenbroek-Hutten MMR. Deviations in daily physical activity patterns in patients with the chronic fatigue syndrome: A case control study. *J Psychosom Res* 2011; 71: 129–135.

153. Meeus M, van Eupen I, van Baarle E, et al. Symptom fluctuations and daily physical activity in oatients with chronic fatigue syndrome: A case-control study. *Arch Phys Med Rehabil* 2011; 52: 1820–1826.

9 Physical activity and sickle cell disease

Introduction

Normal responses of the spleen to physical activity were reviewed in Chapter 7. This chapter looks at issues in the clinical management of athletes where the risk of splenic rupture is increased because of sickle cell disease. A person with sickle cell disease has abnormalities in the molecular structure of his or her haemoglobin, and this can affect the function of the spleen and other visceral organs, particularly during physical activity.

There are normally three types of haemoglobin: haemoglobin A (the most common variety, formed by two alpha and two beta chains), haemoglobin A1 (formed by two alpha and two delta chains) and haemoglobin F (formed by two alpha and two gamma chains, and characteristic of very young children). In sickle cell disease, a mutation of DNA sequencing causes valine to be substituted for glutamic acid as the sixth amino acid on the beta chain of haemoglobin, thus converting haemoglobin-A to the variant haemoglobin-S. Homozygotes who inherit the genetic abnormality from both birth parents develop sickle cell disease, with an associated anaemia, and many major health issues. Heterozygotes who inherit the abnormality from one birth parent develop the largely recessive sickle cell trait. The heterozygotes are able to transmit the condition to their offspring, and their red cells contain a varying proportion of haemoglobin-S, with a potential for adverse effects upon capillary blood flow.

A leakage of potassium ions from sickle cells confers some protection against malaria,[1] and this may explain why the prevalence of sickle cell trait is as high as 10–40% in Equatorial Africa.[2] About 100,000 people in the US also have sickle cell disease, including 1 in 500 African Americans and 1 in 36,000 Hispanic Americans.[3] The heterozygous condition is much more common, affecting 8–9% of African Americans,[4, 5] about 1.5% of the total US population and perhaps 200 million people worldwide.[6] There are substantial inter-individual differences in clinical course of the condition, reflecting the fact that several abnormal genes contribute to and moderate manifestations of the disease.[7]

The clinical prognosis for those with homozygous sickle cell disease is not good. About 1% of US children with sickle cell disease die during the first three years of life, and the survivors face 75,000 hospitalizations per year, at an annual economic cost of $475 million.[3] Sickling-induced episodes of vascular occlusion can lead to infarction of the spleen, haematuria and a rhabdomyolytic breakdown of muscle tissue, with a potential for ischaemic damage to bone, brain, lung and gut.[8] Leakage of potassium ions from the breakdown of red cells and ischaemic muscle may also precipitate death due to an excessive accumulation of potassium in the blood.[8] Acute exacerbations of the disease (sickling crises) are frequent. Other complications include an increased risk of infections, defective development of bone marrow and bone necrosis, hypertension, chronic kidney disease, stroke and episodes of severe pain. Pulmonary involvement (the acute chest syndrome) can be fatal. Athletes with sickle cell trait also seem to face a small increase in the risk of exercise-related death, and some organizations such as the US National Football League thus make sport participation contingent upon either the demonstrated absence of sickle cell trait or the signing of a comprehensive waiver.

This chapter looks first at the physiopathology of sickling and its impact upon physical performance and other aspects of health. Risks, diagnostic procedures and potential preventive measures are then considered. Finally, attention is directed to policy implications, particularly the likely number of critical incidents, the costs and negative consequences of widespread athletic screening and the extent of benefits from prohibiting sport involvement.

Physiology and pathology of sickle cell trait

At rest, heterozygous sickle cell carriers show some abnormal blood characteristics, including an increase in viscosity.[9–11] The red cells are also less readily deformed than in a normal person,[9, 12] the shear force needed to separate aggregated red cells is increased[12] and there is a rise in plasma levels of the adhesion molecule-1 that binds red and white cells to the vascular endothelium.[6, 13, 14] Often, these changes are small and of no clinical importance, but the increase of blood viscosity is substantial in a third of individuals with the sickle cell trait.[10] Moreover, physical activity leads to a greater decrease in red cell deformability than that seen in normal individuals.[15]

Sickling during a brief physical effort such as a progressive maximal exercise test may affect only 1% of cells,[16, 17] and the working capacity of the typical sickle cell carrier thus remains essentially normal. Moderate physical activity is not harmful to the heterozygote;[18] it does not increase serum myoglobin levels more than would be expected in a normal person,[19] it does not increase blood viscosity[20] and it may even reduce red cell aggregation 30–60 hours after activity has ceased.[21]

Any type of oxidative stress accelerates the sickling process, and physical training is helpful to a person with sickle cell trait in that it reduces the oxidative stress associated with a given absolute intensity of effort.[22, 23] If there is a co-existence of α-thalassaemia, this blunts the problem of oxidative stress in individuals with sickle cell disease.[24] Muscle biopsy data suggest that a person with sickle cell trait has a greater number of blood vessels and a greater than normal vascular tortuosity, but a reduced capillary density.[25] Possibly, these changes facilitate the circulation of more viscous blood through the muscles. The vascular tortuosity persists if the affected individuals engage in an aerobic training programme.[26]

The adverse changes seen in sickle cell trait carriers are much more pronounced in homozygotes. In one sample from Lagos, the haemoglobin concentration averaged only 7.9 g/100mL, but white cell and platelet counts were twice as high as in control subjects.[27] Moreover, the abnormal haemoglobin had a reduced affinity for oxygen, compounding the effects of anaemia.[28]

Those with sickle cell disease are vulnerable to sickle cell crises, which typically occur several times per year; such episodes lead to a blockage of the blood supply to vital organs and the haemolysis of red cells. The sickling process is marked by the appearance of red cells with an abnormal shape and diminished flexibility as the deoxygenated form of haemoglobin S undergoes polymerization. Exercise can provoke sickling, also causing activation of white cells and platelets and other changes that favour local coagulation.[6, 47] Exposure to high altitudes, the lactic acidosis of extreme exertion, muscle hyperthermia and red cell dehydration can all exacerbate sickling.[48] The process can develop within two minutes *in vitro*, but it is less certain how far it can occur *in vivo*, except under extreme conditions; the red cells take only one to two seconds to pass through the body's capillary system, and deoxygenation is usually only partial by the time that the blood has reached the veins.[49]

Impact of sickling upon physical performance and health

Functional capacity in sickle cell disease

Sickle cell disease is often associated with poor physical and mental health,[30, 32] a low level of habitual physical activity,[34, 35] cardiac enlargement, non-specific ECG changes and an impaired physical performance[33, 37-45] (Table 9.1).

One study looking at the effects of transfusion concluded that any small loss of aerobic performance in sickle cell disease reflected repeated haemolytic crises and a resulting anaemia, rather than the immediate circulatory effects of changes in blood viscosity.[28] However, maximal oxygen intake is reduced by a greater amount than would be anticipated from anaemia alone, implying other derangements of oxygen uptake.[46] Muscular pain may limit habitual physical activity, giving rise to a pessimistic mood and a substantial use of pain-killing medications such as opioids.[31] Increased sympathetic nerve activity may also trigger vaso-occlusive crises.[62, 66] However, when lying supine or following a tilt test the autonomic response of patients with sickle cell disease was less than that of normal individuals,[36] and brief periods of moderate exercise did not augment autonomic activity in a manner that could trigger a vaso-occlusive crisis.[62]

Homozygotes show a substantial retardation of normal growth,[29] and thus rarely seek permission to participate in high-performance athletics.

Table 9.1 Effects of sickle cell disease upon health and physical performance

Author	Population	Test	Findings	Comments
Overall health				
Henderson et al.[29]	63 children with sickle cell disease	Height and body mass	25% of children below 5th percentile for growth norms	
Connes et al.[30]	Review article		Exercise limitations from anemia, pulmonary vascular or parenchymal disease or congestive heart failure	
Anie et al.[31]	21 adults with sickle cell disease	Self-monitoring	Patients needing to use opioids are less active, more pessimistic and face greater disruption of normal living	
Artz et al.[32]	145 adults with sickle cell disease	SF-12 physical and mental health questionnaire	Length of hospital stay related to poor physical rather than poor mental health	Mental health corresponded to national norms
Adebayo et al.[33]	41 adults with sickle cell anaemia	Percussion, ECG, self-paced walking test	Cardiac enlargement, non-specific electrocardiographic changes, slow walking speed	
Habitual physical activity				
Barden et al.[34]	20 girls, 16 boys aged 11 years with sickle cell disease	Doubly labelled water	Active energy expenditure decreased	Increased resting energy expenditure
Buchowski et al.[35]	28 adolescents with sickle cell anaemia	Tri-axial accelerometry	Active energy expenditure decreased	Increased resting energy expenditure
Charlot et al.[36]	22 cases of sickle cell anaemia,	Questionnaire	Active energy expenditure less than a half of normal	Reduced activity of autonomic nervous system
Physical performance				
Millis et al.[37]	15 girls with sickle cell disease, 15 controls	Times for 20, 40 yd swims and 100 yd potato race	All times impaired relative to size matched controls	Suggested as due to left ventricular dysfunction
Dedeken et al.[38]	46 children with sickle cell disease	Self-paced walking test	14/46 had slow walking speed	Poor performance correlated with silent infarction

Table 9.1 continued

Author	Population	Test	Findings	Comments
Halphen et al.[39]	39 children with sickle cell disease	6 min walk distance	86% of age-related norm	Performance negatively correlated with past history of acute chest syndrome
Hostyn et al.[40]	46 children with sickle cell disease	6 min walk distance	Values less than age-related norms	Effect less if thalassaemia +ve
Liem et al.[41]	77 children and young adults with sickle cell disease	6 min walk distance and cycle ergometry	29/30 had low peak oxygen intake	Low scores related to anaemia and recurrent acute chest syndrome
Ohara et al.[42]	21 adults with sickle cell disease	6 min walk distance	Results below predictions for both men and women	Impairment correlated with poor lung function
Waltz et al.[43]	42 children with sickle cell disease	6 min walk distance	Score 75% of age- and size-related norm	Poor performance related to anaemia, low foetal haemoglobin and low red cell deformability
van Beers et al.[44]	44 adults with sickle cell disease	Cycle ergometry, pulmonary function tests, tricuspid regurgitation	Peak oxygen intake low in 83% of cases, mainly due to anaemia	
Moheeb et al.[45]	Schoolboys aged 9–12 yr: 50 sickle cell disease, 509 sickle cell trait, 50 controls	5 min treadmill running exercise	Sickle cell disease group had higher heart rates and higher lactate concentrations	Sickle cell disease group smaller, higher % body fat
Liem et al.[46]	60 children and young adults with sickle cell anaemia	Cycle ergometry	Maximal oxygen intake reduced	Effect persists after adjustment for anaemia

Functional capacity in sickle cell trait

Most heterozygotes have an aerobic power, anaerobic power and exercise tolerance matching that of healthy controls[52, 54, 57, 67] (Table 9.2). In general, there is no compromise of aerobic[58] or anaerobic[50] performance, although one report noted that sickle cell trait limited the achievements of top competitors in a semi-marathon event.[53]

Table 9.2 Effects of sickle cell trait upon physical performance

Author	Population	Test	Findings	Comments
Athletic performance				
Marlin et al.[50]	3 of 16 West Indian sprinters had sickle cell trait	Analysis of sprint records	Those with sickle cell trait achieved best performances	
Bilé et al.[51]	34 of 122 national champions with sickle cell trait	Analysis of records for throwing and jumping champions	Sickle cell trait appeared to contribute to outstanding performance	
Le Gallais et al.[52]	13 of 129 Ivory Coast athletic champions with sickle cell trait	Analysis of athletic records	Those with sickle cell trait performed well in sprint events, but achieved fewer endurance records	
Le Gallais et al.[53]	123 runners with sickle cell trait of 1506 semi-marathon participants	Competitive involvement of cases and race results	Proportion of cases similar to general population; race performance of cases also matched population	But only 1 case with thalassaemia reached international level
Aerobic performance				
Alpert et al.[16]	48 cases of sickle cell trait aged 4–21 yr, 184 controls	Progressive cycle ergometer test	Lower peak working capacity in cases than in controls	4 cases showed equivocal ischaemia on ECG
Robinson et al.[54]	16 sickle cell males, 16 controls	Progressive treadmill test	No significant differences of maximal oxygen intake or heart rates	
Weisman et al.[55]	22 sickle cell trait males, 15 controls	7 weeks basic army training at 1270 m	Slightly lower initial maximal oxygen intake in cases; difference disappeared over training, no medical complications	

Table 9.2 continued

Author	Population	Test	Findings	Comments
Connes et al.[56]	6 athletes with sickle cell trait, 9 cases with associated a-thalassaemia and 10 controls	Cycle ergometer test	Larger slow component to oxygen on-transient in cases with and without α-thalassaemia	Possible cause lower muscle flow, added fibre recruitment or increased cardiac loading
Shasky et al.[57]	Review		Exercise capacity near normal	Sudden death in sickle cell trait rare, associated with rhabdomyolysis in heat or at altitude
Marlin et al.[58]	7 subjects with sickle cell trait, 8 controls	Incremental cycle ergometer test	Normal ventilatory and lactate thresholds	
Sara et al.[59, 60]	8 male sickle cell trait cases, 8 controls	Lactate levels in whole blood, plasma and red cells	Maximal oxygen intake and ventilatory thresholds unchanged, lactate distribution normal; maximal lactate across red cell membrane fast in sickle cell anaemia	
Oyono-Enguéll et al.[61]	11 double heterozygous cases, 7 controls	20 minute cycle ergometer test	Lower exercise tolerance in cases	
Hedreville et al.[62]	Seven patients with sickle cell anaemia	Temporal and spatial analyses of heart rate variability	Moderate exercise does not increase sympathetic activation	

Anaerobic performance

Connes et al.[63]	7 male athletes with sickle cell trait, 7 controls	Five 6 sec cycling sprints	Peak work unchanged but earlier decrement of performance in repeated sprints	
Hue et al.[64]	16 cases of sickle cell trait, 180 normal subjects	Field tests of explosive muscular performance	Performance similar for sprint, long jump and shuttle-run, but cases excelled for jump and reach test	
Bilé et al.[65]	9 males with sickle cell trait, 9 controls	Cycle ergometer force/velocity test	No inter-group difference	

Given that inheritance influences many aspects of athletic performance, it is not surprising that sickle cell trait is associated with success in some types of competition. In particular, it is associated with a high proportion of type II muscle fibres, thus boosting achievements demanding explosive force, anaerobic activity[50, 51] and anaerobic power.[64] However, runners with sickle cell trait rarely win in events of 800 m or longer,[65] and performance is poorer than controls in 30 minute laboratory endurance tests.[61]

Few individuals with sickle cell trait are discouraged from athletic competition.[52] Proportions of affected individuals on athletic teams usually match numbers in the general population,[68] and indeed 11 athletes with sickle cell trait competed in the 1968 Olympics at an altitude of around 2249 m without incident.[69] A 31-year review of 2462 athletic deaths in the US found that only 23 (about 1%) occurred in individuals with the sickle cell trait,[70] as expected from the current prevalence of the condition in the US population (1.5%). However, one NFL competitor with sickle cell trait (Ryan Clark) suffered a splenic infarction when playing American football in the Denver stadium (at an altitude of 1610 m) in 2007, and sickle cell trait has been reported as a leading cause of death among African Americans during military training and sports partici-pation.[71]

One study of heterozygotes aged 4–21 years found a low maximal heart rate and peak cycle ergometer work capacity relative to controls, although there was no electrocardiographic evidence that exercise had induced cardiac ischaemia.[16] Other investigators have noted a normal peak aerobic power and ventilatory threshold,[54, 72] although with a lesser build-up of lactate[51] and a larger slow com-ponent to the oxygen on-transient.[56] The performance of heterozygotes on repeated force/velocity tests also shows no difference from that of controls,[65] and single sprint ability matches that of their peers, although there is an earlier onset of fatigue with repeated sprints.[63] Lactate distribution and clearance are in general normal,[59] although lactate transport across the red cell membrane occurs faster than normal.[60] Finally, the response to basic military training seems normal.[55]

Specific risks of physical activity with sickle cell trait

Vascular auto-regulation can compensate for some degree of intravascular red cell sickling and coagulation,[73] and despite the possible hazards of altered blood flow dynamics during sleep,[74] sickle cell carriers can lead normal lives, with a normal life span[75] and morbidity.[76–78] Moderate physical activity (15 minutes of cycle ergometry at the first ventilatory threshold) had little effect on blood coagulation relative to a control group,[18] and the usual markers of coagulation were unchanged by three progressive exercise tests undertaken with short (10-min) rest intervals.[79] But if heterozygotes are faced by adverse circumstances such as a hot environment, dehydration and/or hypoxia, there is a risk of more extensive sickling, with activation of neutrophils and increased circulating levels of adhesion molecules.[79, 80] Resulting complications (Table 9.3) remain rare,[75] but

Table 9.3 Potential hazards faced by individuals with sickle cell trait during prolonged physical activity under challenging conditions

- splenic infarction
- muscle damage and exertional rhabdomyolysis
- muscle compartment syndrome
- cardiac dysfunction
- haematuria and impaired kidney function
- renal medullary carcinoma
- haemorrhagic stroke
- venous thrombosis
- pulmonary embolism
- sudden death

include splenic infarction, exertional rhabdomyolysis, cardiac dysfunction, renal problems (exercise haematuria, loss of renal concentrating power and medullary carcinoma) and vascular occlusions (haemorrhagic stroke, venous thrombosis and pulmonary embolism);[81] about a quarter of sickling episodes have a fatal outcome.[82]

Splenic infarction

Sustained and vigorous activity at high altitude can occasionally provoke a splenic infarction in patients with the sickle cell trait.[1, 83, 84] Polymerization of the haemoglobin S and formation of sickle cell-shaped red cells is liable to occur at altitudes above 3500 m.[85–87] In one study, sickling in arm-vein blood increased from a resting value of 1.5% to 8.5% after two to five minutes of vigorous arm cranking at a simulated altitude of 4000 m,[86] however, infarction can only occur if the spleen is still functional. Often, previous infarctions have led to what is in effect an auto-splenectomy.[67] Many people with sickle cell trait have enlarged spleens, with multiple small infarctions.[88]

Splenic infarction can occur without altitude exposure.[89] Polymerization of the haemoglobin S is also induced by hyperthermia[90–92] acidosis and dehydration,[12, 93] particularly if the individual is in poor physical condition relative to the effort that is being undertaken.[94] Other factors that encourage sickling are an increase of oxidative stress and the release of inflammatory mediators. However, the risk is reduced if hydration is well maintained,[93] and Goldsmith and associates[69] have queried whether the 10% sickling commonly observed when exercising under adverse conditions is in itself enough to explain the clinical findings.

Splenic infarction typically presents as a severe mid-line or upper quadrant abdominal pain, followed by nausea, vomiting, respiratory splinting and collapse.[1, 6, 95] Infarction has sometimes occurred after only a few minutes of sprinting drills. Debate continues on the merits of splenectomy versus conservative treatment[87, 96] (see Chapter 8). The infarct is usually self-limiting and often responds well to hydration, analgaesics, oxygen and antibacterial vaccines.[87] However, splenectomy may be needed if there is evidence of extensive necrosis.[1]

One early report documented 15 splenic infarcts that were apparently precipitated by flying in aircraft with unpressurized cabins.[97] More recently, several individuals have undertaken short commercial flights in aircraft pressurized to an altitude of about 2500 m within 48 hours of splenic infarction, apparently without any worsening of their condition.[98]

Exertional rhabdomyolysis

Exertional rhabdomyolysis can develop in anyone who exercises at a high intensity relative to their physical condition. The release of myoglobin during the breakdown of muscle tissue causes an associated myoglobinuria. In 5–7% of cases, the ferrihaemate that is released from myoglobin in an acidic environment reaches a sufficient concentration to damage the renal tubules, leading to progressive renal failure.[99] Manifestations of renal damage include an increase in serum potassium that causes muscle weakness, abnormalities of cardiac rhythm and a possibility of cardiac arrest, and decreases of calcium ion concentrations that induce muscular tremors and weakness of cardiac contraction. Even if a fatal outcome can be avoided, prolonged dialysis is often needed until renal function recovers.[100]

Individuals with sickle cell trait seem at particular risk of developing exertional rhabdomyolysis.[101, 102] One estimate suggested it was 200 times more likely in individuals with sickle cell trait,[103] although it is often difficult to be certain whether the cause was sickling disease or simply the performance of severe exercise under arduous conditions. The rhabdomyolysis reflects ischaemic blockage of the muscle microcirculation by an agglutination of sickling cells.[104] One reviewer suggested that those with sickle trait have difficulty in conserving water, and that this increases their vulnerability to dehydration, thus predisposing to sickling.[105] The blockage of the local blood supply causes extensive muscle necrosis and multiple muscle compartment syndromes as well as exertional rhabdomyolysis.[106] Tissue pressures in the affected compartments rise to 30–80 mm Hg, rather than the normal 0–15 mm Hg, compounding tissue necrosis.[107] Four cases of fatal exertional rhabdomyolysis were encountered among US military trainees between 1970 and 1974; all were in individuals with sickle cell trait.[108, 109]

Genetic variants other than sickle cell trait are sometimes responsible for exertional rhabdomyolysis.[110] In fatal cases, autopsy has generally revealed an accumulation of sickle cells in the spleen, liver and kidneys,[48] but it is less clear how much of the sickling occurred before death.[111] The main arguments for antemortem sickling are a patchy rather than a generalized distribution around the body,[111, 112] and that postmortem treatment with either formaldehyde or glutaraldehyde does not induce sickling if the tissues are fixed rapidly.[113] Hypotension during circulatory collapse could contribute to muscle ischaemia and thus tissue breakdown.[71]

A rapid exertional rhabdomyolysis has been said to account for some 5% of sudden deaths in sports.[104] Seven fatal incidents of exertional rhabdomyolysis were seen in 136 non-traumatic deaths; all occurred in African Americans athletes with sickle cell trait, although a causal relationship to the anomaly remained unproven. More recently, 15 deaths in football players and some sudden deaths in other sports have again been attributed to exertional rhabdomyolysis.[48]

Cardiac dysfunction

Cardiac dysfunction is seen mainly in sickle cell homozygotes. It is probably associated with intravascular haemolysis and progressive obstruction of the coronary blood vessels. The tricuspid regurgitation velocity is increased, as is mortality.[114] Pulmonary hypertension and tricuspid regurgitation point to a high risk of sudden death.[115]

Renal problems

Microinfarctions can cause ischaemic damage to the kidneys, with acute tubular necrosis, a loss of renal concentrating ability, defects in urinary acidification and decreased potassium excretion.[116] Exercise haematuria and bacturia can be followed by renal papillary necrosis and even medullary carcinoma.[69, 77, 117, 118] The tendency to sickling is exacerbated in the renal capillaries, where there is a low pH, a low oxygen tension and an osmotic pressure gradient that progressively dehydrates the red cells.

Gross haematuria may persist for two weeks after a sickling episode.[119] The left kidney is most commonly implicated because it is larger and has a higher venous pressure than the right kidney. Occasionally, the immediate renal blood loss can cause a significant anaemia.[116] While bleeding persists, hydration must be maintained to avoid clotting of the red cells in the urethra. Bed rest and a blood transfusion may be needed. Occasionally, it may become necessary to administer a synthetic vasopressin (desmopressin) to increase clotting factors, or the anti-fubrinolytic agent ε-aminocaproic acid or to consider ureteroscopic intervention to apply a balloon or cauterize the site of bleeding.[120]

Metaplasia is provoked by repeated ischaemic damage and regeneration of the renal medullary cells, and the risk of renal medullary carcinoma is thus increased in sickle cell carriers.[75, 116]

Vascular problems

Sickling gives a ten-fold increase in the risk of a haemorrhagic stroke.[121] Minor strokes often pass undetected, but if repeated, they can lead to a cumulative decline of cognitive function.[122] One report described severe cognitive dysfunction with disorientation and amnesia following the collapse of a sickle cell trait participant in a 5000 m ski race.[123] One year earlier this same individual had collapsed with severe abdominal pain during another cross-country event.

A case control study found a four-fold increase in the incidence of sickle cell trait among athletes with venous thrombo-embolism, and a two-fold increase among those developing a pulmonary embolism.[124] In one instance, a retinal vein thrombosis precipitated sudden and painful blindness in an athlete with sickle cell trait who had just completed a 138 km cycle race across mountainous terrain in a tropical environment (35°C, 60% relative humidity).[125]

Some authors have described autonomic disturbances, abnormal capillary blood flow and sudden death[126] in individuals with sickle cell trait even during sleep, but others argue that the evidence supporting sickling episodes while sleeping is not convincing.[127]

Overall risk

Homozygotes with overt sickle cell disease must expect painful sickling episodes, a reduced quality of life, pulmonary hypertension and orthopaedic or neurologic complications[128]. If pulmonary hypertension has developed, the 2-year mortality is as high as 50%.[129] However, the risk of vigorous physical activity for those with sickle cell trait is more controversial (Table 9.4). There are concerns about

Table 9.4 Evidence of association between sickle cell trait and sudden death during rigorous military exercises and athletic competition

Author	Population sample	Activity	Risk in those with sickle cell trait
Military recruits			
Jones et al.[108]	4000 military recruits	Basic military training	4 deaths – all had sickle cell trait
Kark et al.[92]	2 million military recruits	Basic military training	39.8-fold increase in sudden unexplained deaths
Drehner et al.[118]	3 million US Air Force recruits	Basic training	23.5-fold increase in risk of non-traumatic deaths
Eckhart et al.[134]	Military autopsies in US over 25 years		12 of 38 idiopathic deaths associated with sickle cell trait
Scoville et al.[135]	US recruits over 25 years	Heat-related deaths	14 of 31 associated with sickle cell trait
Athletes			
Harmon et al.[136]	NCAA football competitors	Exercise-related deaths	37-fold increase in risk
Eichner[82]	NCAA Division I players	10-year review	10 of 16 deaths attributed to sickle cell trait (16–21-fold excess)
Harris[70]	US athletes	Sudden death registry	0.9% attributed to sickle cell trait

venous thrombo-embolism and renal complications[130] but the overall danger to health seems low. People with sickle cell trait apparently show no increases in hospital admissions, morbidity or mortality.[77, 78] Reports have been criticized for a small sample size and thus a lack of statistical power to detect risks, but in some studies the person-years experience of sickle cell trait has been substantial (for example, 2396 person-years[131] and 4018 person-years[132]). A more important weakness is that most of the individuals concerned have led a sedentary life, and such data do not establish the safety of athletic competition for those with sickle cell trait, particularly under demanding environmental conditions.

The issue is not easy to resolve, since sudden death during exercise is rare and its cause is often obscure. Possibly, some of the fatalities traditionally attributed to hypertrophic cardiomyopathy could in fact have been due to sickling.[104, 133] The diagnosis of a sickling-related death is based largely on its reported pattern.[70] This includes severe rhabdomyolysis, metabolic acidosis, acute renal failure and disseminated intravascular coagulation occurring over a period of 8–24 hours.[57]

Jones et al.[108] were the first to suggest that sickle cell trait posed a risk during vigorous physical activity. They noted that among 4000 recruits engaged in basic military training, the four who sustained exercise-related deaths all had the sickle cell trait. Their observations stimulated much larger studies of military personnel. A retrospective study of 2 million US army recruits found that between 1977 and 1981 the risk of sudden unexplained death was 27.6 times greater in black recruits and 39.8 times greater in all recruits with haemoglobin AS,[92] but that the risk was similar for black and white recruits if the sickle cell trait was absent. Again, in some 3 million US Air Force recruits, the average death rate of 2.8/100,000 rose 23.5 fold to a total of 7 deaths in individuals with sickle cell trait.[118] Further, a 25-year review of US military autopsies found that a disproportionate 12 of 38 cases of idiopathic deaths during exercise were linked to presence of the sickle cell trait.[134] Another study of non-traumatic deaths in US recruits from 1977–2001 noted that 14 of 31 heat-related deaths were in individuals with sickle cell trait, and all 26 deaths in African Americans with sickle cell trait were exercise related.[135] Based on these findings, it was concluded that sickle cell trait accounted for around 0.3% of exercise-related deaths.[2, 69] Despite recent attempts to increase the safety of basic training, a substantial number of recruits with sickle cell trait are still dying after performing activities such as the Cooper 2.4 km running test.[137]

Athletic organizations have had a similar experience to the US military. A four-year study of NCAA football competitors found five cases of exertional death in athletes with sickle cell trait, a risk 37 times higher than that for athletes without the sickle cell anomaly,[136], and a ten-year review attributed 10 of 16 deaths in NCAA Division I to sickle cell trait, a 16–21-fold excess.[82]. Finally, 23 of 2462 entries in the athletes' sudden death registry[70] were attributed to sickle cell trait (0.9%), although 7 of the fatalities were drawn from the 271 African Americans in the register. Prospective trials are still needed. Although the current findings suggest that the sickle cell trait poses some risk to athletes, they could also be explained by linked abnormality or co-existent disease.[130] Small case series have suggested associations between malignant hyperthermia, variants in the ryamodine receptors that regulate calcium release and coexistent haemoglobin AS.[138] Abnormalities in the gene controlling the cardiac sodium-pumping channel may also predispose to sudden death.[139] The high proportion of type II muscle fibres found in many black athletes further modifies exercise responses.[69] Finally, black recruits may initially be less fit than their white counterparts, or they may exercise harder when they are evaluated in their attempts to gain a military commission.[140]

Ajayi[121] argued that sickle cell trait should be considered a disease state rather than a benign condition. To date, policy decisions on the need for athletic screening have been based largely rather alarming risk ratios suggesting a substantial disadvantage to those with sickle cell trait, but they obscure the fact that even under very adverse circumstances (untrained individuals performing very demanding exercise in hot and humid conditions), the absolute number of deaths among those with sickle cell trait remains small. The risks, already quite low, could be greatly attenuated by better control of heat stress and exercise intensity in those who are initially untrained, with benefit to all recruits.[6]

Diagnostic approaches to sickle cell trait

Given the concern that sickle cell trait can precipitate major illnesses and even sudden death, there has been interest in developing simple and reliable tests to identify the sickle cell anomaly. Athletes are usually classified simply as positive or negative. However, the risk is not as simple as this binary classification might suggest; ancillary factors can modify expression of sickle cell-related disorders.[7] The blood leucocyte concentration affects coagulation and thus the incidence of acute chest syndrome and cerebral infarction, a higher concentration of foetal haemoglobin attenuates sickling, and nitric oxide bioavailability influences the vascular adhesion of red cells during sickling.[141]

Table 9.5 Sensitivity and specificity of tests for the diagnosis of sickle cell trait

Author	Test	Sensitivity	Specificity	Comment
Aluoch et al.[143]	Microscopy of peripheral blood smear	76%	99.7%	Patients with sickle cell anaemia; gold standard cellulose-acetate paper electrophoresis
Hicks et al.[144]	Solubility test	99%	100%	487/493 sickle cell trait, compared relative to electrophoresis
Hicks et al.[144]	Metabisulphite	97%	99.9%	487/493 sickle cell trait, compared relative to electrophoresis
Hicks et al.[144]	Sickledex	98.9%	100%	487/493 sickle cell trait, compared relative to electrophoresis

Available tests vary in their cost, sensitivity and specificity (Table 9.5). The "solubility test", based on the relative insolubility of deoxyhaemoglobin-S in an aqueous solution[6] can cost as little as $10, but the fee for a haemoglobin electrophoresis test[142] ranges from $30–150.[136] The simplest diagnostic option is to examine a peripheral blood film; this has a sensitivity of 76% and a specificity of 99.7%.[143] Hicks and associates[144] evaluated the success of other screening methods in a sample of 4243 people, 487 of whom had the sickle cell trait and 6 of whom had sickle cell disease. All of the procedures evaluated were relatively satisfactory. The standard meta-bisulphite test gave 3% of false negative and 0.07% false positive results. The solubility test fared somewhat better, with 1% false negative and 0% false positive results, and cellulose-acetate electrophoresis gave 100% sensitivity and specificity. The methods currently recommended are electrophoresis (thin-layer isoelectric focusing) or high-performance liquid chromatography, both of which are reported as having an "extremely high" sensitivity and specificity.[145] High-performance liquid chromatography can detect as little as 0.5% of a haemoglobin variant in a blood sample.[146, 147]

Potential for preventive measures

Given the high sensitivity and specificity of current tests, some physicians have proposed that universal sickle cell screening should be carried out at birth. However, at least 50 heterozygotes with sickle cell trait are identified for every homozygote, and the negative personal consequences of being diagnosed with the sickle cell trait as yet remain unclear.[145] Further, even if universal birth screening were to be adopted, occasional cases of sickle cell trait would probably remain undetected because of clerical errors such as mislabeled specimens, blood transfusion prior to screening or the inability to locate affected infants after their discharge from hospital.

The possibility of an exercise-related death in an athlete with sickle cell trait depends upon the intensity of training and competition relative to the individual's initial status. Because competition was more intense in older age groups, one report estimated that the risk of sickle cell deaths was 66 times higher in university than in high school football athletes, although at 0.57 per 100,000 deaths the incidence of sickling deaths in the university group still remained relatively low.[148]

Habitual physical activity such as eight hours of soccer training per week[94] apparently offers some protection against sickling, in part by reducing an individual's relative intensity of effort when performing any given task. Oxidative stress plays a major role in sickling, and the accumulation of reactive species may lead to endothelial activation, with an increased adherence of red cells to the vascular linings.[149] Physical training reduces the oxidative stress associated with a given bout of physical activity, and this also attenuates the risk of sickling.[22] Fluid ingestion sufficient to maintain body mass is another important precaution;[150, 151] well-hydrated subjects showed no evidence of sickling during 45 minutes of brisk treadmill walking at a temperature of 33 °C, whereas their peers showed at least 5% sickling if they performed the same exercise but no fluid was provided.[93] Dehydration apparently has particularly adverse effects in those with the sickle cell trait.[90] Control subjects showed only small increments of blood viscosity over the course of a soccer game, even if no fluids were provided. However, in players with sickle cell trait, a game without fluids increased what was initially a high blood viscosity, although this could be normalized quite easily by the *ad libitum* provision of fluids.[151] Further, playing a match without water increased red cell rigidity in players with sickle cell trait, whereas the provision of *ad libitum* fluids decreased rigidity.[150] Blood viscosity also increased during 40 minutes of exercise at 55% of peak aerobic power in those with sickle cell trait if they were deprived of water,[11] and even a brief bout of exercise at 110% of maximal oxygen intake increased blood viscosity.[47]

Paradoxically, the sickle cell trait does not seem to increase the risk of exertional heat stroke.[67] However, the risks of heat-related death for all athletes can be mitigated by the sensible precautions of adequate heat acclimatization[67] and maintenance of hydration.[93] In known sickle cell trait exercisers, intensities of training should be reduced, and longer periods of rest and recovery intervals allowed. Supplemental oxygen should also be readily available, particularly if athletes are exercising at altitude.[152] Above all, athletes should be encouraged to set their own pace during training and to cease exercising if symptoms develop.

The complications of sickling have been said to increase eight-fold from the late teens to the late 20s.[92, 135, 153] This could reflect an age-related loss of physical condition, or the cumulative influence of such factors as repeated incidents of renal papillary necrosis and poorer regulation of fluid balance; in any event, greater caution should be shown when planning exercise programmes for older athletes with the sickle cell trait.

Nutritional deficiencies, particularly an inadequate intake of zinc, may contribute to occlusive crises in sickle cell trait.[154] Vitamin D supplements may also reduce pain and thus contribute to greater physical activity and quality of life in such individuals.[155]

Administration of hydrourea appears to improve physical functioning and the health-related quality of life in children with sickle cell disease;[156, 157] this drug appears to stimulate production of foetal-type haemoglobin and reduce the production of haemoglobin S.

Finally, those who are providing medical care at an athletic event should become familiar with the warning signs of sickling, keeping a careful watch kept for lower extremity or low back pain, cramp or spasm, muscle weakness and fatigue, difficulty in recovering from exercise, shortness of breath and/or a slow collapse.[152]

Areas for further research

There is a need to identify unidentified risk factors, whether genetic or non-genetic, that increase the risk of complications in athletes with the sickle cell trait.[158, 159] It would be helpful to explore further why certain sports and certain forms of physical conditioning are particularly risky. One useful line of enquiry would be to examine how far small but cumulative renal infarcts limit the regulation of hydration in those with the sickle cell trait. Further studies are also needed to determine whether increased levels of adhesion molecules such as the L and P selectins pose a particular risk for sickle cell carriers.[112] Establishment of a national or international registry of athletes with sickle cell trait would help to answer many of these questions.

Practical implications and conclusions

The recessive sickle cell trait is much more commonly encountered than the homozygous condition of sickle cell disease. Sickle cell trait has little influence upon morbidity and mortality in normal daily life, but there is some risk of sickling when undertaking very vigorous exercise at high altitude or in the heat with fluid deprivation. In many jurisdictions, infants are now screened for sickle cell trait at birth. This allows the early prescription of antibiotics to curtail the potential risk of bacterial infections.[160] However, information on sickle cell status is not always available when a young adult wishes to engage in sport, and even if such information is available, it remains debatable how far it should influence habitual physical activity. Vigorous controversy continues on the ethics of sickle cell trait screening among adolescents and adults.[5, 161–164] The US National Athletic Trainers Association concluded that there was a strong case for screening if data had not been collected at birth.[165] In the absence of testing as an infant or the signing of a comprehensive written waiver, the NCAA also began required testing of sickle cell status for Division I competitors in 2010, and this requirement was extended to Division III competitors as of 2014–2015. This was largely a defensive response to litigation from the relatives of an athlete with sickle cell trait who died of exertional rhabdomyolysis during a football practice.[75, 162]

Despite NCAA policy statements, a 2011 survey found that because of costs, few colleges and universities were undertaking comprehensive sickle cell screening.[166] Given the relatively low risk that heterozygotes would develop complications,[130] it was argued that decisions should be based not on the seemingly alarming risk ratios found when contrasting the experience of black and white athletes but upon a careful cost–benefit analysis, looking at the likely number of lives that would be saved by a given policy.[140] Further, it was recommended that the analysis should consider not only the immediate diagnostic costs, but also the likelihood that testing would extend the individual's life and any negative economic consequences such as denial of participation in a major sports team.

Health economists commonly argue that a procedure can be considered as cost effective if one person-year of life can be saved for less than $50,000. Harmon et al.[136] made such an analysis for collegiate athletes who were participating in NCAA football over the period 2004–2008. The sample was large (2 million athlete-years), and most of the 72 deaths (52/72) were due to trauma; only 5 deaths were associated with sickle cell trait. All of the sickle cell related incidents were in black players, and all occurred during conditioning rather than competition. One weakness in their calculation was the assumption of a simple but effective $5 test; in fact, a reliable analysis, based on electrophoresis, would more likely cost $150 per athlete. It was further assumed that the chosen test had 100% sensitivity and specificity in preventing death, and that the prevention of sudden exercise-related death would extend an athlete's life by 50 years. On this basis, the cost of preventing one death over five years among NCAA athletes would range from $40,580 for black footballers to $23,907,984 for competitors in all sports, irrespective of race,[136] and with 50 years of survival, the costs per life-year saved would range from an acceptable $812 for black footballers to an excessive $478,160 for all athletes. If the sensitivity and specificity of the test were to be assured by use of a more sophisticated electrophoretic test, the cost per life-year would range from $24,360 for the black footballer to an astronomic $1,444,800 for all athletes. Another criticism, even with electrophoretic testing, is that the diagnosis is limited to identification of the sickle cell trait, and it fails to detect other genetic characteristics that could modify the risk of sickling.

It has yet to be demonstrated that a targeted diagnosis can indeed reduce the risk of death relative to the adoption of more general precautions regarding exposure to heat, hypoxia and dehydration that would protect all athletes. Currently, diagnosis does not seem to confer great survival benefit, as athletes with known sickle cell trait continue to die during exercise.[136] Further, the negative personal effects of screening must be considered. Potential consequences include a weakened self-image, parental over-protection, a loss of athletic scholarships, limitations upon employment and increased health insurance premiums.[69, 75, 130, 167–169] Military recruits with sickle cell trait are denied employment as pilots, co-pilots or divers because of potential exposure to hypoxia that could provoke sickling,[170, 171] and many insurance companies have raised premiums for patients with sickle cell trait, despite the demonstration that such individuals have normal morbidity and mortality statistics.[76]

Even enthusiastic proponents have estimated that the universal screening of NCAA Division I student athletes would at most save about seven lives over ten years.[172] A survey conducted by the American Medical Society for Sports Medicine found a preference for a review of medical records and targeted solubility testing focused upon those black athletes who were involved in American football and basketball.[173] Moreover, most respondents indicated that they would still allow sport participation if an athlete or the parents opted out of screening. A case for targeted screening can certainly be made, based on current cost–benefit analyses,[136, 174] but further study is needed to establish that such an approach reduces mortality relative to the alternative option of a more careful management of all athletes, regardless of their genetic background.

References

1.   Franklin QJ, Compeggie M. Splenic syndrome in sickle cell trait: four case presentations and a review of the literature. *Mil Med* 1999; 164(3): 230–233.

2. World Health Organization. *Sickle-cell anaemia: report by the Secretariat.* World Health Organization, Fifty-Ninth World Health Assembly A59/9. Provisional Agenda item 11.4. 2006

3. National Heart, Lung and Blood Institute. *Disease and conditions index. Sickle cell anemia: who is at risk?* Bethesda, MD: US Department of Health and Human Services, National Institutes of Health, National Heart, Lung, and Blood Institute, 2009.

4. Martin JA, Hamilton BE, Sutton PD, et al. Births: final data for 2007. *National Vital Statistics Reports* 2010; 58(24): 1–77.

5. Jordan LB, Smith-Whitley K, Treadwell MJ, et al. Screening US college athletes for their sickle cell disease carrier status. *Am J Prev Med* 2011; 41(6): S406–S412.

6. O'Connor FG, Bergeron MF, Cantrell J, et al. ACSM and CHAMP summit on sickle cell trait: mitigating risks for warfighters and athletes. *Med Sci Sports Exerc* 2012; 44: 2045–2056.

7. Chui DH, Dover GJ. Sickle cell disease: no longer a single gene disorder. *Curr Opin Pediatr* 2001; 13: 1322–1327.

8. Loosemore M, Walsh SB, Morris E, et al. Sudden exertional death in sickle cell trait. *Br J Sports Med* 2012; 46: 312–314.

9. Connes P, Hue O, Hardy-Dessources MD, et al. Hemorheology and heart rate variability: is there a relationship? *Clin Hemorheol Microcirc* 2008; 38(4): 257–265.

10. Tripette J, Alexy T, Hardy-Dessources MD, et al. Red blood cell aggregation, aggregate strength and oxygen transport potential of blood are abnormal in both homozygous sickle cell anemia and sickle-hemoglobin C disease. *Haematologica* 2009; 94(8): 1060–1065.

11. Tripette J, Loko G, Samb A, et al. Effects of hydration and dehydration on blood rheology in sickle cell trait carriers during exercise. *Am J Physiol* 2010; 299(3): H908–H914.

12. Tripette J, Connes P, Beltan E, et al. Red blood cell deformability and aggregation, cell adhesion molecules, oxidative stress and nitric oxide markers after a short term, submaximal, exercise in sickle cell trait carriers. Clin Hemorheol Microcirc 2010; 45(1): 39–52.

13. Connes P, Sara F, Hardy-Dessources, et al. Does higher red blood cell (RBC) lactate transporter activity explain impaired RBC deformability in sickle cell trait? *Jap J Physiol* 2005; 55: 385–387.

14. Monchanin G, Serpero L, Connes P, et al. Effects of progressive and maximal exercise on plasma levels of adhesion molecules in athletes with sickle cell trait with or without alpha-thalassemia. *J Appl Physiol* 2007; 102: 169–173.

15. Tripette J, Hardy-Dessources M-D, Sara F, et al. Does repeated and heavy exercise impair blood rheology in carriers of sickle cell trait? *Clin J Sports Med* 2007; 17: 465–470.

16. Alpert BS, Flood NL, Strong WB, et al. Responses to exercise in children with sickle cell trait. *Am J Dis Childh* 1982; 136: 1002–1004.

17. Ramirez A, Hartley LH, Rhodes D, et al. Morphological features of red blood cells in subjects with sickle cell trait: changes during exercise. *Arch Intern Med* 1976; 136: 1064–1066.

18. Beltan E, Chalabi T, Tripette J, et al. Coagulation responses after a submaximal exercise in sickle cell trait carriers. *Thromb Res* 2011; 127(2): 167–169.

19. Messonnier L, Samb A, Tripette J, et al. Moderate endurance exercise is not a risk for rhabdomyolysis or renal failure in sickle cell trait carriers. *Clin Hemorheol Microcirc* 2012; 51(3): 193–202.

20. Balayssac-Siransy E, Connes P, Tuo N, et al. Mild haemorheological changes induced by a moderate endurance exercise in patients with sickle cell anaemia. *Br J Haematol* 2011; 154(3): 398–407.

21. Waltz X, Hedreville M, Sinnapah S, et al. Delayed beneficial effect of acute exercise on red blood cell aggregate strength in patients with sickle cell anemia. *Clin Hemorheol Microcirc* 2012; 52(1): 15–26.

22. Chirico EN, Martin C, Faës C, et al. Exercise training blunts oxidative stress in sickle cell trait carriers. *J Appl Physiol* 2012; 112: 1445–1453.

23. Charrin E, Aufradet E, Douillard A, et al. Oxidative stress is decreased in physically active sickle cell SAD mice. *Br J Haematol* 2015; 168(5): 747–756.

24. Faës C, Martin C, Chirico EN, et al. Effect of α-thalassaemia on exercise-induced oxidative stress in sickle cell trait. *Acta Physiol* (Oxf) 2012; 205(4): 541–550.

25. Vincent L, Feasson L, Oyono-Enguelle S, et al. Remodeling of skeletal muscle microvasculature in sickle cell trait and alphathalassemia. *Am J Physiol* 2010; 298(2): H375–H384.

26. Vincent L, Oyono-Enguéll S, Féasson L, et al. Effects of regular physical activity on skeletal muscle structural, energetic, and microvascular properties in carriers of sickle cell trait. *J Appl Physiol* 1985; 113: 549–556.

27. Akinbami A, Dosunmu A, Adediran A, et al. Haematological values in homozygous sickle cell disease in steady state and haemoglobin phenotypes AA controls in Lagos, Nigeria. *BMC Res Notes* 2012; 5: 396.

28. Charache S, Bleeker RR, Bross DS. Effects of blood transfusion exercise capacity in patients with sickle cell anaemia. *Am J Med* 1983; 74: 757–784.

29. Henderson RA, Saavedra JM, Dover GJ. Prevalence of impaired growth in children with homozygous sickle cell anemia. *Am J Med Sci* 1994; 307(6): 405–407.

30. Connes P, Machado R, Hue O, et al. Exercise limitation, exercise testing and exercise recommendations in sickle cell anemia. *Clin Hemorheol Microcirc* 2011; 49(1–4): 1561–1563.

31. Anie KA, Steptoe A. Pain, mood and opioid medication use in sickle cell disease. *Hematol J* 2003; 4(1): 71–73.

32. Artz N, Zhang J, Meltzer D. Physical and mental health in adults hospitalized with sickle cell disease: impact on resource use. *J Nat Med Assoc* 2009; 101: 139–144.

33. Adebayo RA, Balogun MO, Akinola NO, et al. The clinical, electrocardiographic and self-paced walking exercise features of Nigerians with sickle cell anaemia presenting at OAUTHC, Ile-Ife. *Nigerian J Med* 2002; 11(4): 170–176.

34. Barden EM, Zemel BD, Kawchak DA, et al. Total and resting energy expenditure in children with sickle cell disease. *J Pediatr* 2000; 136: 73–79.

35. Buchowski MS, Townsend KM, Williams R, et al. Patterns and energy expenditure of free-living physical activity in adolescents with sickle cell anemia. *J Pediatr* 2002; 140: 86–92.

36. Charlot K, Moeckesch B, Jumet S, et al. Physical activity level is not a determinant of autonomic nervous system activity and clinical severity in children/adolescents with sickle cell anemia: A pilot study. *Pediatr Blood Cancer* 2015; 62(11): 1962–1967.

37. Millis RM, Baker FW, Ertugrul L, et al. Physical performance decrements in children with sickle cell anaemia. *J Natl Med Assoc* 1994; 86: 113–116.

38. Dedeken L, Chapusette R, Lé PQ, et al. Reduction of the six-minute walk distance in children with sickle cell disease is correlated with silent infarct: results from a cross-sectional evaluation in a single center in Belgium. *PLoS One* 2014; 9(9): e108922.

39. Halphen I, Elie C, Brousse V, et al. Severe nocturnal and postexercise hypoxia in children and adolescents with sickle cell disease. *PLoS One* 2014; 9(5): e97462.
40. Hostyn SV, Carvalho WB, Johnston C, et al. Evaluation of functional capacity for exercise in children and adolescents with sickle-cell disease through the six-minute walk test. *J Pediatr* (Rio J) 2013; 89(6): 588–594.
41. Liem RI, Nevin MA, Prestridge A, et al. Functional capacity in children and young adults with sickle cell disease undergoing evaluation for cardiopulmonary disease. *Am J Hematol* 2009; 84: 645–649.
42. Ohara DG, Ruas G, Walsh IA, et al. Lung function and six-minute walk test performance in individuals with sickle cell disease. *Braz J Phys Ther* 2014; 18(1): 79–87.
43. Waltz X, Romana M, Hardy-Dessources M-D, et al. Hematological and hemorheological determinants of the six-minute walk test performance in children with sickle cell anemia. *PLoS One* 2013; 8(10): e77830.
44. van Beers EJ, van der Plas MN, Nur E, et al. Exercise tolerance, lung function abnormalities, anemia, and cardiothoracic ratio in sickle cell patients. *Am J Hematol* 2014; 89(8): 819–824.
45. Moheeb H, Wali YA, El-Sayed MS. Physical fitness indices and anthropometric profiles in schoolchildren with sickle cell trait/disease. *Am J Hematol* 2007; 82: 91–97.
46. Liem RI, Reddy M, Pelligra SA, et al. Reduced fitness and abnormal cardiopulmonary responses too maximal exercise testing in children and young adults with sickle cell anemia. *Physiol Rep* 2015; 3(4): e12338.
47. Connes P, Sara F, Dominique M, et al. Effects of short supramaximal exercise on hemorheology in sickle cell trait carriers. *Eur J Appl Physiol* 2006; 97: 143–150.
48. Anzalone ML, Green VL, Buja M, et al. Sickle cell trait and fatal rhabdomyolysis in football training: a case study. *Med Sci Sports Exerc* 2010; 42: 3–7.
49. Mozzarelli A, Hofrichter J, Eaton WA. Delay time of hemoglobin S polymerization prevents most cells from sickling in vivo. *Science* 1987; 237: 500–506.
50. Marlin I, Etienne-Julan M, Le Gallais D, et al. Sickle cell trait in French West-Indian sprint athletes. *Int J Sports Med* 2005; 26: 622–625.
51. Bilé A, Le Gallais D, Mercier J, et al. Sickle cell trait in Ivory Coast athletic throw and jump champions, 1956–1995. *Int J Sports Med* 1998; 19: 215–219.
52. Le Gallais D, Lonsdorfer J, Bogui P, et al. Point: Sickle cell trait should be considered asymptomatic and as a benign condition during physical activity. *J Appl Physiol* 2007; 103: 2137–2141.
53. Le Gallais D, Préfaut C, Mercier J, et al. Sickle cell trait as a limiting factor for high-level performance in a semi-marathon. *Int J Sports Med* 1994; 15: 399–402.
54. Robinson JR, Stone WJ, Asendorf AC. Exercise capacity of black sickle cell trait males. *Med Sci Sports* 1976; 8: 244–245.
55. Weisman IM, Zeballos RJ, Martin TW, et al. Effects of army basic training in sickle cell trait. *Arch Intern Med* 1987; 317: 781–787.
56. Connes P, Monchanin G, Perrey S, et al. Oxygen uptake kinetics during heavy submaximal xercise: Effect of sickle cell trait with or without alpha-thalassemia. *Int J Sports Med* 2005; 27(7): 517–525.
57. Shasky DJ, Green GA. Sports haematology. *Sports Med* 2000; 29(1): 27–38.
58. Marlin L, Connes P, Antoine-Jonville A, et al. Cardiorespiratory responses during three repeated incremental exercise tests in sickle cell trait carriers. *Eur J Appl Physiol* 2008; 102: 181–187.

59. Sara F, Hardy-Dessources M-D, Marlin L, et al. Lactate distribution in the blood compartments of sickle cell carriers during incremental exercise and recovery. *Int J Sports Med* 2006; 27: 436–443.

60. Sara F, Connes P, Hue O, et al. Faster lactate transport across red blood cell membrane in sickle cell trait carriers. *J Appl Physiol* 2006; 100: 427–432.

61. Oyono-Enguéll S, Le Gallais D, Lonsdorfer A, et al. Cardiorespiratory and metabolic responses to exercise in HbSC sickle cell patients. *Med Sci Sports Exerc* 2000; 32(4): 725–731.

62. Hedreville M, Charlot K, Waltz X, et al. Acute moderate exercise does not further alter the autonomic nervous system activity in patients with sickle cell anaemia. *PLoS One* 2014; 9(4): e95563.

63. Connes P, Racinais S, Sara F, et al. Does the pattern of repeated sprint ability differ between sickle cell trait carriers and healthy subjects? *Int J Sports Med* 2006; 27: 937–942.

64. Hue O, Julan ME, Blonc S, et al. Alactic anaerobic performance in subjects with sickle cell trait and hemoglobin AA. *Int J Sports Med* 2002; 23: 174–177.

65. Bilé A, Le Gallais D, Mercier B, et al. Anaerobic exercise components during the force-velocity test in sickle cell trait. *Int J Sports Med* 1996; 17(4): 254–258.

66. Hédreville M, Barthélemy J-C, Tripette J, et al. Effects of strenuous exercise on autonomic nervous system activity in sickle cell trait carriers. *Auton Neurosci Basic Clin* 2008; 143: 68–72.

67. Kark JA, Ward FT. Exercise and hemoglobin S. *Sem Hematol* 1994; 31(3): 181–225.

68. Murphy JR. Sickle cell hemoglobin (Hb AS) in black football players. *JAMA* 1973; 225(8): 981–982.

69. Goldsmith JC, Bonham VL, Joiner CH, et al. Framing the research agenda for sickle cell trait: building on thecurrent understanding of clinical events and their potential implications. *Am J Hematol* 2012; 87(3): 340–346.

70. Harris KM, Haas TS, Eichner ER, et al. Sickle cell trait associated with sudden death in competitive athletes. *Am J Cardiol* 2012; 110: 1185–1188.

71. Mitchell BL. Sickle cell trait and sudden death: bringing it home. *J Nat Med Assoc* 2007; 99(3): 300–305.

72. Marlin I, Sara F, Antoine-Jonville S, et al. Ventilatory and lactic thresholds in subjects with sickle cell trait. *Int J Sports Med* 2007; 28: 916–920.

73. Baskurt OG, Meiselan HJ. Point/counterpoint: comments. *J Appl Physiol* 2007; 103: 2412.

74. Boucher JH. Point/counterpoint: comments. *J Appl Physiol* 2008; 104: 1242.

75. Bonham VL, Dover GJ, Brody LC. Screening student athletes for sickle cell trait: a social and clinical experiment. *N Engl J Med* 2010; 363(11): 997–999.

76. Ashcroft MT, Desai P. Mortality and morbidity in Jamaican adults with sickle cell trait and with normal haemoglobin followed up for twelve years. *Lancet* 1976; (ii): 784–786.

77. Heller P, Best WR, Nelson RB, et al. Clinical implications of sickle-cell trait and glucose-6- phosphate dehydrogenase deficiency in hospitalized black male patients. *N Engl J Med* 1979; 300: 1001–1005.

78. Gima AS, Bemis EL. Absence of major illnesses in sickle cell trait: results from a controlled study. *J Nat Med Assoc* 1975; 67: 216–219.

79. Connes P, Hue O, Tripette J, et al. Blood rheology abnormalities and vascular cell adhesion mechanisms in sickle cell trait carriers during exercise. *Clin Hemorheol Microcirc* 2008; 39: 179–184.

80. Bergeron MF. Point/counterpoint: comments. *J Appl Physiol* 2007; 193: 2142.
81. Tsaras G, Owusu-Ansah A, Boateng FO, et al. Complications associated with sickle cell trait: a brief narrative review. *Am J Med* 2009; 122: 507–512.
82. Eichner ER. Sickle cell trait in sports. *Curr Sports Med Rep* 2010; 9(6): 347–351.
83. Funakowshi H, Takada T, Miyahara M, et al. Sickle cell trait as a cause of splenic infarction while climbing Mt. Fuji. *Intern Med* 2010; 49: 1827–1829.
84. Abeysekera WYM, de Silva WDD, Pinnaduwa SS, et al. Acute massive splenic infarction with splenic vein thrombosis following altitude exposure of a Sri Lankan male with undetected sickle cell trait. *High Alt Med Biol* 2012; 13(4): 288–290.
85. Gupta M, Lehl SS, Singh K, et al. Acute splenic infarction in a hiker with previously unrecognised sickle cell trait. *Br Med J Case Rep* 2013; doi:101136/bcr-2013-008931.
86. Martin TW, Weisman IM, Zeballos RJ, et al. Exercise and hypoxia increase sickling in venous blood from an exercising limb in individuals with sickle cell trait. *Am J Med* 1989; 87(1): 48–56.
87. Sheikha A. Splenic syndrome in patients at high altitude with unrecognized sickle cell trait: splenectomy is often unnecessary. *Can J Surg* 2005; 48: 377–381.
88. Ouyang DL, Kohrt HE, Gurza D, et al. Massive splenic infarct in a collegiate football player with hemoglobin SC disease. *Clin J Sports Med* 2008; 18: 89–91.
89. Gitlin SD, Thompson CB. Non-altitude-related splenic infarction in a patient with sickle cell trait. *Am J Med* 1989; 87: 697–698.
90. Connes P. Hemorheology and exercise: effects of warm environments and potential consequences for sickle cell trait carriers. *Scand J Med Sci Sports* 2010; 20(3 Suppl.): S48–S52.
91. Hedreville M, Connes P, Romana M, et al. Central retinal vein occlusion in a sickle cell trait carrier after a cycling race. *Med Sci Sports Exerc* 2009; 41(1): 14–18.
92. Kark JA, Posey DM, Schumacher HR, et al. Sickle cell trait as a risk factor for sudden death in physical training. *N Engl J Med* 1987; 317(13): 781–787.
93. Bergeron MF, Cannon JG, Hall EL, et al. Erythrocyte sickling during exercise and thermal stress. *Clin J Sports Med* 2004; 14(6): 354–356.
94. Aufradet E, Monchanin G, Oyonno-Engelle S, et al. Habitual physical activity and endothelial activation in sickle cell trait carriers. *Med Sci Sports Exerc* 2010; 42(11): 1987–1994.
95. Eichner ER. Sickle cell considerations in athletes. *Clin Sports Med* 2011; 30(3): 537–549.
96. Owusu-Ofuri S, Hirst C. Splenectomy versus conservative management for acute sequestration crises in people with sickle cell disease. Cochrane database 2002; *Syst Rev* 4: CD003425.
97. Green RL, Huntsman RG, Serjeant JR. Sickle cell and altitude. *BMJ* 1971; 4(5787): 593–595.
98. Norii T, Freeman TH, Alseidi A, et al. Pressurized flight immediately after splenic infarction in two patients with the sickle cell trait. *Aviat Space Environ Med* 2011; 82: 58–60.
99. Soni SN, McDonald E, Marino C. Rhabdomyolysis after exercise. *Postgrad Med J* 1993; 94: 128–132.
100. Shelmadine BD, Baltensperger A, Wilson RL, et al. Rhabdomyolysis and acute renal failure in a sickle cell trait athlete: a case study. *Clin J Sports Med* 2013; 23: 235–237.
101. Harrelson GL, Fincher AL, Robinson JB. Acute exertional rhabdomyolysis and its relationship to sickle cell trait. *J Athl Train* 1995; 30(4): 309–312.

102. Makaryus JN, Catanzaro JN, Katona KC. Exertional rhabdomyolysis and renal failure in patients with sickle celltrait: Is it time to change our approach? Hematology. *Am Soc Hematol Educ Prog* 2007; 12(4): 349–352.

103. Gardner JW, Kark A. Fatal rhabdomyolysis presenting as mild heat illness in military training. *Mil Med* 1994; 159(2): 160–163.

104. Van Camp SP, Bloor CM, Mueller FO, et al. Nontraumatic sports death in high school and college athletes. *Med Sci Sports Exerc* 1995; 27(5): 641–647.

105. Sherry P. Sickle cell trait and rhabdomyolysis: case report and review of the literature. *Mil Med* 1990; 155: 59–61.

106. Way A, Ganesan S, McErlain M. Multiple limb compartment syndromes in a recruit with sickle cell trait. *J R Army Med Corps* 2011; 157(2): 182–183.

107. Dincer HE. Compartment syndrome and fatal rhabdomyolysis in sickle cell trait. *Wisc Med J* 2005; 10(6): 67–71.

108. Jones SR, Binder RA, Donowho EM. Sudden death and sickle-cell trait. *N Engl J Med* 1970; 282: 323–325.

109. Koppes GM, Daly JJ, Coltman CA, et al. Exertion-induced rhabdomyoplysis with acute renal failure and disseminated intravascular coagulation in sickle cell trait. *Am J Med* 1977; 63: 313–317.

110. Deuster PA, Contreras-Sesvold CL, O'Connor FG, et al. Genetic polymorphisms associated with exertional rhabdomyolysis. *Eur J Appl Physiol* 2013; 113: 1997–2004.

111. Wirthwein DP, Spotswood SD, Barnard JJ, et al. Death due to microvascular occlusion in sickle-cell trait following physical exertion. *J Forensic Sci* 2001; 46(2): 399–401.

112. Dudley AW, Waddell CC. Crisis in sickle cell trait. *Hum Pathol* 1991; 22(6): 616–618.

113. Ham TH, Dunn RF, Sayre RW. Physical properties of red cells as related to effects in vivo I. Increased rigidity of erythrocytes as measured by viscosity of cells altered by chemical fixation, sickling and hypertonicity. *Blood* 1968; 32: 847–861.

114. Gordeuk VR, Minniti CP, Nouraie M, et al. Elevated tricuspid regurgitation velocity and decline in exercise capacity over 22 months of follow up in children and adolescents with sickle cell anemia. *Haematologia* 2011; 96(1): 33–40.

115. Gladwin MT, Barst TJ, Gibbs JS, et al. Risk factors for death in 632 patients with sickle cell disease in the United States and United Kingdom. *PLoS One* 2014; 9(7): e99489.

116. Ataga KI, Orringer EP. Renal abnormalities in sickle cell disease. *Am J Hematol* 2000; 63: 205–211.

117. Diggs LW. The sickle cell trait in relation to the training and assignment of duties in the armed forces: III. Hyposthenuria, hematuria, sudden death, rhabdomyolysis, and acute tubular necrosis. *Aviat Space Environ Med* 1984; 55(5): 358–364.

118. Drehner D, Neuhauser KM, Neuhauser TS, et al. Death among basic US Air Force trainess, 1956 to 1996. *Mil Med* 1999; 12: 841–847.

119. Eichner ER. Hematuria: a diagnostic challenge. *Phys Sportsmed* 1990; 18(11): 53–63.

120. Kiryluk K, Jadoon A, Gupta M. Sickle cell trait and gross hematuria. *Kidney Internat* 2007; 71(7): 706–710.

121. Ajayi AA. Should the sickle cell trait be reclassified as a disease state? *J Intern Med* 2005; 18: 463.

122. Gold JI, Johnson CB, Treadwell MJ, et al. Detection and assessment of stroke in patients with sickle cell disease: Neuropsychological functioning and magnetic resonance imaging. *Pediatr Hematol Oncol* 2008; 25: 409–421.

123. Helzlsouer KJ, Hayden FG, Rogol AD. Severe metabolic complications in a cross-country runner with sickle cell trait. *JAMA* 1983; 249(6): 777–779.
124. Austin H, Key NS, Benson JM, et al. Sickle cell trait and the risk of venous thromboembolism among blacks. *Blood* 2007; 110(3): 908–912.
125. Hedreville M, Connes P, Romana M, et al. Central retinal vein occlusion in a sickle cell trait carrier after a cycling race. *Med Sci Sports Exerc* 2009; 41(1): 13–17.
126. Connes P, Martin C, Barthelemy JC, et al. Nocturnal autonomic nervous system activity impairment in sickle cell trait carriers. *Clin Physiol Funct Imaging* 2006; 26: 87–91.
127. Le Gallais D. Comment on Point/Counterpoint: Sickle cell trait should/should not be considered asymptomatic and as a benign condition during physical activity. *J Appl Physiol* 2009; 106: 349.
128. Dommergues J-P, Gimeno L, Galacteros F. Un pédiatre à l'écoute de jeunes adultes drépanocytaires. [A pediatrician listening to young adults affected with sickle cell disease.] *Arch Pédiatr* 2007; 14: 1115–1118.
129. Castro O, Hoque M, Brown BD. Pulmonary hypertension in sickle cell disease: cardiac catheterization results and survival. *Blood* 2003; 101: 1257–1261.
130. Key NS, Derebail VK. Sickle cell trait: novel clinical significance. *Hematology Am Soc Hematol Educ Prog* 2010; 1: 418–422.
131. Hoiberg A, Ernst J, Uddin DE. Sickle cell trait and glucose-6-phosphate dehydrogenase. Effects on health and military performance in black navy enlistees. *Arch Int Med* 1981; 141: 1485–1488.
132. Stark AD, Janerich DT, Jereb SK. Follow-up study of individuals with haemoglobin AS and AA. *Int J Epidemiol* 1980; 9: 325–328.
133. Maron BJ. Sickle cell trait and sudden death in athletes: reply. *JAMA* 1996; 276(18): 1472.
134. Eckart RE, Scoville SL, Campbell CL, et al. Sudden deaths in young adults: A 25-year review of autopsies in military recruits. *Ann Int Med* 2004; 141(11): 829–834.
135. Scoville SL, Gardner JW, Magill AJ, et al. Nontraumatic deaths during US armed forces basic training, 1977–2001. *Am J Prev Med* 2004; 26(3): 205–212.
136. Harmon KG, Drezner JA, Klossner D, et al. Sickle cell trait associated with a RR of death of 37 times in national collegiate athletic association football athletes: a database with 2 million athlete-years as the denominator. *Br J Sports Med* 2012; 46: 325–330.
137. Eichner ER. Preventing exertional sickling the right way, the wrong way and the army way. *Curr Sports Med Rep* 2013; 12(6): 352–353.
138. Sambuughin N, Capacchione J, Blokhin A, et al. The ryanodine receptor type 1 gene variants in African American men with exertional rhabdomyolysis and malignant hyperthermia susceptibility. *Clin Genetics* 2009; 76: 564–568.
139. Burke A, Creighton W, Mont E, et al. Role of SCN5A Y1102 polymorphism in sudden cardiac death in blacks. *Circulation* 2005; 112: 798–802.
140. Stovitz SD, Shrier I. Sickle cell trait, exertion-related death and confounded estimates. *Br J Sports Med* 2014; 48: 285–286.
141. Sharan K, Surrey S, Ballas S, et al. Association of T-786C eNOS gene polymorphism with increased susceptibility to acute chest syndrome in females with sickle cell disease. *Br J Haematol* 2004; 124: 240–243.
142. Pauling L, Itano HA, Singer SJ, et al. Sickle cell anemia, a molecular disease. *Science* 1949; 110: 543–548.

143. Aluoch JR. The presence of sickle cells in the peripheral blood film. Specificity and sensitivity of diagnosis of homozygous sickle cell disease in Kenya. *Trop Geogr Med* 1995; 47(2): 89–91.

144. Hicks EJ, Griep JA, Nordschow CD. Comparison of results for three methods of hemoglobin S identification. *Clin Chem* 1973; 19(5): 533–535.

145. US Preventive Services Task F. Screening for sickle cell disease in newborns. Recommendation statement. *Am Fam Phys* 2008; 77(9): 1300–1302.

146. Ducrocq RP, Pascaud O, Bevier A, et al. Strategy linking several analytical methods of neonatal screening for sickle cell disease. *J Med Screen* 2001; 8: 8–14.

147. Eastman DW, Wong R, Liao CL, et al. Automated HPLC screening of newborns for sickle cell anemia and other hemoglobinopathies. *Clin Chem* 1996; 42(5): 704–710.

148. Boden BP, Breit, I, Beachler JA, et al. Fatalities in high school and college football players. *Am J Sports Med* 2013; 41: 1108–1116.

149. Faës C, Balayssac-Siransy E, Connes P, et al. Moderate endurance exercise in patients with sickle cell anaemia: effects on oxidative stress and endothelial activation. *Br J Haematol* 2014; 164(1): 124–130.

150. Diaw M, Diop M, Mbengue A, et al. Évaluation de la déformabilité érythrocytaire des sujets porteurs de trait drépanocytaire au cours d'un match de football: effet de l'hydratation ad libitum [Evaluation of erythrocyte deformability in subjects with sickle cell trait during a soccer game: effect of hydration ad libitum]. *Bull Soc Pathol Exot* 2013; 106: 95–99.

151. Diaw M, Samb A, Diop S, et al. Effects of hydration and water deprivation on blood viscosity during a soccer game in sickle cell trait carriers. *Br J Sports Med* 2014; 48(4): 326–331.

152. Inter-Association Task F. The Inter-Association task force for preventing sudden death in secondary school athletics programs: best-practice recommendations. *J Athl Train* 2013; 48(4): 546–553.

153. Kark JA, Martin SK, Canik JJ, et al. Sickle cell trait as an age-dependent risk factor for sudden death in basic training. *Ann NY Acad Sci* 1989; 565: 407–408.

154. Martyres DJ, Vijenthira A, Barrowman N, et al. Nutrient insufficiencies/deficiencies in children with sickle cell disease and its association with disease severity. *Pediatr Blood Cancer* 2016; 63(6): 1060–1064.

155. Osunkwo I, Ziegler TR, Alvarez J, et al. High dose vitamin D therapy for chronic pain in children and adolescents with sickle cell disease: results of a randomized double blind pilot study. *Br J Haematol* 2012; 159(2): 211–215.

156. Thornburg CD, Calatroni A, Panepinto JA. Differences in health-related quality of life in children with sickle cell disease receiving hydroxyurea. *J Pediatr Hematol Oncol* 2011; 33(4): 251–254.

157. Wali YA, Moheeb H. Effect of hydroxyurea on physical fitness indices in children with sickle cell anemia. *Pediatr Hematol Oncol* 2010; 28(1): 43–50.

158. Kuypers FA, Marsh AM. Research in athletes with sickle cell trait: just do it. *J Appl Physiol* 2012; 112: 1433.

159. Tripette J, Hardy-Dessources M-D, Romana M, et al. Exercise-related complications in sickle cell trait. *Clin Hemorheol Microcirc* 2013; 55: 29–37.

160. Abkowitz JL, O'Connor FG, Deuster PA, et al. Sickle cell trait and safe athletic participation: the way forward. *Curr Sports Med Rep* 2014; 13(3): 192–193.

161. Aloe A, Krishnamurti K, Kladny B. Testing of collegiate athletes for sickle cell trait: what we, as geneticcounselors, should know. *J Genet Couns* 2011; 20: 337–340.

162. National Collegiate Athletic Association. Protocol decided for sickle cell testing. Online www.ncaa.org/health-and-safety/medical-conditions/sickle-cell-trait. Accessed 27 June 2015.

163. Secretary's Advisory Committee H. Screening US College athletes for their sickle cell disease carrier status. Online www.hrsa.gov/advisorycommittees/mchb advisory/heritabledisorders/recommendations/correspondence/briefingcarrier-status.pdf. 2010. Accessed 8 August 2016.

164. O'Connor TE, Skinner IJ, Kiely P, et al. Return to contact sports following infectious mononucleosis: the role of serial ultrasonography. *Ear, Nose Throat J* 2011; 90(8): E21–E24.

165. National Athletic Trainers Association. Consensus statement: sickle cell trait and the athlete. Paper presented at the Annual Meeting of the National Athletic Trainers' Association; 27 June 2007, Anaheim, CA.

166. Jung AP, Selmon PB, Lett J, et al. Survey of sickle cell trait screening in NCAA and NAIA institutions. *Phys Sportsmed* 2011; 39(1): 58–65.

167. Johnson LN. Sickle cell trait: an update. *J Nat Med Assoc* 1982; 74(8): 751–787.

168. Rutkow IM, Lipton JM. Some negative aspects of state health departments' policies related to screening for sickle cell anemia. *Am J Publ Health* 1974; 64: 217–221.

169. Thompson AA. Sickle cell trait testing and athletic participation: a solution in search of a problem? *Hematology Am Soc Hematol Educ Prog* 2013; 2013: 632–637.

170. Brodine CE, Uddin DE. Medical aspects of sickle hemoglobin in military personnel. *J Nat Med Assoc* 1977; 69(1): 29–32.

171. Vigilante JA, DiGeorge NW. Sickle cell trait and diving: review and recommendations. *Undersea Hyperbar Med* 2014; 41(3): 223–228.

172. Tarini BA, Brooks MA, Bundy DG. A policy impact analysis of the mandaory NCAA sickle cell trait screening program. *Health Services Res* 2012; 47(1)Part II: 448–461.

173. Acharya K, Benjamin HJ, Clayton EW, et al. Attitudes and beliefs of sports medicine providers to sickle cell trait screening of student athletes. *Clin J Sports Med* 2011; 21: 480–485.

174. Koopmans J, Cox LA, Benjamin H, et al. Sickle cell trait screening in athletes: pediatricians' attitudes and concerns. *Pediatrics* 2011; 128: 477–483.

10 Physical activity, benign prostate hyperplasia and prostatitis

Introduction

Physical activity is associated with a clinically useful reduction in the risk of benign prostatic hyperplasia. It is also of interest as a potential palliative treatment in chronic prostatitis.

Benign prostatic hyperplasia is a non-cancerous enlargement of the prostate gland. There is an increased growth of both glandular epithelial cells and stromal cells, with the formation of distinct nodules. As the nodules become larger, they impinge on the urethra, increasing resistance to emptying of the bladder, and the condition is no longer benign due to an augmented risk of urinary and prostate infections. Hyperplasia of the prostate can begin at an age as early as 30 years; 50% of men show some prostatic enlargement by the age of 50 years, and 75% by the age of 80 years.[1] About a half of those affected note significant urinary problems and a quarter require surgical treatment. Because of inflammation and/or an increase in size of the prostate, serum levels of prostate specific antigen may rise, but not to the levels considered diagnostic of prostatic cancer.

The influence of habitual physical activity upon benign prostatic hyperplasia has attracted less attention than its possible role in the prevention of prostate carcinoma (Chapter 11). Nevertheless, a growing number of studies of suggest a reduction of risk with either occupational or leisure activity, possibly because of associated changes in growth hormone levels (Table 10.1). In studying the effects of physical activity, evidence of prostate hypertrophy has been sought in the onset of lower urinary tract symptoms, a need for prostatic surgery, a combination of increased prostate weight, symptoms and a reduced urinary flow rate or the reaching of specific scores on standardized prostate symptom questionnaires.

Occupational activity and prostate hyperplasia

Three investigations have examined the risk of benign prostatic hyperplasia in relation to occupational activity; one found an advantageous trend and the other two a significant reduction of risk for those engaged in heavy, physically demanding employment.

Lacey et al.[2] compared 206 men with prostatic hyperplasia requiring surgery and 471 age-matched controls. All were classified by occupational titles. After co-varying for age, marital status, education, body mass index, energy intake and waist/hip ratio, there was a trend to reduced risk favouring those who were involved in heavy work at age 40–49 years (odds ratio 0.6 [0.4–0.87]), but no benefit was seen with heavy work at 20–29 years of age (odds ratio 1.1, not statistically significant).

Dal Maso et al.[3] studied 1369 histologically confirmed cases of benign prostatic hyperplasia and 1451 hospital controls. After controlling data for age, study centre and the subject's level of education, a multivariate analysis compared risks between individuals with heavy/strenuous and light occupations. At ages 15–19 and 30–39 years, the odds ratios of 0.6 (0.4–0.8) significantly favoured physically active workers, and at age 50–59 years the odds were still 0.7 (0.5–0.9). Lagiou et al.[4] compared 184 surgically treated cases of benign prostatic hyperplasia with 246 hospital controls. A blinded assessment of the physical demands of occupation was made for each participant. After allowing for the effects of age and educational attainment, the odds ratio for those engaged in heavy work was 0.59, with a significant inverse trend of risk (p = 0.04).

Recreational activity and prostate hyperplasia

Thirteen investigations have related recreational activity to the risk of benign prostate hyperplasia. One report found an adverse effect of physical activity, and two gave inconsistent results, but the remaining ten reports pointed to a beneficial outcome, statistically significant in seven of the ten trials.

Lacey et al.[2] compared 206 men requiring surgery for benign prostatic hyperplasia with 471 age-matched controls. After allowing for age, marital status, educational attainment, body mass index, energy intake and waist/hip ratio, the two groups were compared in terms of the volume of moderate, vigorous and all physical activity (MET-h/wk). This analysis may have been compromised by co-varying the data for reported energy intake. The results pointed to a significant *adverse* effect of physical activity at age 20–29 years (odds ratios 1.6 and 1.9 [p = 0.01]), but physical activity at age 40–49 years had no significant effect upon risk (odds ratios 1.4, 1.3).

Hong et al.[5] completed a cross-sectional study of men aged 50–79 years. Three frequencies of physical activity were identified (less than twice per week, three to five times per week and nearly every day). After co-varying the data for age, chronic bronchitis, prostate serum antigen and alcohol consumption, physical activity showed no consistent association with benign prostatic hyperplasia, as defined by the International Prostate Symptom Score (IPSS), prostate volume or urinary flow rate (odds ratios of 1.0, 0.48 and 1.73, respectively). Kristal et al.[6] followed 5667 men for 7 years, to end-points of either surgical treatment or an IPSS score >14 on at least two items. After co-varying for age, ethnicity, smoking, diabetes mellitus and the initial IPSS score, physical activity was not associated with either the total IPPS score or with the incidence of severe cases requiring surgical attention.

Gann et al.[7] completed a case-control study on participants in the physicians' health study; 320 individuals who developed benign prostatic hyperplasia over 9 years were compared with 320 who did not. After co-varying data for diastolic blood pressure and alcohol consumption, there was a non-significant trend to a lower odds ratio in individuals active >5 times per week versus those who exercised rarely or never (odds ratio of 0.7 [0.32–1.51]). In this study, hyperplasia was unrelated to blood levels of testosterone, dihydrotestosterone or androstenedione, but there was a trend for increasing risk with oestradiol levels and a weak inverse trend linking risk to oestrone levels. Rohrman et al.[8] studied 1723 twin pairs, collecting information on those who developed moderate or severe urinary tract symptoms; after adjusting for age, smoking, alcohol consumption and zygosity, the odds ratio of moderate or severe urinary tract symptoms showed a suggestive but non-significant odds ratio favouring the more physically active of the twin pairs (0.60 [0.34–1.08]). Rohrman et al.[9] also compared 279 men with lower urinary tract symptoms versus 599 controls. After co-varying for age, ethnicity, waist circumference, smoking and alcohol consumption, the odds ratio of finding at least three components of the metabolic syndrome in those with symptoms of benign prostatic hyperplasia was 1.80 (1.11–2.94); by implication, this group also tended to a low level of habitual physical activity.

Dal Maso et al.[3] compared those who took less than two hours of active recreation per week with those taking more than five hours per week. The odds ratios significantly favoured the more active individuals, with odds ratios of 0.5 (0.4–0.7) at age 15–19 years, 0.6 (0.5–0.8) at 30–39 years and 0.7 (0.5–0.8) at 50–59 years. Joseph et al.[10] used the IPSS to evaluate 708 African-American men. Introducing age, income, smoking, alcohol consumption, heart disease, hypertension and diabetes mellitus as co-variates, the odds ratio favoured those who engaged in sufficient vigorous physical activity to work up a sweat (0.61 [0.44–0.85]). Meigs et al.[11] followed 1709 men initially aged 40–70 years for 9 years, looking for the onset of symptoms or a need for lower urinary tract surgery. After controlling for age, marital status, waist/hip ratio, alcohol consumption, hypertension, heart disease and medication use, a comparison of the most active quartile (energy expenditure >3.6 MJ/day) with the least active (<0.5 MJ/day) yielded an odds ratio of 0.5 (0.3–0.9) for the more active individuals. Platz et al.[12] followed 30,364 health professionals for 8 years; during this time, 1890 underwent surgery for benign prostatic hyperplasia and 1853 developed severe urinary tract symptoms. Comparing the highest versus the lowest quintile of physical activity (>33.8 vs. <3.0 MET-h/wk), after co-varying for age, ethnicity, smoking and alcohol consumption, the odds ratio for those requiring surgery was 0.76 (0.64–0.90), and for those with severe lower urinary tract symptoms it was 0.79 (0.62–1.00). Prezioso et al.[13] questioned 1033 men; after allowing for age, body mass index, smoking and alcohol consumption, a high level of reported physical activity was associated with lower prostate volumes (p = 0.04) and a lower IPSS score (p = 0.008), with a diminished frequency of incomplete bladder

Table 10.1 Habitual physical activity and a reduced risk of benign prostatic hyperplasia

Author	Sample	Activity	Findings	Comments
Occupational activity				
Dal Maso et al.[3]	1369 histologically confirmed BPH, 1451 hospital controls	Occupation (heavy vs. light activity)	OR 0.6 (0.4–0.8) age 15–19 and 30–39, 0.7 (0.5–0.9) age 50–59 year	Data controlled for age, study centre and educational level
Lacey et al.[2]	206 men with BPH requiring surgery, 471 age-matched controls	Occupational titles, heavy vs. sedentary work	OR 1.1 age 20–29 (ns), 0.6 (0.4–0.87) age 40–49 yr	Age, marital status, education, BMI, energy intake, waist/hip ratio
Lagiou et al.[4]	184 surgically treated cases, 246 hospital controls	Blinded classification of occupations (high vs. low activity)	OR 0.59, p = 0.04 for trend	Age and educational level
Recreational activity				
Dal Maso et al.[3]	1369 histologically confirmed BPH cases, 1451 hospital controls	>5h/wk vs. <2 h/wk recreational activity	OR 0.5 (0.4–0.7) age 15–19, 0.6 (0.5–0.8) age 30–39, 0.7 (0.5–0.8) age 50–59	Data controlled for age, study centre and educational level
Gann et al.[7]	Participants in physicians' health study; 320 developing BPH over 9-yr follow-up, 320 controls	Exercise (>5 times/wk vs. rarely/never)	OR 0.7 (0.32–1.51)	Co-variates diastolic blood pressure and alcohol consumption
Hong et al.[5]	Cross-sectional study of 641 men aged 50–79. BPH defined by IPSS, prostate volume and bladder outflow rate	Exercise <2/wk, 3–5/wk, nearly every day	Inconsistent effect of exercise (OR 1.0, 0.48, 1.73 for 3 categories)	Co-variates age, chronic bronchitis, PSA, alcohol consumption
Joseph et al.[10]	708 African-American men, IPSS	Engaging in vigorous physical activity sufficient to work up a sweat	OR 0.61 (0.44–0.85)	Co-variates age, income, smoking, alcohol consumption, heart disease, hypertension and diabetes mellitus

Table 10.1 continued

Author	Sample	Activity	Findings	Comments
Kristal et al.[6]	5667 men followed for 7 yr, to treatment or IPSS score >14 on 2 items	Sedentary vs. highly active	No effect of physical activity on risk of total or severe BPH symptoms	Co-varied for age, ethnicity, smoking, diabetes mellitus, initial IPSS score
Lacey et al.[2]	206 men with BPH requiring surgery, 471 age-matched controls	Moderate or vigorous energy expenditure (MET-h/wk). All activity, high vs. sedentary	OR 1.6 age 20–29 (p = 0.01), 1.4 (ns) age 40–49; OR 1.9 age 20–29 (p = 0.01), 1.3 (ns) age 40–49	Age, marital status, educational level, BMI, energy intake, waist/hip ratio
Meigs et al.[11]	1709 men aged 40–70 followed for 9 yrs, to symptoms or surgery	Top vs. bottom quartile of physical activity, kJ/day	>3.6 vs. <0.6 kJ/day, OR 0.5 (0.3–0.9)	Age, marital status, waist/hip ratio, alcohol consumption, hypertension, heart disease, medication use
Platz et al.[12]	1890 men who underwent surgery, 1853 with symptoms (8-yr follow-up of 30,364 health professionals)	Highest vs. lowest quintile of physical activity (>33.8 vs. <3.0 MET-h/wk)	OR surgery 0.76 (0.64–0.90), severe symptoms 0.79 (0.62–1.00)	Age, ethnicity, smoking, alcohol consumption
Prezioso et al.[13]	Lower urinary tract symptoms in 1033 men	Reported physical activity	Physical activity associated with lower frequency of incomplete bladder emptying, repeated urination, intermittence and urgency	Age, BMI, smoking, alcohol consumption
Rohrman et al.[9]	279 men aged >60 with lower urinary tract symptoms vs. 599 controls	Men with at least 3 components of metabolic syndrome	OR 1.80 (1.11–2.94)	Age, ethnicity, waist circumference, smoking, alcohol consumption
Rohrman et al.[8]	1723 twin pairs with information on moderate/severe urinary tract symptoms	High vs. low physical activity score	OR 0.60 (0.34–1.08)	Age, smoking, alcohol consumption, zygosity

Table 10.1 continued

Author	Sample	Activity	Findings	Comments
Safarinejad[14]	Cross-sectional survey of 8466 men aged >40, noting prostate size, urine flow and IPSS	Reported physical activity	OR 0.4 (p = 0.01)	Multivariate adjusted
Williams[15]	28,612 runners followed for 7.7 yrs, with 1899 physician-reported cases	Distance run/ week, fastest 10 km time	OR ~0.64 in terms of distance and times	Age, diet, alcohol consumption, BMI (all non-smokers)

Notes: ns = non-significant; BMI = body mass index; BPH = benign prostate hyperplasia; IPSS = International Prostate Symptom Score; MET = metabolic equivalent; OR = odds ratio; PSA = prostate serum antigen.

emptying, repeated urination, intermittence and urgency. Safarinejad[14] completed a cross-sectional survey of 8466 Iranian men over the age of 40 years. Prostate size, urine flow and prostatic symptom score were inversely related to reported physical activity, with a multivariate adjusted odds ratio of 0.4 (p = 0.01). Williams[15] followed 28,612 non-smoking runners for an average of 7.7 years, accumulating 1899 physician-reported cases of benign prostatic hyperplasia. Physical activity levels were categorized in terms of distance run per week and the fastest 10 km times, and by both criteria, after adjusting for age, diet, alcohol consumption and body mass index, a significant odds ratio of ~0.64 favoured those who were the most deeply involved in distance running.

Conclusions regarding benign prostate hyperplasia

The data generally support the idea of benefit from habitual physical activity, with a significant decrease in the risk of benign prostatic hyperplasia in seven studies of recreational activity and two of occupational activity, and positive trends in three recreational and one occupational investigations, against only one study showing an adverse effect and two reports with inconsistent findings. Possibly, beneficial effects arise through a modulation of growth hormones, although such changes would require a substantial volume of endurance activity. Further research on possible mechanisms of benefit is needed as a guide to those planning exercise programmes. Although many authors have included a substantial number of co-variates in their analyses, there remains some possibility that the reported associations between physical activity and a low risk of benign prostatic hyperplasia could have been produced by associated unmeasured variables rather than by physical activity itself.

Physical activity and chronic prostatitis

Prostatitis is an inflammation of the prostate gland that occurs in a substantial proportion of older men. One review based on 10,617 subjects found a prevalence of 8.2%,[16] and others have set prevalence at 9 to 17%.[17] In 90–95% of cases, the prostatitis occurs without obvious bacterial cause. However, chronic prostatitis may result from urinary tract infections that have spread to the prostate gland. If a bacterial infection has developed, early treatment with intravenous antibiotics is required. There is often an enlarged prostate, a back-up of urine into the prostatic tissue, chemical irritation and/or problems with the nerve supply to the lower urinary tract.

Although chronic prostatitis is often treated by a prolonged course of anti-biotics, before embarking upon such an intervention it is important to determine the sensitivity of the micro-organisms involved, as they are often resistant to most antibiotics. Treatment may have only limited long-term success, leaving the patient with chronic pelvic pain, depression and a poor quality of life. Given the well-recognized ability of exercise to elevate mood state, there is interest in the symptomatic benefits that affected individuals can derive from increased habitual physical activity, even if the chronic prostatitis is not entirely remedied.

Giubilei et al.[18] recruited 231 men aged 20–50 years who had chronic prostat-itis and associated complaints of pelvic pain. A half of the group was assigned to an aerobic training programme (40 minutes of walking at 70–80% of maximal heart rate 3 times/week) and a half to a placebo stretching and motion program-me. At 16 weeks, those assigned to the aerobics programme had a more favourable score than the controls in terms of the National Institutes of Health prostatitis symptom index, quality of life and pain scores as assessed by a visual analogue. However, there are large placebo effects associated with most methods of treating prostatitis,[19] and the intensity and duration of effort used in this study seems rather low to have induced any substantial secretion of mood-elevating endorphins. Further studies are thus needed before the symptomatic benefits of aerobic activity can be asserted with confidence.

Areas for further research

Evidence suggesting a reduced risk of benign prostatic hyperplasia in physically active individuals is fairly consistent, but further research on mechanisms is needed. Many authors have included a substantial number of co-variates in their analyses, and there remains some possibility that the apparent benefits of an active lifestyle could have been produced by associated but unmeasured variables.

Given the lack of effective long-term treatments for chronic prostatitis, there is a need to repeat and expand the observations of Giubilei et al.[18] suggesting that aerobic exercise may offer an effective method of alleviating symptoms and to ascertain mechanisms. Is aerobic activity simply inducing a general elevation of mood state or is there some more fundamental basis for the enhanced quality of life among exercisers?

Practical implications and conclusions

There is growing evidence that regular physical activity is helpful in reducing the risk of benign prostatic hyperplasia, with its attendant complications. The mechanisms of benefit remain to be elucidated. However, there is little epidemiological evidence suggesting that moderate physical activity has any adverse effect upon the health of the prostate. Thus, the probable favourable impact of exercise upon the course of prostate hyperplasia seems yet one more reason to recommend regular physical activity to sedentary populations. The pelvic pain of chronic prostatitis can be a major cause of poor health, but the mood-elevating effects of prolonged endurance exercise could offer a helpful symptomatic treatment for this problem.

References

1. Verhamme K, Dieleman JP, Bleumink GS, et al. Incidence and prevention of lower urinary tract symptoms suggestive of benign prostatic hyperplasia in primary care: the Triumph project. *Eur Urol* 2002; 42(4): 323–328.
2. Lacey JV, Deng J, Dosemeci M, et al. Prostate cancer, benign prostate hyperplasia and physical activity in Shanghai, China. *Int J Epidemiol* 2001; 30: 341–349.
3. Dal Maso L, Zucchetto A, Tavani A, et al. Lifetime occupational and recreational physical activity and prostatic hyperplasia. *Int J Cancer* 2006; 118: 2632–2635.
4. Lagiou A, Samoli E, Georgila C, et al. Occupational physical activity in relation with prostate cancer and benign prostate hyperplasia. *Eur J Cancer Prev* 2008; 17: 336–339.
5. Hong J, Kwon D, Yoon H, et al. Risk factors for benign prostatic hyperplasia in South Korean men. *Urol Int* 2006; 76: 11–19.
6. Kristal AR, Arnold KB, Schenk JM, et al. Race/ethnicity, obesity, health-related behaviors and the risk of symptomatic benign prostatic hyperplasia: results from the prostate cancer prevention trial. *J Urol* 2007; 177: 1395–1400.
7. Gann PH, Hennekens CH, Longcope C, et al. A prospective study of plasma hormone levels, nonhormonal factors, and development of benign prostate hyperplasia. *Prostate* 1995; 26: 40–49.
8. Rohrman S, Fallin MD, Page WF, et al. Concordance rates and modifiable risk factors for lower urinary tract symptoms in twins. *Epidemiology* 2006; 17: 419–427.
9. Rohrman S, Smit E, Giovannucci E, et al. Association between markers of the metabolic syndrome and lower urinary tract symptoms in the Third National Health and Nutrition Examination Survey (NHANES III). *Int J Obesity* 2005; 29: 310–316.
10. Joseph MA, Harlow DD, Wei JT, et al. Risk factors for lower urinary tract symptoms in a population-based sample of African American men. *Am J Epidemiol* 2003; 157: 906–914.
11. Meigs JB, Mohr B, Barry MJ, Collins MM, et al. Risk factors for clinical benign prostatic hyperplasia in a community-based population of aging men. *J Clin Epidemiol* 2001; 54: 935–944.
12. Platz E, Kawachi I, Rimm EB, et al. Physical activity and benign prostatic hyperplasia. *Arch Intern Med* 1998; 158: 2349–2356.
13. Prezioso D, Catuogno C, Galassi P, et al. LIfestyle in patients with LUTS suggestive of BPH. *Eur Urol* 2001; 40(Suppl 1): 9–12.

14. Safarinejad MR. Prevalence of benign prostatic hyperplasia in a population-based study in Iranian men 40 years old or older. *Int Urol Nephrol* 2008; 40: 921–931.

15. Williams PT. Effects of running distance and performance on incident benign prostatic hyperplasia. *Med Sci Sports Exerc* 2008; 40(10): 1733–1739.

16. Krieger JN, Lee SWH, Jeon J, et al. Epidemiology of prostatitis. *Int J Antimicro-bAgents* 2008; 31(Suppl. 1): S85–S90.

17. Nickel JC, Downey J, Hunter D, et al. Prevalence of prostatitis-like symptoms in a population based study using the National Institutes of Health chronic prostatitis symptom index. *J Urol* 2001; 165(3): 842–845.

18. Giubelie G, Mondaini N, Minervi A, et al. Physical activity of men with chronic prostatitis/chronic pelvic pain syndrome not satisfied with conventional treatments: could it represent a valid option? The physical activity and male pelvic pain trial: a double-blind, randomized study. *J Urol* 2007; 177: 159–165.

19. Cohen JM, Fagin AP, Hariton E, et al. Therapeutic intervention for chronic prostatitis/chronic pelvic pain syndrome (CP/CPPS): a systemtaic review and meta-analysis. *PLoS One* 2012; 7(8): e41941.

11 Physical activity and prostate cancer

Introduction

This final chapter looks at the value of physical activity in the prevention and management of prostate cancer. Prostate cancer is second only to lung cancer as a cause of cancer morbidity and mortality in male patients. Known modifiable risk factors include the level of male hormones, diet, obesity, smoking, alcohol consumption, sexually transmitted diseases, vasectomy and occupational exposures to toxins such as cadmium and agricultural pesticides.[1] There is also growing evidence of a reduced risk of prostate cancer in physically active individuals. Potential beneficial actions of exercise could include the prevention of obesity, an increased natural killer cell count, a greater ability to counter oxidant stress and the reduction in testosterone levels that is frequently seen in endurance competitors.[2] Exercise programmes also play an important role in management following the successful treatment of prostate cancers by androgen deprivation therapy and/or surgery.

Role of physical activity in preventing prostate cancer

A systematic review[3] noted that early studies were retrospective; two reports found an association between heavy occupational work and the risk of prostate cancer, and a third report found an increased risk among those who had once been enrolled in university athletic teams. Between 1989 and 2001, 13 cohort studies used incident prostate cancer as the end-point. Of these, nine showed an association between exercise and a decreased risk of prostate cancer. Generally, these studies allowed for several important co-variates. Five of 11 case-control studies conducted between 1988 and 2002 also reported an association between high levels of physical activity and a decreased risk of prostatic cancer. In all, 16 of 27 studies through the year 2002 reported a 10–30% reduction of risk in the most active men, with a statistically significant benefit in 9 of the 16 analyses favouring the most active individuals. It was suggested that the inconsistency of trial outcomes reflected in part the weakness in physical activity assessments and in part issues in the diagnosis of prostatic cancer (such as reliance on increased levels of prostate-specific antigens rather than on a histological confirmation of clinically important disease). A further potential difficulty complicating occupational analyses is the association between heavy work and a lower socio-economic status, with less frequent medical examinations and thus a lesser likelihood of an early diagnosis of prostate cancer.[4]

Given the practical importance of containing prostate cancer, many further investigations have now looked at the preventive value of regular physical activity. Despite some duplication of reports, there have now been around 80 investigations. As with cancer in other parts of the body, associations have been sought with the physical demands of occupation, reported leisure activity (sometimes in the same population sample as in an occupational study), sport involvement and attained levels of physical fitness. This considerable volume of research encourages belief in the value of exercise, but we still lack incontrovertible proof of protection from a physically active lifestyle.

Occupational activity and risk of prostate cancer

In occupational analyses, a worker has typically maintained a relatively known level of physical activity at work for many years, including the period 10–30 years prior to diagnosis, when carcinogenesis is likely to have begun. The intensity of occupational effort has generally been moderate, but this activity has usually been maintained for four to five hours per day, thus accumulating a substantial total energy expenditure over the course of a working week. However, heavy physical employment has sometimes involved also exposure to industrial carcinogens. Moreover, there have often been large socio-economic differences between heavy and sedentary workers, influencing the employee's area of residence and issues of lifestyle such as diet, smoking habits and alcohol consumption. Some (but not all) investigations have attempted to allow for such confounding influences by covariance analysis. In recent years, mechanization and automation have reduced the energy costs of what were once physically demanding occupations, and this limits the possibility of future studies based upon the individual's job classification.

Retrospective and prospective cohort studies

There have been at least 19 cohort studies relating occupation to the risk of prostate cancer (Table 11.1). The findings are sometimes nuanced, with differing responses in sub-groups identified *post hoc*, but the conclusions from seven investigations have been essentially negative, six have identified a possible favourable tren, and six have demonstrated a significant reduction of risk of prostate cancer in the most active workers.

Among the seven negative reports, Paffenbarger et al.[5] followed 2665 longshoremen for 12 years, during which time 30 of the group developed a prostate cancer. Despite the small number of neoplasms, relative risks of carcinogenesis were classified in relation to four levels of work (heavy, moderate, light-to-moderate and light). Age-adjusted risk ratios showed no significant inter-

Table 11.1 Physical demands of occupation and the risk of developing prostate cancer

Author	Sample	Activity measure	Findings	Comments
Cohort studies				
Albanes et al.[11]	95 cases of PC in 5141 men over 10-yr follow-up	Very active vs. quite inactive	RR 1.3 if quite inactive (ns)	Age adjusted
Clarke & Whittemore [12]	5377 men followed for 17–21 yr, 201 cases of PC	Very active vs. inactive	RR for inactive 1.75 (1.12–2.67), p = 0.05 for trend (effect greater in African-Americans)	Adjusted for age, education, ethnicity and family history
Grotta et al.[13]	13,109 Swedish men followed for 13 yr, 904 cases of PC	Low vs. high level of occupational activity	HR 0.81 (0.61–1.07, ns)	Adjusted for age, education, smoking, BMI, alcohol consumption, diabetes mellitus
Hartman et al.[6]	29,133 men followed for up to 9 yr, 317 cases of PC	Sedentary vs. walkers vs. walkers/lifters vs. heavy labourers	RR 1.0, 0.6, 0.8, 1.2 (ns)	Adjusted for age, urban living, smoking, benign hyperplasia
Hrafnkelsdóttir et al.[14]	24-year follow-up of 8221 Icelandic men	Occupation involves mostly sitting vs. standing vs. on the move	HR 1.0, 0.97, 0.91 (0.79–1.06, ns)	Adjusted for age, height, BMI, diabetes, family history, education, medical check-ups
Hsing et al.[15]	264 cases of PC, occupational title	Sitting time (<2h/d vs. >6h/d), intensity of physical activity (<8, >12 kJ/min)	SIR 0.94 vs. 1.23, p = 0.14; SIR 1.23 vs. 0.92, p = 0.06	No co-variates
Johnsen et al.[7]	127,923 men followed for 8.5 yr; 2458 cases of PC	Sitting, standing or manual work; inactive, moderately inactive, moderately active, active	Occupational activity unrelated to PC	Adjusted for leisure activity, height, weight, marital status and education

Table 11.1 continued

Author	Sample	Activity measure	Findings	Comments
Lund-Nielsen et al.[8]	22,895 Norwegian men followed for 9.3 yr, with 644 cases of PC	High vs. low level of occupational activity	No effect on PC	Multivariate adjusted
Norman et al.[16]	3 cohorts of 43,836, 28,702 and 19,670 prostate cancers	Occupational titles (sedentary to very high level of activity)	RR for sedentary groups 1.11, 1.10 and 1.11 (p = 0.0001)	Adjusted for age, year of follow-up and area of residence
Orsini et al.[17]	45,887 men followed for 8 yr, 2735 incident cases of PC	4 categories of occupation (mostly sitting vs. heavy manual)	RR = 0.72 (0.57–0.90) p for trend 0.007; effects smaller for advanced and fatal cancers	Adjusted for leisure activity, age, smoking, alcohol consumption, education, diet, energy intake, waist/hip ratio, diabetes mellitus
Paffenbarger et al.[5]	2665 longshoremen followed for 12 yr, 30 cases of PC	Heavy, moderate, light-to-moderate, light work	Inconsistent RR (1.0, 0.14, 1.41, 1.54, ns)	Age adjusted, small number of cases
Parent et al.[18]	449 incident cases of PC	High vs. low lifetime occupational activity (METs)	OR 0.54 (0.31–0.95) favouring active work	
Putnam et al.[9]	101 cases of PC in 1572 initially cancer free men followed for 4 yr	Very active, moderately active or inactive at work	Risk of PC unrelated to occupational activity	Adjusted for age
Severson et al.[10]	8006 Japanese men on Oahu; 205 cases of PC	Self-estimate of job energy demands	Risk of PC unrelated to job activity	
Thune & Lund[19]	220 cases of PC in 53,242 Norwegians followed for 16.3 yr	4-level classification of work, sedentary to heavy manual	RR for heavy manual work 0.81 (0.50–1.30)	Age, BMI, geographic region of residence
Vena et al.[20]	430,000 men in Washington State, 8116 deaths from PC	4-level classification of occupational activity	PMR low = 109, high = 93 (p = 0.05)	

Table 11.1 continued

Author	Sample	Activity measure	Findings	Comments
Zeegers et al.[21]	58,279 men aged 55–69 yr, 1386 cases of PC over 9.3 yr	Occupational activity (energy expenditure, sitting time)	Unrelated to PC	Adjusted for age, alcohol consumption, BMI, energy intake, family history, education

Case-control studies

Author	Sample	Activity measure	Findings	Comments
Bairati et al.[22]	64 cases of PC, 5456 cases of benign prostate hyperplasia aged >45 yr	Ever had sedentary job or light work; 0, 1–49%, >50% of career spent in sedentary or light work	OR 2.0 (1.1–3.6); 1.0, 1.7, 2.8 (trend, p = 0.007)	Adjusted for age, education, total energy intake, smoking, use of vitamin supplements
Brownson et al.[23]	Missouri cancer registry, 2878 cases of PC, controls are cancers at other body sites	High vs. moderate vs. low occupational activity	OR 1.0, 1.1, 1.5 (1.2–1.8), p <0.01	Adjusted for age, smoking
Doolan et al.[24]	1436 cases of PC, 1349 matched controls	Finnish job matrix, physical workload tertiles	OR *highest* tertile 1.15 (0.95–1.40, ns)	Adjusted for age, family history, economic resources
Dosemeci et al.[25]	27 cases PC, 2127 hospital controls	<8 kJ/min vs. >12 kJ/min; active at work <2h/day vs. > 6h/day	OR 5.0 (1.1–31.7); OR 3.4 (1.1–10.6)	Adjusted for age and smoking; very small sample
Friedenreich et al.[26]	988 incident cases of PC, 1063 population controls	Energy expenditure <74.2 vs. >161.9 MET-h/ wk	OR 0.90, 0.60–1.22 (ns)	Adjusted for age, region, education, BMI, waist/hip ratio, energy intake, alcohol consumption, family and medical history

Table 11.1 continued

Author	Sample	Activity measure	Findings	Comments
Hosseini et al.[27]	137 cases of PC, 137 neighbourhood controls	Walking to work (<10 vs. >10 h/wk), intensity of work (inactive/ moderately active vs. highly active)	OR 0.7 (0.4–1.2) for longer walk (ns); OR = 6.7 (1.3–35.1) for highly active work (p = 0.02)	Multivariate adjusted
Krishnadasan et al.[28]	362 cases of PC, 1805 matched controls	Low vs. moderate vs. high occupational energy expenditure	OR 0.63 (0.40–1.00, p = 0.06 for trend)	Adjusted for matching variables, pay, trichlorethylene exposure
Lacey et al.[29]	258 cases of PC, 471 age-matched controls	Sedentary, moderate or high occupational energy expenditures at 20–29 yr, 40–49 yr or 12 yrs ago	RR 1.1 (0.7–1.7), 1.3 (0.8–1.9), 0.9 (0.5–1.8) favouring *sedentary* group	Adjusted for age, marital status, education, BMI, energy intake, waist/hip ratio
Lagiou et al.[30]	320 histologically confirmed PC, 246 hospital controls	Low, medium, high level of occupational activity	OR 0.69 (0.40–1.22, ns) for physically demanding occupation	Adjusted for age and education
Le Marchand et al.[31]	452 cases from Hawaii tumour registry, 899 population controls	Time spent in sedentary jobs (0–>54%)	No effect if <70 yrs; if >70 yrs, OR 0.6 (0.4–1.0, p for trend = 0.07)	Adjusted for age and ethnicity
Sass-Kortak et al.[32]	760 PC cases, 1632 telephone controls	Quartiles of lifetime occupational activity	OR 1.33 for active workers (1.02–1.74) p for trend = 0.18	Adjusted for age, family history, sunlight exposure
Strom et al.[33]	176 cases of PC in Mexican-Americans, 176 controls	None/low vs. moderate/ high energy demands of work	Reduced risk in active (OR 0.46, 0.28–0.77, p = 0.003)	Adjusted for age, education, screening, exposure to agricultural chemicals

Table 11.1 continued

Author	Sample	Activity measure	Findings	Comments
Villeneuve et al.[34]	1623 histologically confirmed cases of PC, 1623 controls	4-level classification of work (sitting to strenuous)	Significant benefit from activity in teens or early 20s (OR 0.6, 0.4–0.9), ns 30s, 50s or 2 yr before interview	Adjusted for age, area of residence, smoking, alcohol consumption, BMI, diet, income, family history
Wiklund et al.[35]	1449 incident cases of PC, 1118 population controls	MET-h/day of lifetime occupational activity, <11.8 to >19.8	OR 0.84 (0.61–1.15), ns; trend to benefit from active employment	Adjusted for age, region, education, BMI, alcohol consumption, family history, diabetes mellitus, energy intake

Notes: ns = not significant; HR = hazard ratio; PC = prostate cancer; OR = odds ratio; PMR = proportionate mortality ratio; RR = relative risk or rate ratio; SIR = standardized incidence ratio

category trend (1.0, 0.14, 1.41, 1.54, ns). Hartman et al.[6] observed 29,133 men for up to 9 years. There were 317 incident cases of prostate cancer in their study. Risk was contrasted between those who were employed in sedentary occupations and those whose jobs required walking, combinations of walking and lifting, or heavy labour. After adjusting data for age, urban living, smoking and a history of benign prostatic hyperplasia, the relative risk of prostate cancer showed no association with the physical demands of work (respective risk ratios of 1.0, 0.6, 0.8 and 1.2). Johnsen et al.[7] followed 127,923 men for an average of 8.5 years, accumulating 2458 cases of prostate cancer. Data were controlled for leisure activity, height, body mass, marital status and educational attainment. The individual's occupational activity (whether classed as sitting, standing or manual work, or as inactive, moderately inactive, moderately active and active) bore no relationship to the risk of prostate cancer, although *advanced* prostate cancer was seen less frequently in those with a high level of occupational activity (p = 0.024). Lund-Nielsen et al.[8] observed 22,895 Norwegian men for 9.3 years, finding 644 incident cases of prostate cancer. Occupational activity was classed as high or low, and after adjustment for co-variates, there was no association between energy expenditures at work and prostate cancer. Putnam et al.[9] found 101 cases of prostate cancer in a sample of 1572 initially cancer-free men who were followed for 4 years. In this study, employment was classified as very active, moderately active or inactive, but after controlling for age, the incidence of prostate cancer was unrelated to the energy demands of work. Severson et al.[10] questioned 8006 Japanese men living on the island of Oahu, Hawaii; 205 had developed prostate cancer. A self-estimate of the physical demands of employment was unrelated to their risk of this condition. Zeegers et al.[21] followed 58,279 Dutch men initially aged 55–69 years over a period of 9.3 years, encountering 1386 cases of prostate cancer. Occupational activity was classed in terms of energy expenditure and sitting time, and after allowance for age, alcohol consumption, body mass index, total energy intake, family history and education, no association was found between the physical demands of occupation and the risk of prostate cancer.

Of the 6 investigations pointing to a possible trend, Albanes et al.[11] observed 95 cases of prostate cancer in 5141 men who had been followed for an average of 10 years. Comparing those who very active with those who were quite inactive at work, the age-adjusted relative risk for the sedentary employees was 1.3, but given the relatively small total number of cases, the trend to a 30% disadvantage was not statistically significant. Grotta et al.[13] followed 13,109 Swedish men for a total of 13 years, finding 904 cases of prostate cancer. There was a weak and non-significant trend to benefit from a high level of occupational activity after adjusting data for age, education, smoking, body mass index, alcohol consumption and diabetes mellitus (a hazard ratio for the physical workers of 0.81 [0.61–1.07]). Hrafnkelsdóttir et al.[14] carried out a 24-year follow-up of 822 Icelandic men. Occupational activity was classed as mostly sitting, standing or "on the move". The hazard ratios, adjusted for age, height, body mass index, diabetes mellitus, family history, education and medical check-ups showed a weak trend favouring those who were engaged in more demanding work (respective values of 1.0, 0.97 and [for the most active group] 0.91 [0.79–1.06, ns]). Hsing et al.[15] obtained occupational titles on 264 cases of prostate cancer, calculating standardized incidence ratios (SIR) for prostate cancer in relation to both the anticipated sitting time and energy expenditures at work, apparently without using any co-variates. The SIR was 0.94 for those who were seated less than 2 hours per day, compared with 1.23 for those sitting longer than 6 hours per day (p = 0.14), and in terms of estimated energy costs the SIR was 1.23 for those with work-place expenditures averaging <8 kJ/min, compared with 0.92 for those expending >12 kJ/min (p = 0.06). Thune and Lund[19] examined 220 cases of prostate cancer in 53,242 Norwegians who had been followed for an average of 16.3 years. A four-level classification of the physical demands of occupation (ranging from sedentary to heavy manual) found a trend to an advantageous risk ratio (0.81 [0.50–1.30]) in those who were engaged in heavy physical work, after adjusting data for age, body mass index and geographic region of residence.

Among the 6 investigations observing statistically significant evidence of benefit, Clarke and Whittemore[12] followed 5377 men for 17–21 years, accumulating 201 incident cases of prostate cancer. Controlling data for age, educational attainment, ethnicity and family history, the relative risk of inactive vs. active employment was 1.75 (1.12–2.67, p = 0.05 for a trend), apparently with an even greater benefit to heavy workers in the African-American subset of the sample.

Norman et al.[16] examined data for 3 cohorts of 43,836, 28,702 and 19,670 patients with prostate cancer. Occupational titles were categorized from sedentary to a very high level of physical activity, and with adjustment of data for age, year of follow-up and area of residence, a small but highly significant increase of relative risk was seen in sedentary individuals (respective risks for the 3 cohorts of sedentary individuals, 1.11, 1.10 and 1.11 [p = 0.0001]). Orsini et al.[17] followed 45,887 men for 8 years, accumulating 2735 incident cases of prostate cancer. Four categories of employment were recognized (ranging from mostly sitting to heavy manual work). After allowing for leisure activity, age, smoking, alcohol consumption, educational attainment, diet, energy intake, waist/hip ratio and diabetes mellitus, the risk ratio favoured active workers (0.72 [0.57–0.90], p for trend = 0.007). However, the advantage was smaller for individuals with advanced or fatal cancers. Parent et al.[18] questioned 449 incident cases of prostate cancer on their lifetime occupational energy expenditures (high vs. low, estimated in METs); the odds ratio for this sample strongly favoured those in active employment (0.54 [0.31–0.95]). Vena et al.[20] obtained data on 430,000 men in Washington State, including 8116 men who died from prostate cancer. A four-level classification of occupational activity was made, and although the findings were not altogether consistent from decade to decade and did not show clear trends, a comparison of the overall proportional mortality between those with low (109) and high (93) occupational demands showed a clear advantage to the heavy workers (p <0.05).

Case-control studies

Of 15 case-control studies, 5 found either no effect or a trend to a higher risk of prostate cancer in individuals with heavy employment. Doolan et al.[24] compared 1436 cases of prostate cancer with 1349 matched controls, using the Finnish job matrix to classify occupational workload into tertiles of physical demand. After adjusting for age, family history and economic resources, the odds ratio for developing prostate cancer tended to be higher in those individuals with the highest energy expenditures (odds ratio 1.15 [0.95–1.40]). Hosseini et al.[27] related 137 cases of prostate cancer to 137 neighbourhood controls. Although a binary classification of the time study participants spent walking to work (<10 vs. >10 h/wk) trended to a reduce risk for those with a longer active commute (odds ratio 0.7 [0.4–1.2] ns), a comparison between those with inactive or moderately active employment and those with highly active work yielded a large multivariate-adjusted odds ratio favouring those with the physically less demanding work (6.7 [1.3–35.1] [p = 0.02]). Lacey et al.[29] compared 258 cases of prostate cancer with 471 age-matched controls. Occupational energy expenditures (classed as sedentary, moderate or high) yielded similar findings whether activity data were examined for the subjects at ages 20–29, 40–49 or 12 years prior to preparation of their report; after adjusting findings for age, marital status, educational attainment, body mass index, energy intake and waist/hip ratio, risk ratios 1.1 (0.7–1.7), 1.3 (0.8–1.9) and 0.9 (0.5–1.8) tended to favour the sedentary vs. the highly active group. Sass-Kortak et al.[32] compared 760 prostate cancer cases with 1632 controls gleaned from telephone listings. Quartiles of lifetime occupational activity adjusted for age, family history and sunlight exposure showed an adverse experience in the most active workers (odds ratio of prostate cancer 1.33 [1.02–1.74], p for trend 0.18). Friedenreich et al.[26] compared data for 988 incident cases of prostate cancer with 1063 population controls in terms of the energy expended at work (less than 74.2 vs. more than 161.9 MET-h/wk). After controlling for age, region, educational attainment, body mass index, waist/hip ratio, energy intake, alcohol consumption, family and medical history, there was no association between prostate cancer and the physical demands of work.

Of the 3 reports with trends suggestive of benefit, Lagiou et al.[30] assigned 320 histologically confirmed cases of prostate cancer and 246 hospital controls between 3 categories of occupational activity (low, medium or high). Following data adjustment for age and educational attainment, there was a non-significant trend (odds ratio 0.69 [0.40–1.22]) suggesting protection from physically demanding work. Le Marchand et al.[31] found 452 cases of prostate cancer in the Hawaii tumour registry. The portion of the lifespan spent in sedentary jobs (from 0% to more than 54%) was compared with that seen in 899 population controls. After adjustment of data for age and ethnicity, the risk of prostate cancer was unaffected by the duration of sedentary employment in those under the age of 70 years, but among those older than 70 years there was a trend for a decreased risk in those with more active jobs (an odds ratio of 0.6 [0.4–1.0, p = 0.07 for trend]). Wiklund et al.[35] compared 1449 incident cases of prostate cancer with 1118 population controls; the average intensity of lifetime occupational activity was classified over a range from less than 11.8 to more than 19.8 MET-h/day, and there was a weak trend to benefit among those with physically demanding occupations (odds ratio 0.84 [0.61–1.15], ns) after controlling data for age, region, educational attainment, body mass index, alcohol consumption, family history, diabetes mellitus and total energy intake.

Seven case-control studies found a significant association of benefit with physically active employment. Bairati et al.[22] compared 64 cases of prostate cancer with 5456 cases of benign prostate hyperplasia. After adjusting data for age, educational attainment, total energy intake, smoking and the use of vitamin supplements, the odds ratio associated with ever having had a sedentary job or light work was 2.0 (1.1–3.6). Classifying subjects on the basis of spending 0%, 1–49% or >50% of one's career in sedentary or light work, the respective odds of developing prostate cancer were 1.0, 1.7 and 2.8 (trend, p = 0.007). The benefit was even greater for those whose longest-held job had involved high or very high rates of energy expenditure (an odds ratio of 0.2 [0.1–0.7] for a highly active vs. a sedentary job). Brownson et al.[23] drew 2878 cases of prostate cancer from the Missouri cancer registry, comparing the reported level of occupational activity (a high vs. a moderate vs. a low physical demand) with that of controls having other types of cancer. Respective odds ratios for the 3 categories of work, after controlling for age and smoking, were 1.0, 1.1 and 1.5 (1.2–1.8), with a statistically significant trend favouring the more active employees (p <0.01). Darlington et al.[50] drew a comparison between the experience of 752 cases of prostate cancer aged 50–84 years who had been selected from the Ontario cancer registry, and that of telephone listing controls. Subjects were asked about undertaking strenuous occupational activity in their mid-teens, early 30s and early 50s. After adjusting data for age, educational attainment, body mass index, family history and occupation, strenuous physical activity by men in their 50s was associated with a reduced the risk of prostate cancer (an odds ratio of 0.8 [0.6–0.9]), but benefit was not statistically significant if the heavy work had been performed during the other age periods. Dosemeci et al.[25] contrasted occupations between a small sample of 27 cases of prostate cancer and 2127 hospital controls; after adjusting for age and smoking habits, significant adverse odds were found for men having a low energy expenditure at work (less than 8 kJ/min vs. more than 12 kJ/min) and for those spending a low proportion of their working day in physical activity (less than two hours vs. more than six hours) with respective odds ratios of 5.0 (1.1–31.7) and 3.4 (1.1–10.6). In a nested case-control study, Krishnadasan et al.[28] rated occupational energy expenditures as low, moderate or high in 362 cases of prostate cancer and 1805 matched controls. Adjusting data for matching variables, pay and trichlorethylene exposure, there was a strong trend for reduced risk in the more active workers (an odds ratio of 0.63 [0.40–1.00, p = 0.06 for trend]). The benefit was statistically significant for aerospace workers, but not for radiation workers, although the reason for the discordance of outcome between the two types of employment was not explained. Strom et al.[33] compared 176 cases of prostate cancer in Mexican-Americans, with data for 176 matched controls. Occupational activity was rated as none/low vs. moderate/high, and after allowing for the effects of age, educational attainment, cancer screening and exposure to agricultural chemicals, a reduced risk was seen in those with active occupations (an odds ratio of 0.46 [0.28–0.77], p = 0.003). Villeneuve et al.[34] compared 1623 histologically confirmed cases of prostate cancer with 1623 controls. After adjusting data for age, area of residence, smoking, alcohol consumption, body mass index, diet, income and family history, a four-level classification of occupational demand (ranging from sitting to strenuous work) found significant benefit was associated with heavy physical activity in the teens or early 20s (an odds ratio of 0.6, [0.4–0.9]), with parallel but non-significant trends in the 30s, 50s and two years before being interviewed.

Leisure activities and risk of prostate cancer

Patterns of recent leisure activity could theoretically be ascertained by interview or by the use of a personal monitor such as an accelerometer, but because large number of subjects have been involved in many studies of prostate cancer, recourse has usually been to physical activity questionnaires. These instruments have limited accuracy and usually examine current or recent activity, rather than an individual's behaviour 10–30 years previously, when carcinogenesis began.

Retrospective and prospective cohort studies

Of 28 retrospective and prospective cohort studies (Table 11.2), 1 found a strong adverse (but not statistically significant) trend, and in a further 11 there was no association between physical activity and the risk of prostate cancer; 12 reports found trends suggesting some benefit, and 4 found statistically significant evidence of a favorable outcome for active individuals.

Cerhan et al.[54] found a strong trend to an adverse effect in rural Iowa, with a relative risk of 2.7 (0.87–9.9) in those members of a small sample of 71 cases of prostate cancer who reported engaging in vigorous physical activity. The measure of physical activity used in this study was relatively crude, and although data were adjusted for age, body mass index and smoking, no information was obtained on occupational activity or exposure to agricultural toxins. Among the 11 investigations with neutral findings, Crespo et al.[36] followed a group of 9824 men initially aged 35–79 years until their death. Data were adjusted for age, educational attainment, urban residence, smoking and body mass index, and no relationship was found between the likelihood of death from prostate cancer and physical activity as assessed by the Framingham index. Giovannucci et al.[37] observed 47,452 health professionals for 8 years, finding 1362 incident cases of prostate cancer. Leisure activity, graded from 1 to 46.8 MET-h per week, was adjusted for age, vasectomy, diabetes mellitus, smoking, energy intake and diet. No significant relationship to prostate cancer was seen, except for a suggestion of less metastatic activity in the more active individuals. Grotta et al.[113] followed 13,109 Swedish men for 13 years, during which time 904 developed prostate cancer. After co-varying data for age, educational attainment, smoking, body mass index, alcohol consumption and diabetes mellitus, the hazard ratio (0.93 [0.76–1.14, ns]) showed little tendency to a lower risk in those with greater leisure activity. Johnsen et al.[7] followed 127,923 men for 8.5 years, accumulating 2458 cases of prostate cancer. With adjustment of data for occupational activity, height, body mass, marital status and education, no association was seen between quartiles of leisure activity (ranging from less than 25 to more than 71 MET-h/wk) and the risk of prostate cancer. Moreover, unlike the occupational data, no significance was seen when the analysis focused simply on the risk of advanced tumours. Lee et al.[40] made one of several examinations of their data on the leisure activity of Harvard alumni, using a questionnaire to estimate quartiles of weekly habitual physical activity (ranging from less than 4.2 to more than 12.6 MJ) at entry to the study. After allowing for age, body mass index, smoking, alcohol consumption and family history, prostate cancer was found to be unrelated to either the total weekly energy expenditure or the volume of vigorous physical activity. Littman et al.[41] studied 34,757 men who were initially aged 50–76 years, finding 583 incident cases of prostate cancer. An exhaustive study of leisure behaviour looked at MET-h/wk of physical activity, typical walking pace, stair climbing, the amount of high intensity activity and activity performed at earlier ages. Controlling for family history, body mass index and income, none of these analyses found any association with prostate cancer, except in a sub-group over

Table 11.2 Leisure-time physical activity and the risk of developing prostate cancer

Author	Sample	Activity measure	Findings	Comments
Cohort studies				
Albanes et al.[11]	95 cases of PC in 5141 men over 10 yr follow-up	Much vs. little or no recreational exercise	RR for inactive 1.8 (1.1–3.3). p = 0.02 for trend	Age-adjusted
Cerhan et al.[54]	20-yr follow-up of 1050 men initially aged 73.5 yr and cancer free, 71 cases of PC	5-question assessment of physical activity (vigorous, moderately active or inactive)	Risk relative to non-cases: Inactive RR = 1.0, Moderate = 1.9 (0.5–6.5) Vigorous = 2.7 (0.7–9.9)	Adjusted for age, BMI, smoking; no information on occupational activity or agricultural chemicals
Clarke & Whittemore[12]	5377 men followed for 17–21 yr, 201 cases of PC	Much vs. little or none	RR for inactive 1.17 (ns)	Adjusted for age, education, ethnicity and family history
Crespo et al.[36]	9824 men initially aged 35–79 yr followed for mortality	Framingham index (quartiles)	No relationship between physical activity and prostate deaths	Adjusted for age, education, urban residence, smoking, BMI
Giovannucci et al.[37]	47,452 health professionals followed for 8 yr, 1362 incident cases of PC	Leisure activity, 1 vs. 46.8 MET-h/wk	No significant relationship except suggestion of less metastatic activity with vigorous intensity exercise	Adjusted for age, vasectomy, diabetes mellitus, smoking, energy intake, diet
Giovannucci et al.[38]	47,620 health professionals, 14 yr follow-up, 2892 incident cases of PC (482 advanced, 280 fatal)	Vigorous physical activity, 0 vs >29 MET-h/wk	No relationship for all subjects; if >65yr, OR for advanced cancer 0.33 (0.17–0.62)	Age, BMI, smoking, height, family history, diabetes mellitus, ethnicity, non-vigorous activity, energy intake and diet
Grotta et al.[13]	13,109 Swedish men followed for 13 yr, 904 cases of PC	Low vs. high leisure activity	HR 0.93 (0.76–1.14, ns)	Adjusted for age, education, smoking, BMI, alcohol consumption, diabetes mellitus

Table 11.2 continued

Author	Sample	Activity measure	Findings	Comments
Hartman et al.[6]	29,133 men followed for up to 9 yr, 317 cases of PC	Sedentary versus moderate/heavy leisure activity in working men	RR 0.7 (0.46–0.94) favouring active leisure	Adjusted for age, urban living, smoking, benign hyperplasia
Hrafnkelsdóttir et al.[14]	24-year follow-up of 822 Icelandic men	Regular physical activity from age of 20 yrs vs. sedentary	HR 0.93 (0.83–1.07) for active individuals	Adjusted for age, height, BMI, diabetes, family history, education, medical check-ups
Johnsen et al.[7]	127,923 men followed for 8.5 yr; 2458 cases of PC	Quartiles of leisure activity (<25 to >71 MET-h/wk)	Leisure activity unrelated to PC	Adjusted for occup. activity, height, weight, marital status and education
Lee et al.[39]	17,719 Harvard alumni, 419 cases of PC	Activity questionnaire completed on 2 occasions	OR if weekly expenditure >16 MJ 0.12 (0.02–0.89) (only 1 case of PG)	Adjusted for age
Lee et al.[40]	8922 Harvard alumni, 439 developed PC	Physical activity questionnaire completed twice, weekly energy expenditure quartiles (<4.2 MJ– >12.6 MJ)	PC unrelated to total activity or weekly volume of vigorous physical activity	Adjusted for age, BMI, smoking, alcohol consumption, family history
Paffenbarger et al.[5]	16,936 male Harvard graduates followed 12–16 yr, with 36 deaths from PC	Questionnaire-based physical activity index (<2 MJ/wk vs >8 MJ/wk)	Mortality rate 2.7 vs. 1.5/10,000 man-yr (ns)	Adjusted for age, smoking, BMI
Littman et al.[41]	34,757 men initially aged 50–76 yr, 583 cases of PC	MET-h/wk, walking pace, stair climbing, high intensity activity, activity at earlier ages	No association with PC except in sub-group aged >65 yr with normal body mass	Adjusted for family history, BMI, income

Table 11.2 continued

Author	Sample	Activity measure	Findings	Comments
Liu et al.[42]	982 cases of PC in 22,071 physicians over 11 yr	Exercise sufficient to cause a sweat <1/wk. vs. >5/wk	No relationship to PC	Adjusted for smoking, alcohol consumption, height, diabetes mellitus, high cholesterol, hypertension, use of multi-vitamins
Lund-Nielsen et al.[8]	22,895 Norwegian men followed for 9.3 yr, with 644 cases of PC	High vs. low leisure activity	RR 0.80 (0.62–1.03)	Multivariate adjusted
Moore et al.[43]	293,902 men initially aged 50–71 yr followed for up to 8.2 yr, 17,872 cases PC	Exercise at baseline and in adolescence (never/rarely to >5 times/wk)	RR 0.97 (0.91–1.03) p for trend favouring activity during adolescence = 0.03. But no relationships to exercise habits at baseline	Adjusted for age, marital status, education, smoking, medical history, BMI, waist circumference, family history, diet and supplements
Nilsen et al.[44]	29,110 Norwegian men followed for 7 yr, 957 incident cases PC	Score based on frequency, intensity and duration of activity (low vs. high)	Relationship for total cancer ns (RR = 0.86), but for advanced cancer RR = 0.64 (0.43–0.95), inverse trend p = 0.02	Adjusted for age, marital status, education, BMI, smoking, alcohol consumption
Orsini et al.[17]	45,887 men followed for 8 yr, 2735 incident PC	Walking or cycling, 5 categories (hardly ever to >60 min/day)	RR = 0.86 (0.76–0.98) p for trend 0.028; effects greater for advanced (RR = 0.74) and fatal (RR = 0.72) cancers	Adjusted for occupational activity, age, smoking, alcohol consumption, education, diet, energy intake, waist/hip ratio, diabetes mellitus
Parent et al.[18]	449 incident cases of PC	Involvement in sports and outdoor activities	No significant effect on PC	

Table 11.2 continued

Author	Sample	Activity measure	Findings	Comments
Patel et al.[45]	72,174 men, 5503 incident cases of PC over 9 yr	MET-h/wk (<0.7–35) at age 40 and in 1992[45]	No significant effect (but active have fewer aggressive tumours, RR 0.69, 0.52–0.92, p for trend = 0.06)	Adjusted for age, ethnicity, BMI, weight change, energy intake, diet and vitamin use, diabetes mellitus, family and medical history
Platz et al.[46]	46,786 health professionals, 2896 incident cases PC over 14 yr	Vigorous leisure activity <3, >3 MET-h/wk	No relationship to PC	Adjusted for age, family history, BMI, diabetes mellitus, smoking, diet
Putnam et al.[9]	101 cases of PC in 1572 initially cancer free men followed for 4 yr	Very active, moderately active, inactive	Risk of PC unrelated to leisure activity	Adjusted for total energy intake
Severson et al.[10]	8006 Japanese men on Oahu; 205 cases of PC	Framingham index, resting heart rate, self-estimate of moderate or heavy leisure activity	Risk of PC unrelated to Framingham index or resting heart rate; suggestion of benefit from self-assessment (OR 0.77, 0.58–1.01)	Adjusted for age, BMI
Steenland et al.[47]	156 cases of PC in NHANES I survey follow-up	Physical activity: little vs. lots	Suggestion of benefit from activity, OR 1.31 (0.76–2.26, ns)	Adjusted for age, BMI, smoking, alcohol consumption, income
Thune & Lund[19]	220 cases of PC in 53,242 Norwegians followed for 16.3 yr	3-level classification, sedentary to regular training	No effect of leisure activity	Adjusted for age, BMI, geographic region
Wannamethee et al.[48]	Prospective study of 7588 men with 120 incident cases of PC	6-level classification of leisure activity from none to vigorous	Benefit from vigorous activity, OR 0.25 (0.06–0.99, p for trend = 0.06)	Adjusted for age, smoking, alcohol consumption, BMI, social class

Table 11.2 continued

Author	Sample	Activity measure	Findings	Comments
Zeegers et al.[21]	58,279 men aged 55–69 yr, 1386 cases of PC over 9.3 yr	Biking/walking (min/day), gardening (h/week)	Gardening unrelated to PC; biking/ walking <10 vs. >60 min/d, RR 0.85 (0.69–1.05, ns)	Adjusted for age, alcohol consumption, BMI, energy intake, family history, gardening, sport involvement

Case/control studies

Author	Sample	Activity measure	Findings	Comments
Andersson et al.[49]	252 cases of PC, 243 controls	Pubertal activity relative to peers, lower, same or higher	OR = 1.3, 1.0, 0.7 (p for trend 0.13)	Adjusted for age, urbanization, adult farming
Darlington et al.[50]	752 cases from Ontario cancer registry aged 50–84 yr, telephone listing controls	Strenuous activity mid-teens, early 30s, early 50s	Strenuous activity by men in 50s reduced risk (OR 0.8, 0.6–0.9). Other age groups ns	Adjusted for age, education, BMI, family history, occupation
Friedenreich et al.[26]	988 incident cases of PC, 1063 population controls	<78.5 vs. >25.1 MET-h/wk	OR 1.00, 0.80 (0.61–1.04) (p = 0.06 for trend)	Adjusted for age, region, education, BMI, waist/hip ratio, energy intake, alcohol consumption, family and medical history
Jian et al.[51]	130 histologically confirmed PC, 274 controls	Reported MET-h of moderate and total activity (<40 vs >120; <44 vs. >135)	OR 0.20 (0.07–0.62, p = 0.015), 0.39 (0.15–0.99, p = 0.50 for trend)	Adjusted for age, area of residence, education, income, marital status, number of children, years in work force, family history, BMI, energy intake
Lacey et al.[29]	258 cases of PC, 471 age-matched controls	Tertiles of moderate/ vigorous or all physical activity at 20–29, 40–49 and 12 yrs ago	No relationship to PC	Adjusted for age, marital status, education, BMI, energy intake, waist/hip ratio

Table 11.2 continued

Author	Sample	Activity measure	Findings	Comments
Strom et al.[33]	176 cases of PC in Mexican-Americans, 176 controls	Leisure activity <1/wk vs. >1/wk	No effect on risk of PC	
Sung et al.[52]	90 cases of PC, 180 controls	Exercise (yes vs. no) 5–10 yr before diagnosis	*Adverse* effect of exercise (OR 2.16, 1.18–3.96, p = 0.01)	Multivariate adjusted
Villeneuve et al.[34]	1623 histologically confirmed cases of PC, 1623 controls	5-level classification <1/month to >5/week)	No clear relationship to PC	Adjusted for age, area of residence, smoking, alcohol consumption, BMI, diet, income, family history
West et al.[53]	358 cases of PC, 679 controls	Activity questionnaire	No relationship between activity and PC	
Whittemore et al.[54]	1655 cases of PC, 1645 population controls	Activity questionnaire	No relationship between activity and PC	
Wiklund et al.[35]	1449 incident cases of PC, 1118 population controls	MET-h/day lifetime recreational activity, <7.4 to >13.5	OR 1.56 (1.16–2.10), p = 0.006, adverse effect of active leisure	Adjusted for age, region, education, BMI, alcohol consumption, family history, diabetes mellitus, energy intake
Yu et al.[55]	1162 cases of PC, 3124 matched hospital controls	Leisure activity (active, moderate or seldom)	Risk higher in sedentary (OR 1.3, 1.0–1.6 p = 0.03)	Adjusted for age

Notes: ns = non-significant; BMI = body mass index; HR = hazard ratio; MET = metabolic equivalent; OR = odds ratio; PC = prostate cancer; RR = relative risk the age of 65 years who had maintained a normal body mass. In contrast, active older subjects who were overweight had an increased risk of prostate cancer. Liu et al.[42] found 982 cases of prostate cancer when following 22,071 physicians over a period of 11 years. The frequency of taking sufficient physical activity to work up a sweat was categorized from "less than once a week" to "more than five times per week". With adjustment of data for smoking, alcohol consumption, height, diabetes mellitus, high cholesterol, hypertension and the use of multi-vitamins, their findings indicated no effect of physical activity upon the risk of prostate cancer. Parent et al.[18] questioned 449 incident cases of prostate cancer on their involvement in sports and outdoor activities; no significant association with the risk of prostate tumours was seen. Parent et al.[49] found 449 incident cases of prostate cancer among a total of 3730 individuals with various types of cancer. Involvement in sports and outdoor activities was classed as "never", "not often" and "often". Age, socio-economic status, educational attainment, ethnicity, smoking and body mass index were included as co-variates in an analysis that found no significant effect of activity upon the risk of prostate cancer. Platz et al.[46] examined 46,786 health professionals; over 14 years, there were 2896 incident cases of prostate cancer. Noting all periods when leisure activity exceeded 6 METs, a binary classification of the volume of vigorous leisure activity was made (less than vs. more than 3 MET-h/wk). Adjusting data for age, family history, body mass index, diabetes mellitus, smoking and diet, there was no difference in the incidence of prostate cancer between the two halves of the sample. However, an increase of risk was seen in individuals with a high energy intake, suggesting the possibility that some people use any excess of ingested energy for growth of tumour tissue rather than for fat formation. Putnam et al.[9] found 101 cases of prostate cancer in 1572 initially cancer-free men who were followed for 4 years. A three-level classification of leisure activity (very active, moderately active and inactive) was unrelated to the risk of developing prostate cancer after adjusting data for the total energy intake. Thune and Lund[19] observed 220 cases of prostate cancer in 53,242 Norwegians who were followed for 16.3 years. A three-level classification of leisure activity (ranging from sedentary to regular training) found no association with the risk of developing prostate cancer after adjustments of data for age, body mass index and geographic region of residence.

Twelve investigations found suggestive but non-significant trends of benefit in more active individuals. Clarke and Whittemore[12] followed 5377 men for 17 to 21 years, accumulating 201 cases of prostate cancer. Data were adjusted for age, educational attainment, ethnicity and family history, and a cross-sectional comparison was made between those taking much vs. those engaging in little or no recreational activity. The relative risk for the inactive group was 1.17 (not statistically significant), but a much higher risk was found in the relatively small African-American segment of the total sample (RR 3.17 [0.96–10.46, p = 0.08]). Giovannucci et al.[38] analysed findings for US health professionals over a 14-year follow-up. Data were analysed in terms of the amount of vigorous physical activity undertaken. No relationship was found for younger adults, but in those over the age of 65 years, vigorous physical activity was associated with a decreased risk of advanced prostate cancer and a lower Gleason tumour aggressivity score (odds ratio 0.33 [0.17–0.62]). Hrafnkelsdóttir et al.[14] completed a 24-year follow-up of 822 Icelandic men. They tested the benefit associated with engaging in regular physical activity from the age of 20 years, finding a hazard ratio of 0.93 (0.83–1.07) for the active group after adjusting their data for age, height, body mass index diabetes, family history, educational attainment and regular medical check-ups. Paffenbarger et al.[5] followed 16,936 male Harvard graduates for 12 to 16 years; there were only 36 deaths from prostate cancer during this period. Nevertheless, they attempted to relate the mortality rate to a questionnaire-based physical activity index; respective values, adjusted for age, smoking and body mass index, were 2.7 vs. 1.5/10,000 person-years (not statistically significant) in those with weekly energy expenditures of less than 2 MJ vs. more than 8 MJ. Lee et al.[39] made a further examination of data for this same population, applying a physical activity questionnaire on 2 occasions to 17,719 Harvard alumni, including 419 men who had developed prostate cancer. The age-adjusted odds ratio for those who maintained a very high energy expenditure (more than 16 MJ) at both assessments had a value of 0.12 (0.02–0.89), but this figure must be regarded with some scepticism, since it is based on only a single case of prostate cancer in the most active group. Benefit was no longer seen when the cut-point for a high energy expenditure was reduced from 16 to 10 MJ/week.[56] Lund-Nielsen et al.[8] followed 22,895 Norwegian men for 9.3 years, encountering 644 incident cases of prostate cancer. Multi-variate adjustment of a simple binary classification of leisure activity found a trend to benefit from a high level of physical activity (relative risk of prostate cancer 0.80 [0.62–1.03]). Moore et al.[43] examined a very large sample of 293,902 men who were initially aged 50–71 years. During an 8.2-year follow-up, there were 17,872 cases of prostate cancer, 1942 of which were advanced and 513 of which were fatal. After adjusting findings for age, marital status, educational attainment, smoking, medical history, body mass index, waist circumference, family history, diet and use of nutritional supplements, vigorous exercise during adolescence was associated with a small reduction in the relative risk of developing prostate cancer (odds ratio 0.97 [0.91–1.03], p for trend favouring activity during adolescence = 0.03), but exercise at entry to the study was unrelated to the total number of tumours, to advanced lesions or to the number of fatal cases. Nilsen et al.[44] studied 29,110 Norwegian men for 7 years, finding 957 incident cases of prostate cancer. Physical activity was scored based on the frequency, intensity and duration of physical activity (low, medium or high). With statistical allowance for effects of age, marital status, educational attainment, body mass index, smoking and alcohol consumption, physical activity bore no significant relationship to the risk of all prostate cancers (risk ratio = 0.86), but there was a significant inverse trend to a decreased risk of advanced tumours (relative risk = 0.64 [0.43–0.95], trend p = 0.02). Patel et al.[45] followed a sample of 72,174 men, accruing 5503 incident cases of prostate cancer over 9 years. Leisure activity was classified in MET-h/wk (from <0.7 to >35). Following adjustment of data for age, ethnicity, body mass index, changes in body mass, energy intake, diet and vitamin use, diabetes mellitus and family and medical history, no significant association was seen between the volume of leisure activity and the incidence of prostate cancer, but a sub-category of tumours with a high Gleason score for aggressiveness tended to be less prevalent among the more active individuals (risk ratio 0.69 [0.52–0.92], p for trend = 0.06). Severson et al.[10] found 205 cases of prostate cancer among 8006 Japanese men living on the island of Oahu, Hawaii. Leisure activity was assessed by the Framingham index, resting heart rate and a self-estimate of involvement in moderate or heavy leisure activity, all of these indices being adjusted for age and body mass index; the first two measures were unrelated to the risk of prostate cancer, although there was a suggestion of benefit associated with a subjective assessment of engagement in moderate or heavy leisure activity (an odds ratio of 0.77 [0.58–1.01]). Steenland et al.[47] found 156 cases of prostate cancer in a follow-up of participants in the NHANES I survey. Contrasting those taking little physical activity with those taking "lots", there was a weak trend to a lower risk in the more active individuals (an odds ratio of 1.31 [0.76–2.26, ns]) after adjustment of data for age, body mass index, smoking, alcohol consumption and income. Zeegers et al.[21] followed 58,279 men who were initially aged 55–69 years for an average of 9.3 years, accumulating 1386 cases of prostate cancer. Leisure activity was assessed in terms of the time individuals allocated to bicycling or walking, and to gardening. Gardening was unrelated to the risk of prostate cancer, but after controlling for age, alcohol consumption, body mass index, energy intake, family history, gardening and sport involvement, there was a weak trend to benefit from walking and cycling; compared with those who were active for less than 10 min/day, the odds ratio for those making a time allocation of >60 minutes per day to walking and cycling was 0.85 (0.69–1.05, ns).

Among the 4 investigators with statistically significant findings, Albanes et al.[11] found 95 cases of prostate cancer in a sample of 5141 men during a 10-year follow-up of individuals who had been recruited to the NHANES I survey. Comparing those who took much vs. those who engaged in little or no recreational exercise, the age adjusted relative risk was 1.8 (1.1–3.3), with a statistically significant trend favouring those who were more active (p = 0.02). Hartman et al.[6] followed 29,133 men for up to 9 years, finding 317 incident cases of prostate cancer. After adjusting data for age, urban living, smoking and benign prostatic hyperplasia, a comparison of those who were sedentary vs. those who undertook moderate or heavy leisure activity found a relative risk of 0.7 (0.46–0.94) favouring those who engaged in active leisure. Orsini et al.[17] followed 45,887 men for 8 years, accumulating 2735 cases of prostate cancer. Walking and cycling habits were placed into five categories, ranging from "hardly ever" to "more than 60 minutes per day". After adjusting data for a substantial range of co-variates (age, smoking, alcohol consumption, educational attainment, diet, energy intake, waist/hip ratio and diabetes mellitus), the relative risk of prostate cancer in the most active category of subjects was 0.86 (0.76–0.98), with risk decreasing by some 8% for each 30 minutes allocated to daily walking or cycling over the range 30–120 minutes/day. Effects of an active lifestyle were greatest for advanced (RR = 0.74) and fatal (RR = 0.72) tumours. Wannamethee et al.[48] carried out a prospective study of 7588 men, with 120 incident cases of prostate cancer. A six-level classification of leisure activity ranged from "none" to "vigorous". After adjusting data for age, smoking, alcohol consumption, body mass index and social class, there was a substantial benefit associated with participation in vigorous activity (an odds ratio of 0.25 [0.06–0.99], p for trend = 0.06).

Case-control studies

Of 12 case-control studies, 2 found an adverse effect of physical activity, 5 no effect, 2 a positive trend and 3 provided statistically significant evidence of benefit. Sung et al.[52] related 90 cases of prostate cancer to 180 controls, noting exercise participation ("yes" vs. "no") 5 to 10 years prior to the tumour diagnosis. In a multivariate analysis, they observed that exercise was associated with a significant increase in the risk of prostate cancer (an odds ratio of 2.16 [1.18–3.96], p = 0.01). Wiklund et al.[35] compared 1449 incident cases of prostate cancer with 1118 population controls. After adjusting data for age, region, educational attainment, body mass index, alcohol consumption, family history, diabetes mellitus and energy intake, a classification of lifetime recreational activity (from less than 7.4 to more than 13.5 MET-h/day) showed a significant increase of risk in those with the more active leisure (odds ratio 1.56 [1.16–2.10], p= 0.006).

Five investigations found little effect from leisure activity. Lacey et al.[29] asked for information about moderate/vigorous and all physical activity at 3 time points (ages 20–29 and 40–49 years and 12 years prior to the study) in a sample of 258 cases of prostate cancer and 471 age-matched controls. Adjusting data for age, marital status, educational attainment, body mass index, energy intake and waist/hip ratio, the extent of leisure activity was unrelated to the risk of prostate cancer. Strom et al.[33] compared leisure activity (a frequency of less than vs. more than once per week) between 176 cases of prostate cancer and 176 matched controls; the risk of developing prostate cancer was not associated with differences in the frequency of leisure-time physical activity. Villeneuve et al.[34] related data on 1623 histologically confirmed cases of prostate cancer to findings in 1623 controls. A five-level classification of the frequency of leisure-time physical activity (from less than once per month to more than five times per week) showed no clear relationship to the risk of developing prostate cancer, after control of the data for age, area of residence, smoking, alcohol consumption, body mass index, diet, income and family history. West et al.[53] compared 358 cases of prostate cancer with 679 controls; in a survey that focused primarily on diet, subjects were questioned about their physical activity and no relationship was seen between leisure activity and tumour development. In another study where physical activity was not the main emphasis, Whittemore et al.[54] studied 1655 cases of prostate cancer and 1645 population controls; they, also, found no relationship between leisure activity and the development of prostate cancer.

Two studies showed trends suggesting benefit from leisure activity. Andersson et al.[49] compared 252 cases of prostate cancer with 243 controls. The pubertal physical activity of these subjects was rated relative to that of their peers, as lower, the same or higher, and the respective odds ratios for subsequently developing a prostate tumour (adjusted for age, urbanization and adult farming) were 1.3, 1.0 and 0.7 (p for a trend = 0.13), favouring those who were active as adolescents. An association of carcinogenesis with living in a densely populated area was also seen; this may have reflected differences of social class, but there may also have been an adverse effect of inner-city living upon the individual's ability to engage in physical activity as a youth. Friedenreich et al.[26] examined 988 incident cases of prostate cancer and 1063 population controls. Multiple co-variates included age, region, educational attainment, body mass index, waist/hip ratio, energy intake, alcohol consumption and the family and medical history. There was a trend towards a favourable odds ratio (0.80 [0.61–1.04] p = 0.06 for trend) when those with the greatest leisure activity (more than 25.1 MET-h/week) were compared with the least active individuals (less than 8.5 MET-h/wk).

Only three case-control studies showed a significant effect favouring active individuals. Darlington et al.[50] related findings on 752 cases drawn from the Ontario cancer registry to telephone-listing controls, enquiring regarding strenuous physical activity in the mid-teens, early 30s and early 50s. After adjusting data for age, educational attainment, body mass index, family history and occupation, the risk of prostate cancer was lower in those who had undertaken strenuous physical activity in their 50s, but benefit was not significantly associated with physical activity at earlier ages. Jian et al.[51] compared 130 histologically confirmed cases of prostate cancer with 274 controls. After adjusting data for age, area of residence, educational attainment, income, marital status, number of children, years in the work force, family history, body mass index and energy intake, the risk of prostate tumours was more closely related to reports of a low volume of moderate physical activity (less than 40 vs. more than 120 MET-h of moderate activity per week) than to a low total volume of physical activity (less than 44 vs. more than 135 MET-h/week, with respective odds ratios for the more active individuals of 0.20 [0.07–0.62, p for trend = 0.015] and 0.39 [0.15–0.99, p for trend = 0.50]). Yu et al.[55] compared 1162 cases of prostate cancer with 3124 matched hospital controls. They classed the frequency of leisure activity, adjusted for age, as active, moderate or seldom, finding a higher odds ratio (1.3 [1.0–1.6], p = 0.03) in the most sedentary group.

Sport involvement and attained fitness

Studies based on an individual's involvement in organized sport are often based on the behaviour reported during youth or when attending university. This may be a relevant period in terms of carcinogenesis, but there is also the difficulty that by middle age, former university athletes are often less active and more obese than those who were not recognized as athletes while attending university. Comparisons with non-athletes are further complicated in that selection for many sports is based upon body build, which can itself modify the risk of carcino-genesis. A final issue is that an athletes may have abused androgenic steroids, and thus increased their risk of prostate cancer.[57, 58] Another option is to compare attained levels of aerobic fitness among those who have been involved in aerobic fitness programmes for substantial periods. Some have considered the attained level of aerobic fitness as a better index of habitual physical activity than responses to questionnaires, although if reliance is placed upon the individual's attained level of maximal oxygen intake, expressed in mL/[kg.min], this measure is heavily influenced not only by the extent of recent aerobic activity, but also by the individual's accumulation of body fat.

Retrospective and prospective cohort studies

Four cross-sectional and cohort studies of sport and fitness have been published (Table 11.3). Two of these reports found no advantage from sport involvement, but the third saw a reduced risk among individuals with a high attained level of aerobic fitness, and the fourth a dose-related effect from the frequency of sport participation.

Merrill et al.[59] evaluated a somewhat fallible index of carcinogenic change (the prostate serum antigen levels) of 536 participants in a seniors' games who were older than 50 years. The age-adjusted PSA was unrelated to the number of years that subjects had been physically active more than three times per week. Zeegers et al.[21] also found no benefit from community sport involvement (a simple binary classification of participation, "never" vs. "ever") when 58,279 men initially aged 55–69 years were followed for 9.3 years, with the accumu-lation of 1386 cases of prostate cancer. Wannamethee et al.[67] included a question on sports involvement ("none," "more than once per month", "more than once per week" or "more than twice per week" in their prospective study of 7588 men aged 40–59 years; 120 of the group developed prostate cancer, and after adjusting data for age, smoking, alcohol consumption, body mass index and socio-economic status, the relative risks for the 4 categories of involvement were 1.0, 0.98, 0.63 and 0.53 (p for trend = 0.05).

Oliveira et al.[60] obtained data on 12,975 men who had been attending the Cooper Fitness Clinic in Dallas, Texas. Quartile scores on a maximal exercise treadmill test of aerobic fitness were inversely related to the risk of prostate cancer (incidence rates for the 3 higher quartiles of fitness of 1.1; 0.73, ns; and 0.26 [0.10–0.63] relative to the least fit group), after allowing for the effects of age, body mass index and smoking.

Case-control studies

Three case-control studies of involvement in sport all reported substantial *adverse* effects. Hållmarker et al.[61] completed a case-control study of 185,412 partic-ipants in the Swedish Vasaloppet long-distance cross-country ski contest and 184,617 non-participants who were matched for age, sex and county of residence. The 2 groups included 1827 and 1435 cases of prostate cancer, respectively, and

Table 11.3 Sports involvement, attained aerobic fitness and risk of prostate cancer

Author	Sample	Activity measure	Findings	Comments
Cohort studies				
Merrill et al.[59]	PSA levels of 536 participants in seniors' games aged >50 yr	Years active >3 times/wk	Physical activity unrelated to PSA levels	Adjusted for age
Oliveira et al.[60]	12,975 men attending Cooper Fitness Clinic	Quartile scores on maximal exercise treadmill test	Incidence rate inversely related to aerobic fitness [1.1, 0.73, ns; 0.26 (0.10–0.63)]	Adjusted for age, BMI, smoking
Wannamethee et al.[67]	Prospective study of 7588 men aged 40–59 yr, with 120 incident cases of PC	Sporting activity (none, >1/month, >1/week, >2/week)	RR 1.00, 0.98, 0.63, 0.53 (p = 0.05)	Age, smoking, alcohol, BMI, SES
Zeegers et al.[21]	58,279 men aged 55–69 yr, 1386 cases of PC over 9.3 yr	Sport participation (never/ever; frequency; duration, yr)	Sport participation unrelated to PC	Adjusted for age, alcohol consumption, BMI, energy intake, family history, education
Case/control studies				
Hållmarker et al.[61]	185,412 participants in Vasaloppet ski contest and 184,617 non-participants	1827 vs. 1435 cases PC	HR 1.22 (1.13–1.30) favouring non-participants	Non-participants matched for age, sex, and county of residence
Paffenbarger et al.[5]	56,683 university alumni followed >28 years, 104 PC cases vs. controls	Playing university sport >5h/wk	RR 1.20 favouring non-athletes (p = 0.028)	Data adjusted for age, sex and birth year of classmate controls
Polednak[62]	8393 university graduates, 124 PC deaths	Athletes vs. minor athletes vs. non-athletes	Age of PC death 70.9, 74.2, 74.8 (p <0.05)	

Notes: ns = non-significant; BMI = body mass index; PC = prostate cancer; PSA = prostate serum antigen; RR = relative risk; SES = socio-economic status a hazard ratio of 1.22 (1.13–1.30) favoured the non-participants. Paffenbarger et al.[5] followed 56,683 university alumni for 28 or more years, accumulating 104 cases of prostate cancer. These individuals were compared with classmate controls matched for age, sex and birth year. Involvement in university sport for longer than five hours per week was associated with a significant adverse effect (relative risk 1.20 [p = 0.028]). Polednak[62] explored data for 8393 university graduates, comparing the experience of major athletes, minor athletes and non-athletes. In his study, there was a statistically significant trend for the major athletes to die of prostate cancer at a younger age than the other two categories of alumni (70.9, 74.2 and 74.8 years, p <0.05).

Possible mechanisms

The demonstration of likely mechanisms whereby exercise modifies prostate carcinogenesis could reinforce the tentative epidemiological evidence of benefit from regular physical activity and provide useful guidance for those designing preventive programmes. In addition to such general benefits of physical activity as a reduction of obesity and oxidant stress and a modulation of immune responses, prolonged endurance exercise may reduce circulating levels of testosterone and insulin-like growth factors,[57, 63] thus reducing the tendency to growth of small prostate neoplasms. Barnard et al.[64] collected serum from men who were undertaking aerobic exercise five times per week and from sedentary controls; when applied to lymph nodes that were infiltrated with prostate cancer cells, the serum from the exercisers decreased levels of insulin-like growth factor, increased insulin-like growth factor binding protein and increased the extent of apoptosis among the tumour cells. However, it is less certain that the average exerciser reaches the intensity and duration of physical activity where such a humoral response might be anticipated.

Conclusions regarding prostate cancer

Despite a large volume of research and some suggestions of benefit, it is difficult to draw strong conclusions about physical activity and the risk of prostate cancer, particularly as many investigators have drawn conflicting inferences from post-hoc analyses on small sub-groups within their overall populations. In terms of occupational activity, relatively few investigators have co-varied their findings for exposure to toxic chemicals, and often there has been an incomplete allowance for socio-economic and dietary differences between those engaged in sedentary and physically demanding work.

There have been around 81 analyses, 34 based on differences of occupational activity, 40 on leisure behaviour, 6 on involvement in sport and 1 on levels of attained aerobic fitness. However, 16 of these reports have examined both occupational and leisure activity, 1 has covered both sport participation and other forms of active leisure, and in 3 instances there have been repeated analyses of the same data set. Summarizing across the various measures of physical activity,

20 reports found significant benefit in one or more of their analyses and a further 23 found a non-significant trend favouring the more active individuals, but against this must be set 31 analyses finding either no effect or an adverse response with an active lifestyle. The evidence to date is far from conclusive, although it tends to support earlier contentions of that regular physical activity may reduce the risk of prostate cancer by 10–30%. Given the other general health benefits of an active lifestyle, and the small number of analyses that have demonstrated an adverse effect, regular physical activity can thus be recommended as a potentially useful tool in reducing the risk of prostate tumours.

Side-effects of androgen deprivation therapy

In about a half of patients, the immediate treatment of prostate cancer by irradiation or surgery is followed by a two to three year course of androgen deprivation therapy (ADT). The latter has major physical side-effects (Table 11.4), including a persistent decrease in maximal aerobic power[65] and muscle strength[66–75], a 3–5% loss of bone mineral density, an increased risk of fractures,[66, 67, 71, 76–91] and a decrease in the overall quality of life.[65, 66, 70, 74, 92–96] There may also be an increased risk of cardiovascular disease and acute renal injury, possibly due to the breakdown of atherosclerotic plaques.[97] However, most of these side effects are of the type that could be reduced by an increase in physical activity following successful initial treatment of the tumour.

Aerobic performance

Alibhai et al.[65] compared 87 cases who had been receiving ADT for 36 months with 86 cases who were not receiving ADT and 86 matched controls, finding a poorer performance on a simple measure of aerobic function (the six minute walking distance) in those who were receiving ADT.

Muscle strength

Typical responses to ADT have been a decrease in lean body mass and an increase in body fat.[67, 70] Thus, a comparison between 30 cases of prostate cancer who were receiving ADT for 6 months with 25 healthy men found a decrease of skeletal muscle mass and lean tissue in the limbs of the affected individuals, with an associated increase of body fat.[68] Galvao et al.[71] demonstrated that after 36 weeks of ADT, the decrease of lean tissue in 72 cases of prostate cancer was distributed across all body sites (decreases of 5.6, 3.7, 1.4 and 2.4% in the upper and lower limbs, trunk and total body, respectively). Van Londen et al.[75] reported data for 43 men who had been receiving ADT for less than 6 months, 67 cases on chronic ADT, 81 who were not receiving ADT and 53 age-matched controls. The acute ADT group showed lean mass losses of 0.93 kg at 12 months and 1.79 kg after 24 months, although losses at 24 months were smaller in the chronic ADT group. As in the other studies, there were associated increases of fat mass.

Table 11.4 Side-effects associated with the androgen-deprivation treatment of prostate cancer

Author	Sample	Findings	Comments
Aerobic performance			
Alibhai et al.[65]	87 cases of non-metastatic PC receiving ADT for 36 months, 86 matched cases not receiving ADT	6 min walk distance poorer if receiving ADT	Side-effects seen at 12 months persisted at 36 months. No specific rehabilitation programme adopted
Muscular performance			
Alibhai et al.[65]	87 cases of non-metastatic PC receiving ADT, 86 matched cases not receiving ADT for 36 months	Grip strength and timed get-up and go poorer if receiving ADT	Side-effects seen at 12 months persisted at 36 months. No specific rehabilitation programme adopted
Basaria et al.[66]	20 cases of PC treated by ADT, 18 treated cases of PC awaiting ADT, 20 age-matched healthy controls	Reduced upper body strength with ADT	
Berrutti et al.[67]	36 cases of PC with 12 months ADT	Decrease of LBM	Increase of body fat
Boxer et al.[68]	30 cases of PC with 6 months ADT vs. 25 healthy controls	Decrease of muscle mass and lean tissue in limbs with ADT	Associated increase of body fat
Bylow et al.[69]	50 men aged >70 yr treated with ADT	24% had impaired ADL, deterioration of balance, walking and chair stand times	22% had falls within 3 months
Galvao et al.[71]	72 cases of PC, 36 weeks of ADT	Decrease of LBM in upper and lower limb, trunk, total 5.6, 3.7, 1.4, 2.4% respectively	Associated increase of body fat
Levy et al.[73]	23 men <6 months ADT, 12 men >6 months ADT, 13 not receiving ADT	Lean mass decreased with duration of ADT, 4 metre walk velocities slower if on ADT	
Stone et al.[74]	62 men receiving ADT as primary treatment of PC	Loss of muscle bulk and reduction in voluntary muscle function (grip, grip fatigue)	

Table 11.4 continued

Author	Sample	Findings	Comments
van Londen et al.[75]	43 men on ADT <6 months, 67 cases on chronic ADT, 81 not on ADT, 53 age-matched controls	Losses of lean mass of 0.93 kg at 12 months, 1.79 kg after 24 months in acute ADT, smaller loss in chronic ADT group at 24 months	Associated increases of fat mass

Bone strength

Author	Sample	Findings	Comments
Basaria et al.[66]	20 cases of PC treated by ADT, 18 treated cases of PC awaiting ADT, 20 age-matched healthy controls	BMD lower, increased urinary N-telopeptide with ADT	
Berrutti et al.[67]	36 cases of PC with 12 months ADT	Decreased BMD at hip and lumbar spine relative to baseline	
Chen et al.[76]	62 cases of PC, 1–5 yr of ADT, 47 healthy controls	Low BMD (total, trochanter, inter-trochanter and hip sites)	Associated higher percent body fat
Daniell et al.[77]	26 cases of PC with ADT or orchidectomy followed 6–42 months	2.4% and 7.6% decrease of BMD in femoral neck after 1 and 2 yr respectively	Further 1.4–2.6%/yr loss of BMD over yrs 3–8
Galvao et al.[71]	72 men treated by ADT for 36 wks	Decreases of BMD at hip, spine, upper limb, whole body 1.5, 3.9, 1.3, 2.4% respectively, but no change in lower limbs	Associated decrease of lean mass
Greenspan et al.[79]	30 with acute ADT <6 months, 50 with chronic ADT >6 months, 72 no ADT, 43 healthy controls	5- to 10-fold increase in loss of bone mineral relative to no ADT or healthy controls	Bone loss maximal in first year of ADT
Hatano et al.[80]	218 cases of PC treated with ADT for >6 months	6% of cases had bone fractures unrelated to metastasis	Low bone density and increased N-telopeptides in those developing fractures
Kiratli et al.[81]	36 patients with PC, age matched controls; ADT or surgical castration for up to 10 yr	Bone mineral loss continues relative to controls for 10 yr	Effect greater with surgical than with chemical castration

Table 11.4 continued

Author	Sample	Findings	Comments
Maillefert et al.[82]	12 cases of PC receiving ADT for 6, 12 and 18 months	BMD decreased 2.7, 3.9 and 6.6% over 18 months	Increased serum osteocalcin
Malcolm et al.[83]	395 cases of PC receiving ADT followed for average of 66 months	23% developed osteoporosis, 7% developed non-pathological fractures	Osteoporosis related to duration of treatment
Morote et al.[84]	31 cases on ADT, 31 controls not on ADT	Bone mass loss of 2.3–5.6% at 12 months, less severe further loss at 24 months	Major bone loss in Ward's triangle
Oefelein et al.[85]	181 cases of PC on ADT	4% fracture at 5 yr, 20% fracture at 10 yr	Fractures less likely if BMI maintained
Preston et al.[86]	23 men receiving ADT for 24 months, 30 controls	Greatest bone loss in distal arm bones (−9.4% vs. −4.4% in controls)	Less loss in controls at all sites except lumbar spine
Shahinian et al.[88]	50,613 cases of prostate cancer	If case survived >5yr, risk of fracture 19.4% with ADT, 12.6% without ADT	Risk of fracture related to dosage of ADT
Smith et al.[89]	Medical claims from 5% of welfare beneficiaries (3887 non-metastatic cases of PC)	Clinical fracture rate 7.88 per 100 person-years with ADT, 6.51 in matched controls	Confirmed by data for hip and vertebral fractures
Stoch et al.[90]	60 men with PC, 19 of whom were receiving ADT	ADT associated with decreased BMD at various sites, increased N-telopeptides and bone-specific alkaline phosphatases	No bone changes in cases of PC not receiving ADT
Townsend et al.[91]	224 cases of PC treated with ADT	9% of ADT group had 1 or more fractures, mean time to fracture 22 months	Osteoporotic fractures 5%

Quality of life

Author	Sample	Findings	Comments
Alibhai et al.[65]	87 cases of non-metastatic PC receiving ADT, 86 matched cases	36 SF QOL scores poorer if receiving ADT	Side-effects seen at 12 months persist at 36 months. No specific rehabilitation programme adopted

Table 11.4 continued

Author	Sample	Findings	Comments
Basaria et al.[66]	20 cases of PC treated by ADT, 18 treated PC cases awaiting ADT, 20 age-matched healthy controls	Decrease in desire, arousal and erections with ADT, lower QOL (physical function, physical health)	
Dacal et al.[70]	96 men, including short and long term ADT, no ADT and healthy controls	SF-36 questionnaire shows poor physical function, general health and physical health with ADT, unrelated to duration of ADT treatment	Associated lower levels of testosterone and free testosterone with ADT
Fowler et al.[92]	298 men who received ADT following radical prostatectomy compared with 2240 who did not receive ADT	ADT associated with lower scores on all 7 measures of health-related quality of life	
Green et al.[93]	65 patients with PC on ADT for 6 months, 16 community controls	Main impact of ADT is decreased sexual function, with decreased social and role function scores	
Potosky et al.[94]	431 cases of PC treated only by ADT or orchidectomy	Fewer orchidectomy patients rated their health as fair or poor than those receiving androgen suppressant drugs	
Sadetsky et al.[95]	2922 cases of prostate cancer	24-month self-reported quality of life poorer in those receiving ADT	Adverse effects even more marked if ADT is primary therapy
Spry et al.[96]	250 men receiving ADT for 9 months or more	Decrease of global health related quality of life and most function and symptom scales	Recovery in 3 months when ADT halted, slower recovery in older men
Stone et al.[74]	62 men receiving ADT as primary treatment of PC	Significant increase of fatigue severity over 3 months of treatment	28% of fatigue explained by psychological distress; also loss of virility and potency

Notes: ADL = activities of daily living; ADT = androgen deprivation therapy; BMD = bone mineral density; LBM = lean body mass; PC = prostate cancer; QOL = quality of life

Stone et al.[74] followed 62 men who were receiving ADT as a primary treatment of prostate cancer. They observed not only a progressive loss of muscle bulk, but also a decrease of grip strength and a faster fatigue of handgrip. Basaria et al.[66] also found a reduction of upper body strength when 20 cases of prostate cancer who had been treated with ADT were compared with 18 cases who were awaiting such treatment.

Several authors have found functional consequences from the loss of muscle tissue. Alibhai et al.[65] saw not only a reduction of grip strength in those receiving ADT, but also a deterioration in their times for a "get up and go" test, with the poor performance persisting throughout the 36 months of treatment. Bylow et al.[69] found an adverse effect upon performance of the activities of daily living in a quarter of 50 men over the age of 70 years who were treated by ADT, with a deterioration in balance, walking and chair-stand times. Levy et al.[73] reviewed data for 23 men who had received ADT for <6 months, and 12 men who had received ADT for >6 months relative to 13 who were not receiving ADT. The lean tissue mass decreased in proportion to the duration of ADT and 4-metre walk velocities were also slower in those receiving ADT.

Bone mineral density

Many investigations have associated androgen deprivation therapy with a progressive decrease in bone mineral density. Berrutti et al.[67] followed 36 cases of prostate cancer over the course of 12 months ADT; lumbar spine and hip bone mineral density were decreased relative to baseline over the 12 months of observation. Chen et al.[76] compared 62 cases of prostate cancer treated with ADT for 1–5 years; relative to 47 healthy controls; a lower bone mineral density was seen in the trochanter, inter-trochanter, hip and total scores. Daniell et al.[77] noted that in 26 cases treated by ADT or orchidectomy, the decrease of bone mineral density in the femoral neck continued unremittingly, with 2.4% and 7.6% decreases in years 1 and 2, and a further 1.4–2.6%/year loss over years 3–8.

The extent of bone loss seems to vary from one site to another. Preston et al.[86] compared 23 men who had been receiving ADT for 24 months with 30 controls. There was less bone loss in controls at all sites except the lumbar spine. The site of greatest loss was the distal forearm, where respective losses over 2 years were –9.4% and –4.4%. Galvao et al.[71] found decreases of bone mineral density of 1.5, 3.9, 1.3 and 2.4% respectively for the hip, spine, upper limb and whole body in a group of 72 men who were treated by ADT for 36 weeks. Possibly because of some protection from ambulation, this series showed no changes of bone density in the lower limbs. Greenspan et al.[79] measured changes of bone mineral density in 30 men receiving ADT for <6 months, 50 men receiving ADT >6 months, 72 not receiving ADT and 43 healthy controls. The rate of loss of bone mineral with ADT was increased five- to ten-fold relative to those not receiving ADT, with the maximal bone loss occurring during the first year of such treatment. Morote et al.[84] compared 31 cases of prostate cancer on ADT with 31 patients who were not receiving ADT. Those receiving androgen suppression experienced a 2.3–5.6% loss of bone mass at 12 months, and as in the previous study, a less severe loss continued to 24 months. Kiratli et al.[81] studied 36 patients with prostate cancer who received ADT or surgical castration and age matched controls. Bone mineral loss continued relative to controls for ten years, and the effect was greater following surgical treatment than after chemical castration.

Some investigations have demonstrated an increase in markers of bone turnover. Maillefert et al.[82] evaluated 12 cases of prostate cancer who were receiving ADT at 6, 12 and 18 months. There was a progressive decrease of bone mineral density (2.7, 3.9 and 6.6%) and increased serum osteocalcin levels. Basaria et al.[66] found a lower bone mineral density when 20 cases of prostate cancer treated with ADT were compared with 18 men who were awaiting such treatment.; moreover, the ADT group showed an increase of urinary N-telopeptide, another marker of bone turnover. Stoch et al.[90] examined 60 men with prostate cancer, including 19 who were receiving ADT. The ADT group showed a decreased bone mineral density at various sites, and also increased markers of bone turnover (N-telopeptides and bone-specific alkaline phosphatases). Likewise, Hatano et al.[80] reported that 6% of 218 cases of prostate cancer who were treated with ADT for >6 months developed fractures that were unrelated to tumour metastasis. A low bone mineral density and increased N-telopeptide concentrations were found in those developing fractures.

A greater propensity to fracture seems an inevitable consequence of the bone mineral loss. Malcolm et al.[83] followed 395 cases of prostate cancer who received ADT for an average of 66 months; 23% developed osteoporosis and 7% developed non-pathological fractures, with the risk of osteoporosis related to the duration of ADT. The primary end-point for Oefelein et al.[85] was the development of a fracture. In 181 cases of prostate cancer on ADT, 4% had sustained a fracture at 5 years and 20% at 10 years, the risk being lower in those who had conserved their body mass. Shahinian et al.[88] examined data for 50,613 cases of prostate cancer. In those who survived for 5 years or more, the risk of fracture with ADT was 19.6%, compared with 12.6% in those who did not receive such treatment. Moreover, in this series the risk of fracture was correlated with the dose of ADT administered. Smith et al.[89] evaluated medical claims from 5% of welfare beneficiaries (providing 3887 non-metastatic cases of prostate cancer). The overall clinical fracture rate was 7.88 per 100 person-years in those receiving ADT, compared with 6.51 per 100 person-years in matched controls, and this difference was confirmed by specific data for hip and vertebral fractures. Townsend et al.[91] studied 224 cases of prostate cancer who were treated with ADT; 9% of this group had 1 or more fractures within an average of 22 months of beginning treatment. Some of the fractures were due to severe trauma, but 5% were due to osteoporosis.

Although drugs such as alendronate can be given as a preventive measure, their effectiveness is limited and they have undesirable side-effects, so that it is a better tactic to counter the bone loss by a programme of weight-bearing exercise.

Quality of life

Not surprisingly, the loss of aerobic function, muscle strength and bone density are usually accompanied by a deterioration in the quality of life, particularly as reported on the scales for "physical health" and "physical function" on the short form medical health outcomes questionnaire (SF-36). Dacal et al.[70] used the SF-36 to demonstrate a significant deterioration in physical function, general and physical health in men receiving ADT relative to those who did not, although changes did not seem related to the duration of ADT; there were associated lower levels of testosterone and free testosterone. Fowler et al.[92] conducted a large-scale survey of men following radical prostatectomy; 298 individuals who received ADT were compared with 2240 who did not, and ADT was shown to be associated with lower scores on all 7 measures of the health-related quality of life. Potosky et al.[94] evaluated 431 cases of prostate cancer treated only by ADT or orchidectomy. In this study, fewer of the orchidectomy patients rated their health as only fair or poor as compared with those who were receiving a chemical suppressants of androgens. Sadetsky et al.[95] examined 2922 cases of prostate cancer; the 24-month self-reported quality of life was poorer in those receiving androgen suppressants, and they noted that the adverse effect was most marked if androgen deprivation was the primary form of therapy.

At least a part of the low scores on the SF-36 questionnaire seems related to reduced sexual function. Thus, Basaria et al.[66] reported not only a low score for the physical function and physical health scales of the SF-36, but also specific decreases in sexual function that included decreases in desire, arousal and erections, and a reduced score on Watt's scale of sexual function. Green et al.[93] compared 65 cases of prostate cancer receiving ADT for 6 months and 16 community controls. In this study, the main adverse effects of ADT were a decreased sexual function and a decrease in scores for social and role functioning. Spry et al.[96] followed 250 men receiving ADT for 9 months or longer. There was a decrease of global health-related quality of life and reduced scores on most function and symptom scales. Recovery commonly occurred within three months of halting ADT, but was slower in older men. Stone et al.[74] followed 62 men who were receiving ADT as the primary treatment of prostate cancer. A significant increase of fatigue severity was seen over three months of treatment; 28% of this was explained by psychological distress, but there was also a loss of virility and potency. Again, mood-elevating drugs can be prescribed, but an increase of physical activity is a healthier way of countering anxiety and elevating mood state.

Countering the side-effects of androgen deprivation and prostate surgery

Urinary incontinence is a frequent early sequel to either radical prostate surgery or irradiation. Many of the side-effects of subsequent androgen deprivation mirror what might be anticipated from an excessively sedentary lifestyle, and an early countering of the resulting loss of physical function is particularly important in what is typically an elderly population. A restoration of physical condition is likely to contribute not only to general well-being and independence, but also to long-term survival. Reviewers have found at least 25 controlled trials of various exercise programmes during the period of medical treatment (radiation or prostatectomy, androgen deprivation), and several have looked at exercise responses during after-care.[98-100] These analyses have generally pointed to improvements of aerobic and muscular fitness, a reduction of fatigue, less bone demineralization, an enhanced quality of life and a lower risk of urinary incontinence.

We will look at issues of spontaneously chosen habitual physical activity and specific programmes of aerobic and resistance exercise, emphasizing the need to adapt programmes in the light of specific complications of surgery and/or irradiation such as urinary incontinence and exercise-induced diarrhoea.

Habitual physical activity

The spontaneously chosen level of physical activity in patients undergoing treatment for prostate cancer often falls below recommended levels (Table 11.5). Chipperfield et al.[101] evaluated habitual physical activity in 356 men with prostate cancer; activity levels were lower in those receiving ADT than in those treated only by irradiation. Only 42% of the group met national physical activity guidelines, a low level of physical activity being associated with depression, anxiety and the presence of co-morbid conditions. Keogh et al.[102] studied 84 cases of prostate cancer that were receiving ADT. Less than a half of the men reported that they were physically active, although those who were indeed active had a higher quality of life than their sedentary peers. The attitude towards physical activity was the dominant predictor of the intention to be active, and perceived behavioural control was the dominant predictor of actual behaviour.

Livingston et al.[106] assigned 54 cases of prostate cancer receiving ADT to an exercise programme (2 supervised sessions/week for 12 weeks), and 93 men served as usual care controls. The 12-week programme increased the volume of self-reported vigorous activity, with gains in cognitive function and reduced levels of depression; the main unresolved issue was how long the stimulation of physical activity persisted after the patients had completed the immediate intervention.

Several reports have underlined an association between adequate physical activity and health outcomes, although given the cross-sectional nature of the observations, this could imply either benefit from the greater level of physical activity or less severe disease in those who were able to sustain an active lifestyle. Mennen-Winchell et al.[107] used Canada Fitness Survey data to estimate the endurance activity of 96 men who had been treated with ADT for longer than 9 months. The reported absolute level of physical activity averaged 4.6 MET-h/week, and the bone mineral density of the hip and spine was significantly correlated with the volume of reported endurance activity, whether expressed in minutes per week of physical activity or MET-h per week. Self-reported

Table 11.5 Habitual physical activity and response to rehabilitation during and following the treatment of prostate cancer

Author	Sample	Type of physical activity	Findings	Comments
Habitual physical activity				
Boisen et al.[103]	137 cases of PC	Self-selected	Active individuals had better quality of life on WHO scale and lower PSA levels	Cross-sectional comparison
Bonn et al.[104]	4623 men with localized PC followed for 10–15 yr	MET-h/day of walking/cycling, household work and exercise	194 deaths from PC, risk lower if walking/cycling >20 min/d or exercising >1 h/wk	Cross-sectional comparison
Chipperfield et al.[101]	356 men with PC	Adherence to national physical activity guidelines	42% of sample met guidelines; low activity was associated with depression, anxiety and co-morbid conditions	ADT patients less active than those given only irradiation
Kenfield et al.[105]	548 deaths in 2705 cases of PC followed 18 years	Vigorous activity >3 hr/wk vs. <1 hr/wk	61% lower risk of PC death (HR 0.39, 0.18–0.84) in active	
Keogh et al.[102]	84 cases of PC on ADT	"Active" on questionnaire response	Less than half reported they were active; active individuals had higher QOL	Attitude and perceived behavioural control main determinants of physical activity
Livingston et al.[106]	147 cases of PC on ADT, 54 exercised, 93 usual care	Self-reported activity, QOL, anxiety and depression	Exercise programme increased vigorous exercise, cognitive functioning, reduced depression	Duration of study only 12 weeks
Mennen-Winchell et al.[107]	96 men treated with ADT >9 months	Canadian Fitness Survey measure of habitual physical activity	BMD of hip and spine correlated with reported endurance activity (min/wk or MET-h/wk)	Self-reported endurance exercise 4.6 MET-h/wk, Resistance exercise 0.7 MET-h/wk

Table 11.5 continued

Author	Sample	Type of physical activity	Findings	Comments
Richman et al.[108]	1455 cases of localized PC followed ~2 years	Activity, walking duration and pace	117 events (local recurrence, secondary treatments, metastases, deaths) inversely associated with brisk walking	Few engaged in vigorous physical activity
Wolin et al.[109]	589 men undergoing radical prostatectomy for PC	Activity, obesity	Men active >1 h/wk and not obese less likely to be urinary incontinent (RR 0.74, 0.52–1.06)	

Aerobic and/or resistance exercise

Author	Sample	Type of physical activity	Findings	Comments
Buffart et al.[110]	100 cases of PC aged 71.7 yr	6 months supervised aerobic and resistance exercise (2 times/wk), pedometer, exercise prescription, 6 months home programme vs. printed advice	Exercise programme had significant benefits for global QOL, physical function and social function at 6 months	Gains of physical function sustained at 12 months
Cormie et al.[111]	63 cases of PC within 10 days of commencing ADT	3 months supervised aerobic and resistance exercise (32) vs. usual treatment (31)	Exercise preserved lean mass, avoided fat accumulation, greater aerobic power and muscle strength, lower body function, sexual function, less fatigue and psychological distress	
Culos-Reid et al.[112]	100 cases of PC receiving ADT >6 months; 53 in intervention group vs. 47 controls	16 week programme (supervised once/wk, 4 home sessions/ wk)	Significant increases in physical activity, changes in girth and blood pressure, trends to less depression and fatigue in exercise group	Conclusions limited by drop-outs (11/53 in intervention, 23/47 in controls)

Table 11.5 continued

Author	Sample	Type of physical activity	Findings	Comments
Galvao et al.[113]	10 men with localized PC on ADT	20 wk resistance training at 6–12 RM	Muscle strength and endurance increased, gains of forward and backward walking, chair rise time, stair climbing, 400 m walk and balance	
Galvao et al.[72]	57 cases of PC with ADT	12 weeks resistance and aerobic exercise vs. usual care	Increase of lean mass and muscle strength, faster forward and backward walk, less creactive protein, less fatigue and enhanced QOL in exercised group	No adverse events among exercisers
Galvao et al.[114]	100 cases of PC with ADT	6 months supervised exercise and 6 month home programme vs. educational material	Intervention gave increased aerobic performance, muscle mass and strength, self-reported physical functioning	Benefits seen at 6 months, maintained at 12 months with home programme
Hansen et al.[115]	10 cases of PC, 5 receiving ADT	Recumbent, high force eccentric cycle ergometer exercise 3 times/ wk for 12–15 min	Both groups showed enhanced strength and functional mobility (6 min walk distance)	Strength training response not impaired by ADT
Hanson et al.[116]	17 African Americans with PC, on ADT	12 weeks of strength training	Increase of muscle mass (2.7%), strength (28%), QOL (7%), decreased perceived fatigue (38%)	Muscle hypertrophy occurs in absence of testosterone. No control group
Jones et al.[117]	50 cases of PC treated by radical prostatectomy	5 walking sessions/week at 55–100% of peak oxygen intake vs. usual care	Similar reduction of erectile dysfunction in intervention and control group (20, 24%)	

Table 11.5 continued

Author	Sample	Type of physical activity	Findings	Comments
Kvorning et al.[118]	22 healthy but untrained men, 11 treated with ADT for 12 wk	8 wk strength training at 6–10 RM	No change of isometric knee extension in ADT group, untreated men show 10% increase	ADT reduced testosterone level 22.6 to 2.0 nmol/L
Monga et al.[119]	21 cases of PC treated by radiation alone; 11 aerobic exercise, 10 controls	Aerobic exercise 3 times/wk for 8 weeks	Exercised group showed gains in aerobic fitness, strength, flexibility, QOL, physical and social well-being, less fatigue	
Nilsen et al.[120]	58 cases of PC on ADT	28 followed 16 wk high-load strength training, 30 usual care controls	Gains of LBM in upper and lower limbs, but not total LBM; gains of 1-RM strength, sit-to-stand, stair climbing and shuttle walk in exercisers	No change in fat mass in exercisers
Norris et al.[121]	30 cases of PC not receiving ADT	12 weeks of resistance exercise 3 or 2 times/wk	Gains of lower body strength, chair stand time, sit-and-reach and 6 min walk distance greater for 3/wk than for 2/wk group	2/wk more favourable for mental component of QOL
Park et al.[122]	49 cases of PC	Resistance, flexibility and Kegel exercises 2/wk for 12 weeks vs. Kegel exercises alone	Exercise group fared better on strength (except grip), continence (71% vs. 44%) and QOL	
Segal et al.[123]	155 cases of PC on ADT	Resistance exercise 3/wk for 12 wks (n = 82) vs. wait-list controls (n = 73)	Increased levels of upper and lower body fitness, less fatigue, increased QOL in exercisers	No changes in BMI or body fat in exercisers

Table 11.5 continued

Author	Sample	Type of physical activity	Findings	Comments
Segal et al.[124]	121 cases of PC, some receiving ADT	Aerobic exercise vs. resistance exercise vs. usual care	Both aerobic and resistance exercise reduced fatigue; resistance exercise also yielded gains of strength and QOL	Resistance exercise reduced triglycerides and body fat
Windsor et al.[125]	66 cases of localized PC	Aerobic exercise (home-based walking 30 min 3/wk) vs. controls	Improvement of shuttle-run score with no significant increase in fatigue in exercisers	
Winters-Stone et al.[126]	51 cases of PC on ADT	1 yr of impact + resistance exercise (2 supervised sessions, 1 home/wk) vs. placebo stretching exercises	Loss of BMD: 0.4% in exercisers vs. −3.1% in controls	84% 1 yr adherence to exercise, no injuries

Special programmes

Author	Sample	Type of physical activity	Findings	Comments
Bourke et al.[127]	25 patients with advanced PC on ADT, vs. 25 standard treatment	12-week lifestyle programme (aerobic and resistance exercise, dietary advice)	Improved exercise behaviour, diet, energy intake, aerobic tolerance, muscle strength, less fatigue in exercisers	Attrition of exercisers 44% at 6 months, no effect on clinical
Bruun et al.[128]; Uth et al.[129]	Men receiving ADT >6 months, 21 soccer group, 20 controls, 32-wk follow-up	Community-based recreational football (45–60 min, 2–3/wk) vs. standard care	Soccer gave significant advantages in bone density, jump height and stair climbing	2 fibula fractures and 3 muscle or tendon injuries in soccer group
Craike et al.[130]	52 men treated for PC	3 month supervised exercise programme	Adherence 80%; role functioning and hormonal symptoms predicted adherence	Positive perceptions of ability increased adherence
Demark-Wahnefried et al.[131]	543 prostate and breast cancer survivors	Tailored diet and exercise print intervention vs. non-tailored materials	Tailored programme increased exercise (59 vs. 39 min/wk), BMI −0.3 vs. +0.1 kg/m^2	95.6% completed 1-yr intervention

Table 11.5 continued

Author	Sample	Type of physical activity	Findings	Comments
Sajid et al.[132]	19 cases of PC on ADT	Home-based walking/ resistance exercise 5 days/wk vs. technology-mediated home programme vs. usual care for 6 wks	Best response is to home-based programme (increase of 2720 steps/day)	
Santa Mina et al.[133]	10 cases of PC on ADT	60 min group exercise or personal trainer, 3/wk for 8 wk	Suggestion of better response with personal trainer	
Skinner et al.[134]	51 cases of PC	4 sessions of supervised exercise over 4 wk	Gains of strength, 400 m walk, chair stands, walking speed, sit-and-reach, well-being	Uncontrolled study
Uth et al.[135, 136]	57 men receiving ADT >6 months	32 weeks of recreational football 2–3 times/wk vs. standard care	Football gave significant gains in BMD, LBM, muscle strength, maximal oxygen intake, jump height and stair climbing	

Notes: ADT = androgen deprivation therapy; BMD = bone mineral density; HR = hazard ratio; LBM = lean body mass; MET = metabolic equivalent; PC = prostate cancer; PSA = prostate serum antigen; QOL = quality of life; RM = repetition maximum; RR = relative risk

participation in endurance exercise was also associated with greater density of the hip bones as assessed by dual energy x-ray absorptiometry.[107] Others have commented on an association of habitual physical activity with muscular fitness, physical functioning and quality of life in prostate cancer survivors.[72, 100, 137] Thus, a survey of questionnaire respondents (137 of 348 men treated for prostate cancer) made a cross-sectional comparison between those who maintained an adequate level of habitual physical activity and those who did not. It found greater social participation, a better quality of life on the WHO scale and lower prostate serum antigen levels in the more active individuals.[103]

Both a lower overall and a lower prostate-specific mortality have been seen in more active individuals. Bonn et al.[104] followed 4623 men with localized prostate cancer for 10–15 years. A questionnaire assessed activity (MET-h/day invested in walking/cycling, household work and exercise). There were 194 deaths from prostate cancer during the follow-up, with a lower risk lower among those walking/cycling >20 min/day or exercising >1 hour per week. A similar study by Kenfield et al.[105] looked at 548 deaths in 2705 cases of prostate cancer who were followed for 18 years. Survival was compared between those taking more than three hours vigorous activity per week and those spending less than one hour per week. Those taking more vigorous activity had a 61% lower risk of dying from prostate cancer (hazard ratio 0.39 [0.18–0.84]). The same group of investigators (Richman et al.[108]) followed 1455 cases of localized prostate cancer for an average of ~2 years. Over the follow-up, there were a total of 117 events (a local recurrence, a need for secondary treatment, metastases or death). Few of the sample engaged in vigorous physical activity. Nevertheless, disease progression was less likely in men who walked briskly for three or more hours per week, or who engaged in vigorous physical activity more than three hours per week than in those who did not take such exercise (HR = 0.63 [0.32–1.23], p for trend = 0.17).

Urinary incontinence is often a major handicap following radical prostatectomy. Wolin et al.[109] demonstrated that in 589 men who had undergone such treatment there was a trend to a lower risk of incontinence in men who were active for more than one hour per week (relative risk 0.74 [0.52–1.06]). However, incontinence can limit exercise participation, so it is difficult to be sure whether this is cause or effect!

Aerobic and resistance exercise programmes

Many investigators have followed the programmes recommended by consensus groups (a combination of aerobic, resistance, impact and flexibility exercises). However, some have focused uniquely on aerobic or resistance training. Some interventions have continued for as long as a year. In 100 cases of prostate cancer who were receiving ADT, Galvao et al.[114] compared responses in those individuals who received six months of supervised exercise followed by a six-month home programme with the findings in a group who were simply given educational material. The direct exercise intervention enhanced aerobic performance, muscle mass, strength and self-reported physical functioning compared to the comparison group. Benefits were apparent at six months, and were maintained after six further months of home exercises. In another report from the same laboratory, Buffart et al.[110] followed 100 cases of prostate cancer aged an average of 71.7 years for 12 months. A half of the group received six months of supervised aerobic and resistance exercise twice per week, followed by a six-month home programme with a pedometer and a detailed exercise prescription, and the remaining subjects received standard treatment plus some printed advice. At six months, the exercise group showed significant benefit relative to the comparison group in terms of the global quality of life, physical function and social function, and these gains of physical function were sustained at 12 months.

Culos-Reid et al.[112] assigned 53 of 100 cases of prostate cancer who had been receiving ADT for longer than 6 months to a 16 week programme of once-weekly supervised exercise, supplemented by up to 4 home sessions per week. Relative to 47 controls, they showed significant increases in physical activity and reductions of abdominal girth and blood pressure, with trends to less depression and fatigue; however, conclusions were limited by the small sample and a substantial number of drop-outs (11 in the intervention group and 23 among the controls).

The benefits of increased exercise can be realized quite quickly. Thus, Galvao et al.[72] examined 57 cases of prostate cancer who were receiving ADT after 12 weeks of assignment to either a bi-weekly aerobic and resistance exercise programme or usual care. The three-month intervention was sufficient to induce increases of lean mass and muscle strength, faster forward and backward walking speeds, a decrease of one marker of chronic inflammation (c-reactive protein concentrations), less fatigue and an enhanced quality of life. Moreover, there were no adverse events among the exercisers. Cormie et al.[111] examined the benefits of the early initiation of an aerobic and resistance exercise programme. Cases were contacted within 10 days of beginning ADT, with 32 following a 3-month aerobic and resistance exercise programme (twice weekly, supplemented by home exercise), and 31 subjects serving as controls. The exercise programme conserved lean mass and reduced the accumulation of body fat relative to the controls. The exercisers also showed a greater aerobic power and muscular strength, with better lower body function and sexual function, less fatigue and less psychological distress.

Segal et al.[124] compared aerobic exercise with resistance exercise or usual treatment in 121 cases of prostate cancer, some of whom were receiving ADT. Both aerobic and resistance exercise increased aerobic fitness and reduced fatigue relative to usual treatment, but the resistance exercise group also demonstrated gains of strength and quality of life, with a reduction of triglycerides and body fat.

Among studies using only aerobic training, some have found a good response, but in others gains have been disappointing. Monga et al.[119] investigated 21 patients with localized prostate cancer, treated by irradiation alone. Eleven of the group undertook eight weeks of aerobic exercise (three times/week), and despite the short duration of their programme, they showed substantial advantages relative to the ten controls (gains in aerobic fitness, strength, flexibility, quality of life, physical and social well-being, and less fatigue). Windsor et al.[125] examined 66 cases of localized prostate cancer. A half of the group were assigned to a home-based aerobic walking programme (30 minutes of walking, 3 times/week). All of the exercisers maintained at least this minimum activity over the four weeks of radiotherapy. Despite the very brief duration of the intervention, the exercised group showed an improved score on the shuttle run test, with no significant increase of fatigue.

In contrast, Jones et al.[117] studied 50 cases of prostate cancer who had under-gone radical prostatectomy, but apparently were not receiving ADT. A six-months aerobic programme (5 walking sessions/week at 55–100% of peak oxygen intake) led to no greater reduction of erectile dysfunction among the exercisers than that seen in the usual care group.

Among programmes that have focused specifically on resistance training, substantial gains of muscle strength have been observed, despite the low levels of circulating androgens caused by the ADT. Galvao et al.[113] enrolled 10 men with localized prostate cancer who were receiving ADT in a 20 week resistance training at a 6–12 repetition maximum intensity. This induced gains in muscle strength and endurance, forward and backward walking times, chair-stand speed, stair climbing, 400 m walk and balance. Hansen et al.[115] looked at the effects of eccentric training in ten cases of prostate cancer, five of whom were receiving ADT. The programme involved recumbent, high force eccentric cycle ergometer exercise performed for 12–15 minutes, 3 times per week. This regimen enhanced isometric strength and functional mobility, the latter shown by a greater six minute walking distance, whether or not the subject was receiving ADT. Hanson et al.[116] made similar observations on 17 African Americans with prostate cancer who were receiving ADT; 12 weeks of strength training led to an increase of muscle mass (2.7%), strength (28%) and quality of life (7%) and a decreased perception of fatigue (38%), despite the demonstrated suppression of testosterone levels. Nilsen et al.[120] studied 58 cases of prostate cancer on ADT; 28 of the group followed a 16-week high-load strength training programme, and the other 30 men served as usual care controls. Relative to the controls, the strength-training group showed gains of lean body mass in the upper and lower limbs (although not in the total lean mass), gains of 1-RM strength, sit-to-stand times, stair-climbing performance and shuttle-walk scores. Segal et al.[123] evaluated 155 cases of prostate cancer on ADT; 82 were assigned to resistance exercise 3 times per week for 12 weeks, and 73 remained in a wait-list control group. Despite the ADT, the exercised group again showed increased levels of upper and lower body fitness, less fatigue and an increased quality of life.

In contrast to the responses observed in those with prostate cancer, Kvorning et al.[118] carried out a study on 22 healthy but untrained men, administering ADT to 11 of the group for 12 weeks. In this population, strength training (8 weeks at 6–10 RM) increased the isometric knee extension of the controls by 10%, but there was no change of strength in those receiving ADT (where circulating testosterone levels had dropped from 22.6 to 2.0 nmol/L).

Possibly, the gains of muscle strength realized despite ADT in those with prostate cancer may reflect better neuromuscular coordination rather than muscle hypertrophy, since in general there have been no changes of body mass index or body fat in response to the resistance training.

How often should resistance exercise be performed? Unfortunately, the answer is not very clear. Norris et al.[121] assigned 30 cases of prostate cancer who were not receiving ADT to 12 weeks of resistance exercise, performed 2 or 3 times per week. The thrice-weekly group fared better than the twice-weekly group on the physical components of response, including gains of lower body strength, chair-stand times, sit-and-reach distances and the six minute walk distance, but the twice per week group fared better on the mental component of quality of life, including scores for mental health, vitality, emotional role, anxiety, happiness and perceived stress.

The loss of bone mineral density is a major concern with ADT. Winters-Stone et al.[126] thus compared one year of high impact plus resistance exercise (two one-hour supervised and one home session/week) with a placebo programme of light stretching in 51 cases of prostate cancer on ADT. The resistance exercise group showed a one-year adherence of 84%, without injuries, and a substantially smaller decrease in bone mineral density relative to those on the stretching programme (an average loss of only –0.4% vs. –3.1%).

Park et al.[122] evaluated a combination of resistance, flexibility and Kegel exercises vs. Kegel exercises alone in a 12 week biweekly trial. The exercise group fared better on measures of strength (except grip strength), urinary continence (71% vs. 44%, with 24-hour pad weights of 12 vs. 46 g), quality of life and depression scales.

Special considerations in programme design

Unfortunately, vigorous physical activity seems necessary for enhanced outcomes during ADT.[106] Relatively few prostate cancer survivors spontaneously engage in adequate volumes of physical activity.[101] This may be in part because of the symptoms associated with androgen-suppression[130] but another issue is the need to adapt programmes in the light of specific complications such as urinary incontinence and exercise-induced diarrhoea. Some investigators have found good sustained compliance with what seem fairly standard exercise programmes, albeit with some individual tailoring, but others have suggested that motivation can be boosted by novel approaches such as a recreational soccer programme[129] or the use of a personal trainer.

Craike et al.[130] examined factors influencing adherence to a 3-month exercise programme (2 supervised sessions, 1 unsupervised session/week) in 52 men who were undergoing treatment for prostate cancer. Adherence averaged 80% and was influenced by role functioning and hormone-related symptoms, with effects from perceptions of ability increasing adherence.

Bourke et al.[127] compared the response to a 12-week lifestyle programme with standard treatment in 2 groups of 25 men with advanced prostate cancer who were receiving ADT. The 12-week lifestyle programme comprised aerobic and resistance exercise (twice weekly for six weeks, once weekly for a further six weeks, plus self-directed exercise and dietary advice). This regimen improved exercise behaviour, diet, energy intake, aerobic tolerance, muscle strength and reduced fatigue in participants, but it had no effect on clinical disease, and the attrition rate was 44% by six months.

Demark-Wahnefried et al.[131] explored the value of personally tailored mailed recommendations for diet and exercise vs. non-tailored recommendations in a mixed sample of 543 breast and prostate cancer survivors. The personally tailored information led to a larger increase in weekly exercise (59 vs. 39 min) relative to the non-tailored recommendations, and there was also a favourable change in the body mass index of participants (–0.3 vs. +0.1 kg/m²). Moreover, the compliance for the one-year intervention was high (95.6%). Another comparison of a supervised programme of aerobic and resistance exercise with general printed physical activity recommendations found that the former gave greater improvements in global quality of life as well as physical and social functioning, all mediated by improved lower body functioning.[106, 110, 114] Sajid et al.[132] divided 19 cases of prostate cancer on ADT between a home-based walking and resistance exercise programme, a technology mediated programme and usual care. The sample was rather small for clear conclusions, but the home programme appeared to yield the best results, with an increase in step count of 2720 steps/day over the course of the trial.

Skinner et al.[134] examined the effects of a minimal exercise intervention (foursessions of supervised exercise over four weeks) in an uncontrolled study of 51 cases of prostate cancer. They reported gains of muscle strength, 400 m walk times, chair-stand times, walking speed, sit-and-reach and well-being with this very limited intervention.

Bruun et al.[128] and Uth et al.[129] argued for the motivational value of participating in community-based recreational soccer. Men receiving ADT for longer than six months were divided into a soccer group (n = 21) and a usual treatment group (n = 20). Over a 32-week follow-up, the soccer participants gained significant advantages in bone density, jump height and stair climbing relative to standard care, but they sustained two fractures of the fibula and three muscle or tendon injuries. Uth et al.[135, 136] further evaluated the motivational and therapeutic value of recreational soccer (2–3 games/week for 32 weeks) in 57 men who were receiving ADT. Relative to usual-care controls, they showed substantial gains in bone mineral density, along with increases of lean body mass, muscle strength, maximal oxygen intake, jump height and stair-climbing ability.

Santa Mina et al.[133] compared the response to 60 minutes of group exercise, 3 times per week for 8 weeks to the benefits seen with the services of a personal trainer. In ten cases, there was a trend suggesting that the personal trainer was somewhat more effective than group exercise.

Areas for further research

The value of regular physical activity as a means of reducing the risk of prostate cancer is still not proven conclusively. One obstacle to resolving this issue is that even when a large population is followed for a long period, the number of cases of cancer remains quite small. Given the number of studies that have already been carried out, meta-analysis may provide some resolution to this question, but challenges include differences between samples, differing criteria used to identify active individuals and variations in the age at which activity has been evaluated. One alternative may be to study a high-risk group, looking at the effectiveness of increased physical activity in preventing a recurrence of the tumour in those who have completed treatment. Possibly, as mechanisms of carcinogenesis are clarified, it may also become possible to determine which types of physical activity are best suited to modulating the causal agents. It also seems worth following up suggestions from *post-hoc* analyses that susceptibility to exercise is modified by the subject's age or by the aggressivity of the tumour.

The spontaneously chosen level of physical activity amongst those undergoing treatment for prostate cancer is typically below recommended levels for good health, and there is a need for research on tactics to increase habitual physical activity in this population. The gains of strength observed with resistance training in patients who are receiving ADT are intriguing, and studies are needed to examine how far these represent true muscle hypertrophy and how far they simply reflect test learning and greater neuromuscular coordination.

Practical implications and conclusions

Despite many cohort and case control studies, the suggestion that physical activity reduces the risk of prostate cancer has yet to be proven conclusively. About a half of studies show a favourable trend or a statistically significant benefit, commonly with a reduction in risk of 10–30%. Moreover, there is little evidence that moderate exercise has an adverse effect upon prostate health, so that it is good practice to advocate regular exercise while conclusive proof is awaited. The use of ADT following the immediate treatment of prostate cancer unfortunately carries many side-effects, including a reduction of aerobic and muscle power, a demineralization of bone and an impaired quality of life. However, an exercise rehabilitation programme is helpful in countering these adverse effects.

References

1. Friedenreich CM, Thune I. A review of physical activity and prostate cancer risk. *Cancer Causes Control* 2001; 12: 461–475.
2. Hackney AC, Sinning WE, Bruot BC. Reproductive hormonal profiles of endurance trained and untrained males. *Med Sci Sports Exerc* 1988; 20: 60–65.
3. Torti D, Matheson GO. Exercise and prostate cancer. *Sports Med* 2004; 34(6): 363–369.
4. Morote J, Celma A, Planas J, et al. Sedentarismo y sobrepeso como factores de riesgo en la detección del cáncer de próstata y su agresividad [Sedentarism and overweight as risk factors in the detection and aggressivity of prostate cancer]. *Actas Urol Esp* 2014; 38(4): 232–237.
5. Paffenbarger RS, Hyde RT, Wing AL. Physical activity and incidence of cancer in diverse populations: a preliminary report. *Am J Clin Nutr* 1987; 45(1 Suppl.): 712–717.
6. Hartman TJ, Albanes D, Rautalahti M, et al. Physical activity and prostate cancer in the alpha-tocopherol, beta carotene (ATBC) cancer prevention study (Finland). *Cancer Causes Control* 1998; 9: 11–18.
7. Johnsen NF, Tjønneland A, Thomsen BLR, et al. Physical activity and risk of prostate cancer in the European prospective investigation into cancer and nutrition (EPIC) cohort. *Int J Cancer* 2009; 125: 902–908.
8. Lund Nielsen TI, Johnsen R, Vatten LJ. Socio-economic and lifestyle factors associated with the risk of prostate cancer. *Br J Cancer* 2000; 82(7): 1358–1363.

9. Putnam SD, Cerhan JR, Parker AS, et al. Lifestyle and anthropometric risk factors for prostate cancer in a cohort of Iowa men. *Am J Epidemiol* 2000; 10: 361–369.

10. Severson RK, Nomura AMY, Grove JS, et al. A prospective analysis of physical activity and cancer. *Am J Epidemiol* 1989; 130(3): 522–529.

11. Albanes D, Blair A, Taylor PR. Physical activity and the risk of cancer in the NHANES I population. *Am J Publ Health* 1989; 79: 744–750.

12. Clarke G, Whittemore AS. Prostate cancer risk in relationship to anthropometry and physical activity: the National Health and Nutrition Examination Survey I epidemiological follow-up study. *Cancer Epidemiol Biomarkers Prev* 2000; 9: 875–881.

13. Grotta A, Bottai M, Adami H-O, et al. Physical activtiy and body mass index as predictors of prostate cancer. *World J Urol* 2015; 33: 1495–1502.

14. Hrafnkelsdóttir SM, Torfadóttir J, Aspelund T, et al. Physical activity from early adulthood and risk of prostate cancer: a 24-year follow-up study among Icelandic men. *Cancer Prev Res* 2015; 8(10): 905–911.

15. Hsing AW, McLaughlin JK, Zheng W, et al. Occupation, physical activity, and risk of prostate cancer in Shanghai, People's Republic of China. *Cancer Causes Control* 1994; 5: 136–140.

16. Norman A, Moradi T, Gridley G, et al. Occupational physical acvtivity and risk for prostate cancer in a nationwide cohort study in Sweden. *Br J Cancer* 2002; 86: 70–75.

17. Orsini N, Bellocco R, Botti M, et al. A prospective study of lifetime physical activity and prostate cancer incidence and mortality. *Br J Cancer* 2009; 101: 1932–1938.

18. Parent ME, Rousseau MC, El Zein M, et al. Occupational and recreational physical activity during adult life and the risk of cancer among men. *Cancer Epidemiol* 2011; 35(2): 151–159.

19. Thune I, Lund E. Physical activity and the risk of prostate and testicular cancer: a cohort study of 53,000 Norwegian men. *Cancer Causes Control* 1994; 5: 549–556.

20. Vena JE, Graham S, Zielezny M, et al. Occupational exercise and risk of cancer. *Am J Clin Nutr* 1987; 45: 318–327.

21. Zeegers MPA, Dirx MJM, van den Brandt PA. Physical activity and the risk of prostate cancer in the Netherlands cohort study, results after 9.3 years follow-up. *Cancer Epidemiol Biomarkers Prev* 2005; 14(6): 1490–1495.

22. Bairati I, Jarouche R and Meyer Fea. Lifetime occupational physical activity and incidental prostate cancer (Canada). *Cancer Causes Control* 2000; 11: 759–764.

23. Brownson RC, Chang JC, Davis JR, et al. Physical activity on the job and cancer in Missouri. *Am J Publ Health* 1991; 81(5): 639–642.

24. Doolan GW, Benke G, Giles GG, et al. A case control study investigating the effects of levels of physical activity at work as a risk factor for prostate cancer. *Environ Health* 2014; 13: 64.

25. Dosemeci M, Hayes RB, Vetter R, et al. Occupational physical activity, socioeconomic status, and risks of 15 cancer sites in Turkey. *Cancer Causes Control* 1993; 4: 313–321.

26. Friedenreich CM, McGregor SE, Courneya KS, et al. Case-control study of lifetime physical activity and prostate cancer. *Am J Epidemiol* 2004; 159(8): 740–749.

27. Hosseini M, Alinaghi SAS, Mahmoudi M, et al. A case-control study of risk factors for prostate cancer in Iran. *Acat Med Iran* 2010; 48(1): 61–66.

28. Krishnadasan A, Kennedy N, Zhao Y, et al. Nested case-control study of occupational physical activity and prostate cancer among workers using a job exposure matrix. *Cancer Causes Control* 2008; 19: 107–114.

29. Lacey JV, Deng J, Dosemeci M, et al. Prostate cancer, benign prostate hyperplasia and physical activity in Shanghai, China. *Int J Epidemiol* 2001; 30: 341–349.

30. Lagiou A, Samoli E, Georgila C, et al. Occupational physical activity in relation with prostate cancer and benign prostate hyperplasia. *Eur J Cancer Prev* 2008; 17: 336–339.

31. Le Marchand L, Kolonel LN, Yoshizawa CN. Lifetime occupational phyical activity and prostate cancer. *Am J Epidemiol* 1991; 133(2): 103–111.

32. Sass-Kortak AM, Purdham JT, Kreiger N, et al. Occupational risk factors for prostate cancer. *Am J Industr Med* 2007; 50: 568–576.

33. Strom SS, Yamamura Y, Flores-Sandoval FN, et al. Prostate cancer in Mexican-Americans: identification of risk factors. *Prostate* 2008; 68: 563–570.

34. Villeneuve PJ, Johnson KC, Kreiger N, et al. Riskn factors for prostate cancer: results from the Canadian natioinal enhanced cancer surveillance system. *Cancer Causes Control* 1999; 10: 355–367.

35. Wiklund F, Lageros YT, Chang E, et al. Lifetime total physical activity and prostate cancer in a population-based case-control study in Sweden. *Eur J Epidemiol* 2008; 23: 739–746.

36. Crespo CJ, Garcia-Palmieri MR, Smit E, et al. Physical activity and prostate cancer mortality in Puerto Rican men. *J Phys Activ Health* 2008; 5(6): 918–929.

37. Giovannucci E, Leitzmann E, Spiegelman D, et al. A prospective study of physical activity and prostate cancer in male health professionals. *Cancer Res* 1998; 58: 5117–5122.

38. Giovannucci E, Liu Y, Leitzman MF, et al. A prospective study of physical activity and incident and fatal prostate cancer. *Arch Intern Med* 2005; 165: 1005–1010.

39. Lee I-M, Paffenbarger RS, Hsieh C-C. Physical activity and risk of prostatic cancer among College alumni. *Am J Epidemiol* 1992; 135(2): 169–179.

40. Lee I-M, Sesso HD, Paffenbarger RS. A prospective cohort study of physical activity and body size in relation to prostate cancer risk (United States). *Cancer Causes Control* 2001; 12: 187–193.

41. Littman AJ, Kristal AR, White E. Recreational physical activity and prostate cancer risk (United States). *Cancer Causes Control* 2006; 17: 831–841.

42. Liu S, Lee I-M, Linson P, et al. A prospective study of physical activity and risk of prostate cancer in US physicians. *Int J Epidemiol* 2000; 29: 29–35.

43. Moore SC, Peters TM, Ahn J, et al. Physical activity in relation to total, advanced and fatal prostate cancer. *Cancer Epidemiol Biomarkers Prev* 2008; 17(9): 2458–2466.

44. Nilsen TIL, Romundstad PR, Vatten LJ. Recreational physical activity and risk of prostate cancer; a prospective population-based study in Norway (the HUNT study). *Int J Cancer* 2006; 119: 2943–2947.

45. Patel AV, Rodriguez C, Jacobs EJ, et al. Recreational physical activity and risk of prostate cancer in a large cohort of US men. Cancer Epidemiol Biomarkers Prev 2005; 14(1): 275–279.

46. Platz E, Leitzmann MF, Michaud DS, et al. Interrelation of energy intake, body size and physical activity with prostate cancer in a large prospective cohort study. *Cancer Res* 2003; 63: 8542–8548.

47. Steenland K, Nowlin S, Palu S. Cancer incidence in the National Health and Nutrition Survey I follow-up data: diabetes, cholesterol and physical activity. *Cancer Epidemiol Biomarkers Prev* 1995; 4: 807–811.

48. Wannamethee SG, Shaper AG, Walker M. Physical activity and risk of cancer in middle-aged men. *Br J Cancer* 2001; 85(9): 1311–1316.

49. Andersson S-O, Baron J, Wolk A, et al. Early life risk factors for prostate cancer: a population-based case-control study in Sweden. *Cancer Epidemiol Biomarkers Prev* 1995; 4: 187–192.

50. Darlington GA, Kreiger N, Lightfoot N, et al. Prostate cancer risk and diet, recreational physical activity and cigarette smoking. *Chron Dis Canada* 2007; 27(4): 145–153.

51. Jian L, Shen ZJ, Lee AH, et al. Moderate physical activity and prostate cancer risk: a case-control study in China. *Eur J Epidemiol* 2005; 20: 155–160.

52. Sung JF, Lin RS, Pu YS, et al. Risk factors for prostate carcinoma in Taiwan: a case-control study in a Chinese population. *Cancer* 1999; 86(3): 484–491.

53. West DW, Slattery ML and Robison LM, et al. Adult dietary intake and prostate cancer risk in Utah: a case-control study with special emphasis on aggressive tumours. *Cancer Causes Control* 1991; 2: 85–94.

54. Whittemore AS, Kolonel LN, Wu AH, et al. Prostate cancer in relation to diet, physical activity, and body size in blacks, whites, and Asians in the United States and Canada. *J Natl Cancer Inst* 1995; 87: 652–661.

55. Yu H, Harris RE, Wynder EL. Case-control study of prostate cancer and socio-economic factors. *Prostate* 1988; 13: 317–325.

56. Lee I-M, Paffenbarger RS. Physical activity and its relation to cancer risk: a prospective study of college alumni. *Med Sci Sports Exerc* 1994; 26(7): 831–837.

57. Klap J, Schmid M, Loughlin KR. The relationship between total testosterone levels and prostate cancer: a review of the continuing controversy. *J Urol* 2015; 193: 404–415.

58. Noble RL. Androgen use by athletes: a possible cancer risk. *Can Med Assoc J* 1984; 130: 549–550.

59. Merrill RM, Perego UAM, Heiner SW. Age, lifestyle, health risk indicators and prostate specific antigen scores in men participating in the world senior games. *Urol Oncol* 2002; 7: 105–109.

60. Oliveira SN, Kohl HW, Trichopoulos T, et al. The association between cardiorespiratory fitness and prostate cancer. *Med Sci Sports Exerc* 1996; 28(1): 97–104.

61. Hållmarker U, James S, Michaëlsson K, et al. Cancer incidence in participants in a long-distance ski race (Vasaloppet, Sweden) compared to the background population. *Eur J Cancer* 2015; 51(4): 558–568.

62. Polednak AP. College athletics, body size and cancer mortality. *Cancer* 1976; 38: 382–387.

63. Heitkamp HC, Jelas I. Korperlich Activitat zur Primarpravention des Prostata-karzinoms. Mogliche Mechanismen [Physical activity in the prevention of prostate carcinoma. Possible mechanisms]. *Urologe* 2012; 51: 527–532.

64. Barnard RJ, Leung PS, Aronson WJ, et al. A mechanism to explain how regular exercise reduces the risk for prostate cancer. *Eur J Cancer Prev* 2007; 16: 415–421.

65. Alibhai SMH, Breunis H, Timilshina N, et al. Long-term impact of androgen-deprivation therapy on physical function and quality of life. *Cancer Causes Control* 2015; 121: 2350–2357.

66. Basaria S, Lieb J, Tang AM, et al. Long-term effects of androgen deprivation therapy in prostate cancer patients. *Clin Endocrinol* 2002; 56: 779–786.

67. Berrutti A, Dogliotti L, Terrone C, et al. Changes in bone mineral density, lean body mass and fat content as measured by dual energy in patients with prostate cancer without apparent bone metastases given androgen deprivation therapy. *J Urol* 2002; 167: 2361–2367.

68. Boxer RS, Kenny AM, Dowsett R, et al. The effect of 6 months of androgen deprivation therapy on muscle and fat mass in older men with localized prostate cancer. *Aging Male* 2005; 8(3/4): 207–212.
69. Bylow K, Dale W, Mustian K, et al. Falls and physical performance deficits in older patients with prostate c ancer undergoing androgen deprivation therapy. *Urology* 2008; 72: 422–427.
70. Dacal K, Sereika SM, Greenspan SL. Quality of life in prostate cancer patients taking androgen deprivation therapy. *J Am Geriatr Soc* 2006; 54: 85–90.
71. Galvao DA, Spry NA, Taaffe DR, et al. Changes in muscle, fat and bone mass after 36 weeks of maximal androgen blockade for prostate cancer. *BJU Int* 2008; 102: 44–47.
72. Galvao DA, Taaffe DR, Spry N. et al. Combined resistance and aerobic exercise program reverses muscle loss in men undergoing androgen suppression therapy for prostate cancer without bone metastases: a randomized controlled trial. *J Clin Oncol* 2010; 28: 340–347.
73. Levy ME, Perera S, van Londen GJ, et al. Physical function changes in prostate cancer patients on androgen deprivation therapy: a 2-year prospective study. *Urology* 2008; 71: 735–739.
74. Stone P, Hardy J, Huddart R, et al. Fatigue in patients with prostate cancer receiving hormone therapy. *Eur J Cancer* 2000; 36: 1134–1141.
75. van Londen GJ, Levy ME, Perera S, et al. Body composition changes during androgen deprivation therapy for prostate cancer: a 2-year prospective study. *Crit Rev Oncol Hematol* 2008; 68(2): 172–177.
76. Chen Z, Maricic M, Nguyen P, et al. Low bone desity and high percentage body fat among men who were treated with androgen deprivation therapy for prostate cancer. *Cancer* 2002; 95(10): 2136–2144.
77. Daniell HW. Osteoporosis after orchidectomy for prostate cancer. *J Urol* 1997; 157: 439–444.
78. Daniell HW. Osteoporosis due to androgen deprivation therapy in men with prostate cancer. *Urology* 2001; 58(Suppl. 2A): 101–107.
79. Greenspan SL, Coates P, Sereika SM, et al. Bone loss after initiation of androgen deprivation therapy in patients with prostate cancer. *J Clin Endocrinol Metab* 2005; 90: 6410–6417.
80. Hatano T, Oishi Y, Furuta A, et al. Incidence of bone fracture in patients receiving luteinizing hormone relasing hormone agonists for prostate cancer. *BJU Internat* 2000; 86: 449–452.
81. Kiratli BJ, Srinivas S, Perkash I, et al. Progressive decrease in bone density over 10 years of androgen deprivation therapy in patients with prostate cancer. *Urology* 2001; 57: 127–132.
82. Maillefert JF, Sibilia J, Michel F, et al. Bone mineral density in men treated with synthetic gonadotropin-releasing hormone agonists for prostatic carcinoma. *J Urol* 1999; 161(4): 1219–1222.
83. Malcolm JB, Derweesh IH, Kincade MC, et al. Osteoporosis and fractures after androgen deprivation initiation for prostate cancer. *Can J Urol* 2007; 14(3): 3551–3559.
84. Morote J, Orsola A, Abascal JM, et al. Bone mineral density changes in patients with prostate cancer during the first 2 years of androgen suppression. *J Urol* 2006; 175: 1679–1683.
85. Oefelein MG, Ricchuiti V, Conrad W, et al. Skeletal fracture associated with androgen suppression induced osteoporosis: The clinical incidence and risk factors for patients with prostate cancer. *J Urol* 2001; 166: 1724–1728.

86. Preston DM, Torréns JI, Harding P, et al. Androgen deprivation in men with prostate cancer is associated with an increased rate of bone loss. *Prostate Cancer Prostate Dis* 2002; 5: 304–310.
87. Ross RW, Small EJ. Osteoporosis in men treated with androgen deprivation therapy for prostate cancer. *J Urol* 2002; 167: 1952–1956.
88. Shahinian VB, Kuo Y-F, Freeman JL, et al. Risk of fracture after androgen deprivation for prostate cancer. *N Engl J Med* 2005; 352(2): 154–164.
89. Smith MR, Lee WC, Brandman J, et al. Gonadotrophin-releasing hormone agonists and fracture risk: A claims-based cohort study of men with nonmetastatic prostate cancer. *J Clin Oncol* 2005; 23(31): 7897–7903.
90. Stoch SA, Parker RA, Chen L, et al. Bone loss in men with prostate cancer treated with gonadotropin-releasing hormone agonists. *J Clin Endocrinol Metab* 2001; 86: 2787–2791.
91. Townsend MF, Sanders WH, Northway R, et al. Bone fractures associated with luteinizing hormone-releasing hormone agonists used in the treatment of prostate carcinoma. *Cancer* 1997; 79(3): 545–550.
92. Fowler FJ, Collins M, Corkery EW, et al. The impact of androgen deprivation on quality of life after radical prostatectomy for prostate cancer. *Cancer* 2002; 95: 287–295.
93. Green HJ, Pakenham KI, Headley RC, et al. Coping and health-related quality of life in men with prostate cancer randomly assigned to hormonal medication or close monitoring. *Psychooncology* 2002; 11: 401–414.
94. Potosky L, Knopf K, Clegg LX, et al. Quality of life outcomes after primary androgen deprivation therapy: results from the prostate cancer outcomes study. *J Clin Oncol* 2001; 19: 3750–3757.
95. Sadetsky N, Greene K, Cooperberg MR, et al. Impact of androgen deprivation on physical well-being in patients with prostate cancer. *Cancer Causes Control* 2011; 117: 4406–4413.
96. Spry NA, Kristjanson L, Hooton B, et al. Adverse effects of life arising from treatment can recover with intermittent androgen suppression in men with prostate cancer. *Eur J Cancer* 2006; 42: 1083–1092.
97. Crawford ED, Moul JW. ADT risks and side-effects in advanced prostate cancer: cardiovascular and renal injury. *Oncology* 2015; 29(1): 55–58, 65–66.
98. Baumann FT, Zopf EM, Bloch E. Clinical exercise interventions in prostate cancer patients: a systematic review of randomized controlled trials. *Support Care Cancer* 2012; 20: 221–233.
99. Champ CE, Francis L, Klement RJ, et al. Fortifying the treatment of prostate cancer with physical activity. *Prostate Cancer* 2016; Article ID 9462975.
100. Gardner JR, Livingston PM, Fraser SF. Effects of exercise on treatment related adverse effects for patients with prostate cancer receiving androgen- deprivation therapy: a systematic review. *J Clin Oncol* 2014; 32: 335–346.
101. Chipperfield K, Fletcher J, Millar J, et al. Factors associated with adherence to physical activity guidelines in patients with prostate cancer. *Psychooncology* 2013; 22: 2478–2486.
102. Keogh JWL, Shepherd D, Krägeloh CU, et al. Predictors of physical activity and quality of life in New Zealand prostate cancer survivors undergoing androgen-deprivation therapy. *NZ Med J* 2010; 123(1325): 20–28.
103. Boisen S, Krägeloh C, Shepherd D, et al. A cross-sectional comparison of quality of life between physically active and under-active older men with prostate cancer. *J Aging Phys Activ* 2016; 24(4): 642–648.

104. Bonn SE, Sjölander A, Lageross YT, et al. Physical activity and survival among men diagnosed with prostate cancer. *Cancer Epidemiol Biomarkers Prev* 2014; 24(1): 57–64.

105. Kenfield SA, Stampfer MJ, Giovannucci E, et al. Physical activity and survival after prostate cancer diagnosis in the health professionals follow-up study. *J Clin Oncol* 2011; 29: 726–732.

106. Livingston PM, Craike M, Salmon J, et al. Effects of clinician referral and exercise program for men whoi have completed active treatment for prostate cancer: a multicenter cluster randomized controlled trial (ENGAGE). *Cancer Causes Control* 2015; 121(15): 2646–2654.

107. Mennen-Winchell LJ, Grigoriev V, Alpert P, et al. Self-reported exercise and bone mineral density in prostate cancer patients receiving androgen deprivation therapy. *J Am Assoc Nurse Pract* 2014; 26: 40–48.

108. Richman EL, Kenfield SA, Stampfer MJ, et al. Physical activity after diagnosis and risk of prostate cancer progression: data from the cancer of the prostate strategic urologic research endeavor. *Cancer Res* 2011; 71: 3889–3895.

109. Wolin KY, Luly J, Sutcliffe S, et al. Risk of urinary incontinence following prostatectomy: the role of physical activity and obesity. *J Urol* 2010; 183(2): 629–633.

110. Buffart LM, Newton RU, Chinapaw MJ, et al. The effect, moderators, and mediators of resistance and aerobic exercise on health-related quality of; life in older long-term survivors of prostate cancer. *Cancer Causes Control* 2015; 121: 2821–2830.

111. Cormie P, Galvao DA, Spry N, et al. Can supervised exercise prevent treatment toxicity in patients with prostate cancer initiating androgen-deprivation therapy: a randomised controlled trial. *BJU Int* 2015; 115: 256–266.

112. Culos-Reid SN, Robinson JW, Lau H, et al. Physical activity for men receiving androgen depriovation therapy for prostate cancer; benefits from a 16-week intervention. *Support Care Cancer* 2010; 18: 591–599.

113. Galvao DA, Nosaka K, Taaffe DR, et al. Resistance training and reduction of treatment side effects in prostate cancer patients. *Med Sci Sports Exerc* 2006; 38(12): 2045–2052.

114. Galvao DA, Spry N, Denham J, et al. A multicentre year-long randomised controlled trial of exercise training targeting physical functioning in men with prostate cancer previously treated with androgen suppression and radiation from TROG 03.04 RADAR. *Eur Urol* 2014; 65: 856–864.

115. Hansen PA, Dechet CB, Porucznik CA, et al. Comparing eccentric resistance exercise in prostate cancer survivors on and off hormone therapy: a pilot study. *PM R* 2009; 1(11): 1019–1024.

116. Hanson ED., Sheaff EK, Sood S, et al. Strength training induces muscle hypertrophy and functional gains in black cancer prostate cancer patients despite androgen deprivation therapy. *J Gerontol A Biol Med Sci* 2013; 68(4): 490–498.

117. Jones LW, Hornsby WE, Freedland SJ, et al. Effects of nonlinear aerobic training on erectile dysfunction and cardiovascular function following radical prostatectomy for clinically localized prostate cancer. *Eur Urol* 2014; 65: 852–855.

118. Kvorning T, Andersen M, Brixen K, et al. Suppression of endogenous testosterone production attenuates the response to strength training: a randomized, placebo controlled, and blinded interventioin study. *Am J Physiol* 2006; 291: E1325–E1332.

119. Monga U, Garber SL, Thornby J, et al. Exercise prevents fatigue and improves quality of life in prostate cancer patients undergoing radiotherapy. *Arch Phys Med Rehabil* 2007; 88: 1416–1422.

120. Nilsen TS, Raastad T, Skovlund E, et al. Effects of strength training on body composition, physical functioning, and quality of life in prostate cancer patients during androgen deprivation therapy. *Acta Oncol* 2015; 54: 1805–1813.
121. Norris MK, Bell GJ, North S, et al. Effects of resistance training frequency on physical functioning and quality of life in prostate cancer survivors: a pilot randomized controlled trial. *Prostate Cancer Prostate Dis* 2015; 18: 281–287.
122. Park SW, Kim TN, Nam JK, et al. Recovery of overall exercise ability, quality of life, and continence after 12-week combined exercise intervention in elderly patients who underwent radical prostatectomy. *Urology* 2012; 80: 299–305.
123. Segal RJ, Reid RD, Courneya KS, et al. Resistance exercise in men receiving androgen deprivation therapy for prostate cancer. *J Clin Oncol* 2003; 21: 1653–1659.
124. Segal RJ, Reid RD, Courneya KS, et al. Randomized controlled trial of resistance or aerobic exercise in men receiving radiation therapy for prostate cancer. *J Clin Oncol* 2009; 27: 344–351.
125. Windsor PM, Nicol KF, Potter J. A randomized controlled trial of aerobic exercise for treatment-related fatigue in men reciving radical external beam radiotherapy for localized prostate carcinoma. *Cancer* 2004; 101: 550–557.
126. Winters-Stone KM, Dobek JC, Bennett JA, et al. Skeletal response to resistance and impact training in prostate cancer survivors. *Med Sci Sports Exerc* 2014; 46(8): 1482–1488.
127. Bourke L, Doll H, Crank H, et al. Lifestyle intervention in men with advanced prostate cancer receiving androgen suppression therapy: a feasibility study. *Cancer Epidemiol Biomarkers Prev* 2011; 20(4): 647–657.
128. Bruun DM, Bjerre E, Krustrup P, et al. Community-based recreational football: a novel approach to promote physical activity and quality of life in prostate cancer survivors. *Int J Environ Res Public Health* 2014; 11: 5567–5585.
129. Uth J, Schmidt JF, Christensen JF, et al. Effects of recreational soccer in men with prostate cancer undergoing androgen deprivation therapy: study protocol for the "FC Prostate" randomized controlled trial. *BMC Cancer* 2013; 13: 595.
130. Craike M, Gaskin CJ, Courneya KS, et al. Predictors of adherence to a 12-week exercise program among men treated for prostate cancer: ENGAGE study. *Cancer Med* 2016; 5(5): 787–794.
131. Demark-Wahnefried W, Clipp EC, et al. Main outcomes of the FRESH START trial: a sequentially tailored, diet and exercise mailed print intervention among breast and prostate cancer survivors. *J Clin Oncol* 2007; 25(109): 2709–2718.
132. Sajid S, Dale W, Mustian K, et al. Novel physical activity interventions for older patients with prostate cancer on hormone therapy: a pilot randomized study. *J Geriatr Oncol* 2016; 7: 71–80.
133. Santa Mina DF, Ritvo P, Matthew AG, et al. Group exercise versus personal training for prostate cancer patients: a pilot randomized trial. *J Cancer Ther* 2012; 3: 146–156.
134. Skinner TL, Peeters G, Croci I, et al. Impact of a brief exercise program on the physical and psychosocial health of prostate cancer survivors: a pilot study. *Asia-Pacific J Clin Oncol* 2016; doi: 10.1111/ajco.12474 [Epub ahead of print].
135. Uth J, Hornstrup T, Schmidt JF, et al. Football training improves leab body mass in men with prostate cancer undergoing androgen deprivation therapy. *Scand J Med Sci Sports* 2014; 24(Suppl. 1): 105–112.

136. Uth J, Hornstrup T, Christensen JF, et al. Efficacy of recreatioinal football on bone health, body composition and physical functioning in men with prostate cancer undergoing androgen deprivation therapy: 32 week follow-up of the FC prostate randomized controlled trial. *Osteoporosis Int* 2016; 27: 1507–1518.

137. Thorsen L, Courneya KS, Stevinson C, et al. A systematic review of physical activity in prostate cancer survivors: outcomes, prevalence, and determinants. *Support Care Cancer* 2008; 16: 987–997.

Index